4th edition

pharmacology

National Medical Series

In the basic sciences

anatomy, 2nd edition
the behavioral sciences
  in psychiatry, 3rd edition
biochemistry, 3rd edition
clinical epidemiology and
  biostatistics
genetics
hematology
histology and cell biology,
  2nd edition

human developmental anatomy
immunology, 3rd edition
introduction to clinical medicine
microbiology, 2nd edition
neuroanatomy
pathology, 3rd edition
pharmacology, 4th edition
physiology, 3rd edition
radiographic anatomy

In the clinical sciences

medicine, 2nd edition
obstetrics and gynecology,
  3rd edition
pediatrics, 3rd edition
preventive medicine and
  public health, 2nd edition
psychiatry, 3rd edition
surgery, 3rd edition

In the exam series

review for USMLE Step 1,
  3rd edition
review for USMLE Step 2
geriatrics

The National Medical Series for Independent Study

4th edition
pharmacology

Leonard S. Jacob, M.D., Ph.D.

Research Associate, Professor of Pharmacology
Medical College of Pennsylvania and Hahnemann University
Philadelphia, Pennsylvania
Chief Operating Officer
Magainin Pharmaceuticals, Inc.
Plymouth Meeting, Pennsylvania

Williams & Wilkins

Philadelphia • Baltimore • Hong Kong • London • Munich • Sydney • Tokyo

A Waverly Company

Senior Acquisitions Editor: Elizabeth A. Nieginski
Development Editor: Melanie Cann
Managing Editor: Amy G. Dinkel
Production Coordinator: Marette Magargle
Copy Editor: Patricia Nale
Editorial Assistants: Beth Goldner, Carol Loyd
Typesetter: Telecomposition, Inc.
Printer: Port City Press
Binder: Port City Press

Copyright © 1996 Williams & Wilkins

351 West Camden Street
Baltimore, Maryland 21201-2436 USA

Rose Tree Corporate Center
1400 North Providence Road
Building II, Suite 5025
Media, Pennsylvania 19063-2043 USA

Printed in the United States of America

Library of Congress Cataloging-in-Publication Data

Jacob, Leonard S.
   Pharmacology / Leonard S. Jacob. — 4th ed.
     p.   cm. — (The National medical series for independent study)
   Includes index.
   ISBN 0-683-06251-4
   1. Pharmacology—Examinations, questions, etc. I. Title.
II. Series.
     [DNLM: 1. Pharmacology—outlines. 2. Pharmacology—examination
questions. QV 18.2 J15p 1996]
   RM105.J33   1996
   615'.1'076—dc20
   DNLM/DLC
   for Library of Congress   95-23710
                                            CIP

*The Publishers have made every effort to trace the copyright holders for borrowed material. If
they have inadvertently overlooked any, they will be pleased to make the necessary arrange-
ments at the first opportunity.*

96 97 98 99
10 9 8 7 6 5 4 3 2 1

RECYCLED

Dedication

To Dr. Ronald J. Tallarida, mentor, colleague, and friend

Contents

Preface

As stated in the third edition, the success of *NMS Pharmacology* has exceeded my expectations. This continues to be the case!

Because of the exceptional amount of technical knowledge presented to students, focused lectures and reviews are critical. The National Medical Series, with its unique narrative outline format, is an excellent source of the latter.

The fourth edition of *NMS Pharmacology* presents up-to-date treatment regimens for most diseases. Several tables have been added to provide the student with a concise review. Additionally, questions have been added or revised to better prepare the reader for the National Board Examination.

Once again, my hope is that *NMS Pharmacology* will have a positive role in the education of students who are committed to healing sick individuals.

Leonard S. Jacob

Acknowledgments

The writing of the fourth edition was the most challenging technically and the easiest editorially. Melanie Cann's editorial direction and her assistance in keeping the writing clear were appreciated, and I appreciate the editorial support offered by Beth Goldner and Carol Loyd. In addition, I am indebted to my administrative assistant, Sandra Hitner, who catalogued the many journals we receive each week, thus ensuring that the most current therapeutic information could be presented.

I would also like to thank my wife, Terri, and our daughters, Stefanie and Ellen, for their support of my efforts. I am equally proud of their many accomplishments.

Chapter 1
General Pharmacologic Principles

I. **INTRODUCTION. Pharmacology** is the study of the biochemical and physiologic aspects of drug effects, including absorption, distribution, metabolism, elimination, toxicity, and specific mechanisms of drug action. The two main areas of pharmacology are pharmacokinetics and pharmacodynamics.

A. **Pharmacokinetics** refers to the way the body handles drug absorption, distribution, biotransformation, and excretion. Once the pharmacokinetics of a drug is determined, rational dosage regimens can be instituted.

B. **Pharmacodynamics** is the study of the biochemical and physiologic effects of drugs and their mechanisms of action.

II. **PHARMACOKINETICS**

A. **General principles**

1. **Drug transport.** The movement of drug molecules in the body affects absorption, distribution, and excretion. Drugs can cross cellular membranes by passive diffusion, carrier-mediated diffusion, active transport, or endocytosis. The cell membrane, being a bimolecular lipid layer, can also act as a barrier to some drugs.
   a. **Passive diffusion.** Most foreign compounds penetrate cells by diffusing as the **un-ionized moiety** through the lipid membrane. Factors affecting the passage of a molecule through a membrane are the molecule's size and charge, the lipid–water partition coefficient, and the concentration gradient. The two types of passive drug transport are **simple diffusion** and **filtration**.
   (1) **Simple diffusion**
      (a) Simple diffusion is based on **Fick's law:**

$$dQ/dt = (-D)(A)(dc/dx)$$

where dQ/dt is the rate of drug flux (i.e., the change in concentration of a drug within a given time); D is a temperature-dependent diffusion constant of the molecule; A is the area of the absorbing surface; and dc/dx is the concentration gradient.
   (i) The greater the concentration gradient, the greater the rate of absorption.
   (ii) The larger the absorbing surface, the greater the drug flux.
   (iii) The diffusion constant, D, is directly proportional to the temperature and is inversely related to the molecular size.
   (iv) The greater the lipid–water partition coefficient, the greater the drug flux.
      (b) In simple diffusion, molecules cross the lipid membrane in an **uncharged form**. The distribution of the uncharged form is a function of the pK_a of the

compound and the pH of the medium and is expressed by the **Henderson-Hasselbalch equation:**

(i) If the drug is a weak acid:

$$pK_a = pH + \log \frac{\text{concentration of un-ionized acid}}{\text{concentration of ionized acid}}$$

(ii) If the drug is a weak base:

$$pK_a = pH + \log \frac{\text{concentration of ionized base}}{\text{concentration of un-ionized base}}$$

(c) The pH of the medium, therefore, affects the absorption and excretion of a passively diffused drug.

(i) Aspirin and other weak acids are best absorbed in the stomach because of its acidic environment.

(ii) Alkalinic drugs are best absorbed in the small intestine, which has a higher pH.

(iii) Because the pH of urine is acidic, a weakly acidic drug can be extensively reabsorbed into the body from the urine. If the pH of the urine is increased, excretion of the drug can be increased.

(2) **Filtration**

(a) Water, ions, and some polar and nonpolar molecules of low molecular weight can diffuse through membranes, suggesting that **pores** or **channels** may exist.

(b) The capillaries of some vascular beds (e.g., in the kidney) have large pores, which permit the passage of molecules as large as proteins.

b. **Carrier-mediated (facilitated) diffusion**

(1) In this type of transport, movement across the membrane is facilitated by a macromolecule.

(2) The properties of carrier-mediated diffusion are as follows:

(a) It is a saturable process; that is, external concentrations can be achieved in which increasing the external/internal concentration gradient will not increase the rate of influx.

(b) It is selective for the chemical structure of a drug; that is, the carrier mechanism transports only those drugs having a specific molecular configuration.

(c) It **requires no energy**.

(d) It cannot move against a concentration gradient and, therefore, is still a diffusion process.

c. **Active transport**

(1) Active transport is similar to carrier-mediated diffusion in several ways:

(a) Movement across the membrane is mediated by a macromolecule.

(b) It is a saturable process.

(c) It is selective for chemical structure.

(2) Several important features, however, distinguish active transport from diffusion processes:

(a) Active transport **requires metabolic energy;** this is often generated by the enzyme known as Na^+-K^+-ATPase.

(b) It transports molecules against a concentration gradient.

d. **Endocytosis** is a minor method by which some drugs are transported into cells.

(1) A vacuolar apparatus in some cells is responsible for this process.

(2) There exist both **fluid-phase endocytosis** for substances such as sucrose and **adsorptive-phase endocytosis** for substances such as insulin.

2. **Bioavailability** is the relative rate and extent to which an administered drug reaches the general circulation; this is especially important when a drug is administered orally. Factors that influence bioavailability are:

a. Solubility of the drug in the contents of the stomach

b. Dietary patterns

c. Tablet size

d. Quality control in manufacturing and formulation

B. **Absorption** is the rate at which a drug leaves the site of administration and the extent to which this occurs. The absorption of a drug through the mucosal lining of the gastrointestinal tract or through capillary walls depends on the physical and chemical properties of the drug.

  1. **Route of administration** is an important determinant of the rate and efficiency of absorption.

  a. **Alimentary routes** are the most common routes of administration.

  (1) **Examples of alimentary routes** include:

  (a) Oral

  (b) Rectal

  (c) Sublingual

  (d) Buccal

  (2) **Advantages of alimentary administration**

  (a) An alimentary route is generally the safest route of administration. The delivery of the drug into the circulation is slow after oral administration, so that rapid, high blood levels are avoided and adverse effects are less likely.

  (b) The dosage forms available for alimentary administration are convenient and do not require sterile technique.

  (3) **Disadvantages of alimentary administration**

  (a) The rate of absorption varies. This becomes a problem if a small range in blood levels separates a drug's desired therapeutic effect from its toxic effects.

  (b) Irritation of mucosal surfaces can occur.

  (c) Patient compliance is not ensured.

  (d) With oral administration of some drugs, extensive hepatic metabolism may occur before the drug reaches its site of action. This is known as the **first-pass effect**. Passage through the liver and the resulting initial hepatic metabolism are avoided by administering the drug sublingually.

  b. **Parenteral routes** bypass the alimentary tract.

  (1) **Examples of parenteral routes** are:

  (a) Intravenous

  (b) Intramuscular

  (c) Subcutaneous

  (d) Intraperitoneal

  (e) Intra-arterial

  (f) Intrathecal

  (g) Transdermal

  (2) **Advantages of parenteral administration**

  (a) The drug gets to the site of action more quickly, providing a rapid response, which may be required in an emergency.

  (b) The dose can often be more accurately delivered.

  (c) Parenteral administration can be used when the alimentary route is not feasible (e.g., when the patient is unconscious).

  (d) Large volumes can be delivered intravenously.

  (3) **Disadvantages of parenteral administration**

  (a) More rapid absorption can lead to increased adverse effects.

  (b) A sterile formulation and an aseptic technique are required.

  (c) Local irritation may occur at the site of injection.

  (d) Parenteral administration is not suitable for insoluble substances.

  c. **Miscellaneous routes**

  (1) **Topical administration** is useful in the treatment of patients with local conditions; with topical administration, there is usually little systemic absorption. Drugs can be applied to various mucous membranes and skin.

  (2) **Inhalation** provides a rapid access to circulation; it is the common route of administration for gaseous and volatile drugs.

        (c) Tyrosine hydroxylase, which is important in the synthesis of adrenergic neurotransmitters because it hydroxylates tyrosine to dopa (L-β-3, 4-dihydroxyphenylalanine)

        (d) Monoamine oxidase, which is important to the metabolism of catecholamines and serotonin

  b. Reduction occurs in both the microsomal and nonmicrosomal metabolizing systems; it is less common than oxidation.

    (1) Examples of microsomal reduction include nitro (chloramphenicol) and azo (prontosil).

    (2) Examples of nonmicrosomal reduction include aldehyde (chloral hydrate), ketone (naloxone), and quinone (menadione).

  c. Hydrolysis

    (1) Nonmicrosomal hydrolases exist in a variety of body systems, including the plasma. Examples of **nonmicrosomal hydrolases** are:

      (a) Nonspecific **esterases** for drugs, such as acetylcholine, succinylcholine, and procaine

      (b) Peptidases (e.g., proinsulin)

      (c) Amidases for drugs, such as procainamide and indomethacin

    (2) Microsomal hydrolases have also been identified.

  d. Conjugation involves the coupling of a drug or its metabolite with an endogenous substrate, usually inorganic sulfate, a methyl group, acetic acid, an amino acid, or a carbohydrate. Usually, a conjugate is a readily excreted polar substance.

    (1) Glucuronide conjugation is the most common conjugation reaction. It occurs frequently with phenols, alcohols, and carboxylic acids.

      (a) Activated glucuronic acid (uridine diphosphoglucuronic acid; UDP-glucuronide) is formed from glucose 1-phosphate, which then reacts as follows:

$$\text{UDP-glucuronide} + \text{ROH} \rightarrow \text{RO-glucuronide} + \text{UDP}$$

      where ROH is the drug or its metabolite.

      (b) Glucuronides are generally inactive and are rapidly excreted in urine or bile by anionic transport systems.

      (c) Glucuronides eliminated in the bile can be hydrolyzed by intestinal or bacterial β-glucuronidases, and free drug can be reabsorbed. This **enterohepatic recirculation** can greatly extend the action of a drug.

    (2) Other conjugation reactions. All conjugations except glucuronide formation are catalyzed by nonmicrosomal enzymes. These reactions include:

      (a) Sulfate formation, in which phenols, alcohols, and aromatic amines are converted to sulfates and sulfanilates; 3'-phosphoadenosine 5'-phosphosulfate (PAPS) is the sulfate donor (e.g., steroids).

      (b) O-, S-, and N-methylation; S-adenosylmethionine is the methyl donor (e.g., norepinephrine).

      (c) N-acetylation; acetyl coenzyme A is the acetyl donor (e.g., isoniazid).

      (d) Glycine and glutamine conjugation with acids (e.g., salicylic acid)

      (e) Glutathione conjugation (e.g., ethacrynic acid)

3. Factors affecting drug metabolism

  a. Genetics. The most important factor is genetically determined polymorphisms. The acetylation of isoniazid and the hydrolysis of succinylcholine are genetically controlled.

  b. Chemical properties of the drug. Certain drugs may stimulate or inhibit the metabolism of the other drugs (e.g., phenobarbital stimulates the metabolism of diphenylhydantoin).

  c. Route of administration. The oral route, for example, can result in extensive hepatic metabolism of some drugs (the **first-pass effect**).

  d. Diet. Starvation can deplete glycine stores and alter glycine conjugation.

  e. Dosage. Toxic doses can deplete enzymes needed for detoxification reactions.

  f. Age. The liver cannot detoxify drugs, such as chloramphenicol, as well in neonates as it can in adults.

    g. Gender. Young males are more prone to sedation from barbiturates than females.

    h. Disease. Liver disease decreases the ability to metabolize drugs, whereas kidney disease hampers the excretion of drugs.

    i. Species differences. Experimental findings in animals do not necessarily translate to humans.

    j. Circadian rhythm. In rats and mice, the rate of hepatic metabolism of some drugs follows a diurnal rhythm. This may be true in humans as well.

E. **Drug excretion** is the process by which a drug or metabolite is eliminated from the body.

    1. Rate of elimination

        a. For most drugs, **elimination from the blood** follows exponential (first-order) kinetics.

        b. The elimination process can be saturated after high doses of some drugs, and elimination then follows zero-order kinetics. Ethanol is a prototypic example.

        c. For drugs that are eliminated by first-order kinetics, the fractional change in the amount of drug in the plasma or blood per unit of time is expressed by the **half-life** $(t_{1/2})$—or by the **elimination rate constant (k),** which is equal to $0.693/t_{1/2}$.

    2. Routes of elimination

        a. The **kidney** is the most important organ for excretion of drugs. Excretion of drugs and their metabolites via the urine involves three processes:

            (1) Glomerular filtration. Water-soluble and polar compounds are unable to diffuse back into circulation and are excreted unless a specific transport exists for their reabsorption.

            (2) Active tubular secretion. Mechanisms for active tubular secretion exist in the proximal tubule. Drugs such as organic acids (e.g., penicillin, bases, quinine) are transported by these systems.

            (3) Passive tubular reabsorption

        b. The **biliary tract and the feces** are important routes of excretion for some drugs that are metabolized in the liver.

        c. Other routes. Drugs and their metabolites can also be eliminated in expired air, sweat, saliva, tears, and breast milk. Drugs eliminated through these routes tend to be lipid-soluble and non-ionized.

F. **Effect of repeated doses**

    1. A drug accumulates in the body if the time interval between doses is less than four of its half-lives, in which case, the total body stores of the drug increase exponentially to a plateau. This plateau is known as the **steady-state concentration**.

    2. The **average total body store** of a drug at the plateau is a function of the dose, the interval between doses, and the elimination half-life of the drug.

        a. When the drug is administered in intervals that equal its half-life of elimination, the average total body store of the drug is approximately equal to 1.5 times the amount administered.

        b. When the drug is given by constant infusion, the plasma concentration will be within 10% of the desired steady-state concentration after four elimination half-lives.

III. PHARMACODYNAMICS

A. **Mechanisms of drug action**

    1. Receptors. It is believed that most drugs interact with macromolecular components (called receptors) of a cell or an organism to begin biochemical and physiologic changes that produce the drug's observed effects or response. Receptors **bind ligands** and **transduce signals**.

a. Properties of drugs
  (1) Agonists have intrinsic activity; that is, they produce some of the effects of endogenous compounds when they interact with the receptor. Examples include acetylcholine, epinephrine, and histamine.
  (2) Antagonists lack intrinsic activity yet can reduce or abolish the effect of an agonist. Examples include atropine and curare, which inhibit the effects of acetylcholine.
  (3) Partial antagonists possess **some intrinsic activity**.
b. Quantifying effect. In general, the effect (E) is a function of the quantity of the drug–receptor complex (DR), and can be expressed as:

$$E = \alpha \, [DR]$$

  (1) The magnitude of E depends on the amount of DR, which, in turn, depends on the amount of drug given. Once all receptors are saturated, the maximum effect is achieved.
  (2) Alpha (α) is a constant for a given drug and is a partial determinant of whether an effect occurs. It is determined experimentally and is considered to be a **measure of a drug's intrinsic activity;** that is, its inherent ability to produce an effect. If α is a zero, the drug has no intrinsic pharmacologic activity, and, therefore, if the drug binds to the receptor, it must be an effective antagonist.
c. Signal transduction. There are four well-known mechanisms by which receptors produce a pharmacologic response.
  (1) Ligand-gated ion channels are confined to excitable tissue [e.g., central nervous system (CNS), neuromuscular junctions, autonomic ganglia].
    (a) Ligand-gated ion channels regulate the flow of ions through the cellular plasma membrane channels, producing depolarization or hyperpolarization.
    (b) Examples of synaptic transmitters include acetylcholine (at nicotinic receptors), gamma-aminobutyric acid (GABA), glutamate, and glycine.
  (2) G proteins, a group of guanosine triphosphate (GTP) proteins, are **effector proteins** that are regulated by receptors located on the inner face of the plasma membrane. Some hormone peptide receptors and neurotransmitter receptors (e.g., α- and β-adrenergic receptors, muscarinic receptors) depend on G proteins to mediate their actions on cells.
    (a) Effectors. The G protein regulates the activity of enzymes (e.g., adenyl cyclase, phospholipases C and A_2) or ion channels (e.g., Na^+, K^+, Ca^{2+}) to produce a response.
    (b) Subunits. Each G protein contains α, β, and γ subunits. Specificity for receptor–effector coupling lies within the α subunit.
    (c) Termination of signal transmission results from hydrolysis of GTP to guanosine diphosphate (GDP) by GTPase that is intrinsic to the α subunit.
  (3) Intracellular receptors are proteins associated with the nuclear matrix that are activated by steroid hormones [e.g., estrogen, progesterone, glucocorticoids, triiodothyronine (T_3), thyroxine (T_4), vitamin D]. The steroid–receptor complex ultimately increases binding of RNA polymerase and the expression of regulated genes.
  (4) Tyrosine kinase receptors are located on the plasma membrane and are critical to cell growth and differentiation. A variety of growth factors and growth-promoting hormones [e.g., colony-stimulating factors (CSF), epidermal growth factor (EGF), insulin-like growth factor (IGF-1), certain oncogenes] interact with these receptors.
d. Receptor regulation
  (1) Certain receptors when exposed to an agonist repeatedly can become desensitized or down-regulated. For example, β-adrenergic bronchodilators used in the treatment of patients with asthma can become less effective over time when administered at the same concentration. The signal from the stimulated receptor can become depressed, or the receptor itself can be altered.

(2) Supersensitivity of receptors to agonists can occur with chronic administration of an antagonist. For instance, the abrupt discontinuation of propranolol in a patient who had been taking it chronically could precipitate dysrhythmias. Supersensitivity may result from the synthesis of additional receptors (up-regulation).

2. **Gene replacement** introduces a therapeutic gene to correct a genetic defect. Target organs include the liver (to treat hypercholesterolemia, α_1-antitrypsin deficiency, phenylketonuria, hemophilia), the hematopoietic system (to treat immune deficiency disease and hemoglobinopathies), skeletal muscle (to treat muscular dystrophic diseases), the respiratory system (to treat cystic fibrosis), and the central nervous system (CNS) [to treat Parkinson's disease].

   a. **Viral vectors** are created by rendering adenoviruses, adeno-associated viruses, and herpes simplex viruses replication-defective by deleting essential genes. Therapeutic genes and regulator elements (promoters and enhancers) are then inserted into the engineered virus.

      (1) The viral vector infects the target cell, transferring the therapeutic gene without exerting the detrimental effects of the original virus.

      (2) A retroviral vector then integrates into the host genome, causing permanent expression of the therapeutic gene.

   b. **Chemical or physical vectors** include liposome-like delivery and direct injection of a recombinant DNA molecule (consisting of a promoter and a polyadenylation signal) into the target cell's DNA. Advantages of this method include safety and lack of size limits on the therapeutic gene.

   c. **Transplantation.** Bone marrow specimens are obtained from the patient, and genes targeted to bone marrow stem cells are transferred into the bone marrow. The bone marrow is then reintroduced into the patient's body.

3. **Other mechanisms.** Some drugs may combine with small molecules or ions found in the body (e.g., chelating agents) to produce an effect.

B. | **Dose–response relationships**

1. **Quantal dose–response curve**

   a. A **quantal response** is an all-or-none response to a drug and relates to the frequency with which a specified dose of a drug produces a specific response in a population (e.g., death among the mice in a preclinical study or a 20% decrease in blood pressure among the patients in a clinical trial).

   b. The smallest amount of a drug that will produce a quantal response is not the same for all members of a population. If the frequency of response is plotted against the minimum dose necessary to produce the response, the result is often a gaussian distribution. A graphic representation of this gaussian **frequency distribution curve** is shown in Figure 1-1.

   c. The **quantal dose–response curve** is a cumulative graph of the frequency distribution curve (Figure 1-2).

FIGURE 1-1. Frequency distribution curve, plotting the number of patients showing a quantal response to a drug against the minimum dose needed to produce the response.

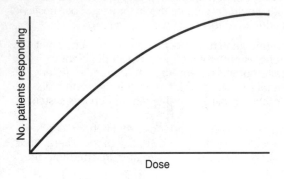

Dose

FIGURE 1-2. Quantal dose–response curve, cumulating the data used in plotting Figure 1-1.

2. **Graded dose–response curve** (Figure 1-3)
   a. As the dosage administered to a single subject or isolated tissue is increased, the pharmacologic effect will also increase (**graded dose–response**).
   b. At a certain dose, the resulting effect will reach a maximum level (**ceiling effect**).
   c. **Efficacy versus potency.** Potency is independent of efficacy, and efficacy is usually more important than potency in selecting drugs for clinical use.
      (1) **Efficacy** is the maximum effect of a drug, $\mathbf{E_{max}}$ (see Figure 1-3).
         (a) Efficacy is independent of the slope or position of the dose–response curve. In Figure 1-3, drugs A and B have equal efficacies (i.e., the same E_{max}).
         (b) Drugs such as aspirin and morphine produce the same pharmacologic effect (analgesia) but have very different levels of efficacy.
      (2) **Potency,** a comparative measure, refers to the different doses of two drugs that are needed to produce the same effect.
         (a) In Figure 1-3, drug A is more potent than drug B because the dose of drug B (D_B) must be larger than the dose of drug A (D_A) to produce a given effect (E_1).
         (b) Meaningful comparisons of potency can be made only when the drugs being compared have log dose–response curves (see III B 3) of the same slope.
         (c) $\mathbf{K_D}$ (the dissociation constant for the drug–receptor complex) and the $\mathbf{ED_{50}}$ [see III B 3 a (1)] are measures of drug potency.

3. **Log dose–response curve**
   a. To construct the log–dose response curve, the log of the dose is plotted on the abscissa and the drug effect on the ordinate. This causes the hyperbolic graded dose–response curve to become sigmoidal. Log dose–response curves for two drugs, A and B, are shown in Figure 1-4.

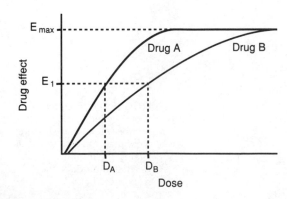

FIGURE 1-3. Graded dose–response curves for two drugs, A and B. E_{max} = maximum effect; D_A and D_B = amount (dose) of drug A and drug B, respectively, needed to produce the drug effect, E_1.

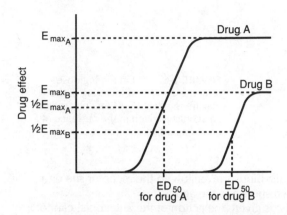

FIGURE 1-4. Log dose–response curves for two drugs, A and B. E_{max} = maximum effect; ED_{50} = smallest dose showing an effect that is 50% of the E_{max}.

(1) The **ED_{50},** the smallest dose showing an effect that is 50% of the maximum, is a measure of drug potency: The smaller the ED_{50}, the greater the potency. Thus, in Figure 1-4, drug A is more potent than drug B.

(2) **Efficacy** is indicated by the **height** of the log dose–response curve. Drug B in Figure 1-4 is less efficacious than drug A; the E_{max} of the two drugs is, therefore, different.

    b. One advantage of plotting on a logarithmic scale is that drugs with the same action at a receptor, but with different potencies, usually show dose–response curves that are parallel.

4. Antagonism between drugs

    a. Pharmacologic antagonism occurs when an antagonist prevents an agonist from interacting with its receptors to produce an effect. This type of antagonism can be either competitive or noncompetitive.

        (1) Competitive antagonism

            (a) Competitive antagonists compete with agonists in a reversible fashion for the same receptor site.

            (b) When the antagonist is present, the log dose–response curve is shifted to the right, indicating that a higher concentration of agonist is necessary to achieve the same response as when the antagonist is absent.

            (c) In the presence of the antagonist, if enough agonist is given, the E_{max} can be achieved, indicating that the action of the antagonist has been overcome. This results in a **parallel shift** of the dose–response curve, as shown in Figure 1-5.

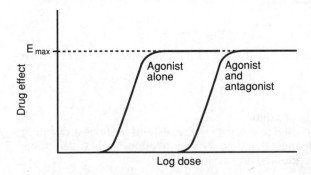

FIGURE 1-5. Shift in the log dose–response curve that occurs when an agonist is administered in the presence of a competitive antagonist.

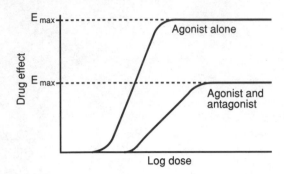

FIGURE 1-6. Shift in the log dose–response curve and lowering of the maximum effect (E_{max}) that occur when an agonist is given in the presence of a noncompetitive antagonist.

(2) Noncompetitive antagonism
  (a) The noncompetitive antagonist binds irreversibly to the receptor site or to another site that inhibits the response to the agonist.
  (b) No matter how much agonist is given, the action of the antagonist cannot be overcome.
  (c) This results in a **nonparallel shift** of the log dose–response curve with a lower E_{max} (Figure 1-6).
b. Physiologic antagonism. With pharmacologic antagonism, the agonist and antagonist compete for the same receptor site. In contrast, with physiologic antagonism, the drugs act independently on two different receptors.
  (1) Physiologic antagonism is exemplified by one drug acting on the sympathetic nervous system causing the heart rate to increase and causing vasoconstriction, while another drug acting on the parasympathetic nervous system decreases the heart rate and causes vasodilation.
  (2) Using physiologic antagonists is generally less preferable than using a receptor-specific antagonist. Because physiologic antagonists work on different receptors, they produce effects that are harder to control than the effects of a receptor-specific antagonist.
c. Antagonism by neutralization (also called **chemical antagonism**) occurs when two drugs combine with one another to form an inactive compound. For example, drugs containing sulfhydryl (—SH) groups, when combined with mercury or arsenic, no longer show agonistic actions.

5. Enhancement of drug effects
  a. Additive drug effects occur if two drugs with the same effect, when given together, produce an effect that is **equal in magnitude** to the sum of the effects when the drugs are given individually:

$$E_{AB} = E_A + E_B \qquad 1 + 1 = 2$$

  b. Synergism occurs if two drugs with the same effect, when given together, produce an effect that is **greater in magnitude** than the sum of the effects when the drugs are given individually:

$$E_{AB} > E_A + E_B \qquad 1 + 1 > 2$$

  c. Potentiation occurs if a drug lacking an effect of its own increases the effect of a second, active drug:

$$E_{AB} > E_A + E_B \qquad 0 + 1 > 1$$

6. Therapeutic index (TI) and margin of safety
  a. The **therapeutic index** is a ratio used to evaluate the safety and usefulness of a drug for an indication. It is a measurement that describes the relationship between doses of a drug required to produce undesired and desired effects.

(1) The formula for the therapeutic index is:

$$TI = \frac{LD_{50}}{ED_{50}}$$

where LD_{50} is the minimum dose that is **lethal** or toxic for 50% of the population, and ED_{50} is the minimum dose that is **effective** for 50% of the population.*

(2) Ideally, the LD_{50} should be a much higher dose than the ED_{50}, so that the therapeutic index would be large.

b. Standard margin of safety. The therapeutic index may be misleading if the log dose–response curves for effectiveness and toxicity have different slopes (i.e., are not parallel). Therefore, the standard margin of safety may be more useful.

(1) The formula for the standard margin of safety is:

$$\frac{(LD_1)}{(ED_{99})} - 1 \times 100$$

(2) The standard margin of safety shows the percentage by which the ED_{99} (the dose effective in 99% of the population) must be increased to cause toxic effects in 1% of the population.

(3) For example, if 100 mg of a drug causes toxicity in 1% of the population and 10 mg is effective in 99%, then the drug's standard margin of safety is $(100/10) - 1 \times 100$, or 900. Therefore, the dose that is effective in 99% must be increased 900% to be toxic to 1% of the population.

---

*The definition for ED_{50} here is for a population rather than a single individual or tissue, and thus it differs from the ED_{50} described in III B 3 a (1).

DIRECTIONS: Each of the numbered items or incomplete statements in this section is followed by answers or by completions of the statement. Select the ONE lettered answer or completion that is BEST in each case.

1. A patient with a systemic infection is being treated with an antibiotic whose elimination half-life ($t_{1/2\beta}$) is 8 hours. To maintain the patient's total body store at 300 mg of the antibiotic, what should the dosage be?

(A) 100 mg every 8 hours
(B) 200 mg every 8 hours
(C) 300 mg every 8 hours
(D) 400 mg every 8 hours
(E) 500 mg every 8 hours

2. The maximum effect (E_{max}) achieved by a drug is a measure of

(A) potency
(B) efficacy
(C) the quantal response
(D) antagonist magnitude
(E) the therapeutic index (TI)

3. Which route of drug administration is most likely to lead to the first-pass effect?

(A) Oral
(B) Sublingual
(C) Intravenous
(D) Subcutaneous
(E) Intramuscular

4. Which of the following statements best describes a drug receptor?

(A) Gamma globulin can bind to a drug and serve as a drug receptor
(B) A drug cannot act unless it is first bound to a receptor
(C) A drug cannot act unless it is first released from a receptor
(D) Drug receptors play a role in the bioavailability of a drug
(E) A drug can act as an antagonist even if it is bound to a drug receptor

DIRECTIONS: Each of the numbered items or incomplete statements in this section is negatively phrased, as indicated by a capitalized word such as NOT, LEAST, or EXCEPT. Select the ONE lettered answer or completion that is BEST in each case.

5. All of the following statements about Fick's law as it pertains to simple diffusion are true EXCEPT

(A) the greater the concentration gradient, the greater the rate of absorption
(B) the smaller the surface area, the greater the drug flux
(C) the greater the lipid–water partition coefficient, the greater the drug flux
(D) diffusion constant is directly proportional to the temperature
(E) diffusion constant is inversely related to the molecular size

6. Correct statements concerning characteristics of a particular route of drug administration include all of the following EXCEPT

(A) intravenous administration provides a rapid response
(B) oral administration requires that the patient be alert
(C) intramuscular administration requires sterile technique
(D) subcutaneous administration may cause local irritation
(E) inhalation provides slow access to the general circulation

7. Properties of drug absorption include all of the following EXCEPT

(A) the route of administration is an important factor affecting drug absorption
(B) the rate of absorption varies after oral administration
(C) after rectal administration, drug absorption follows first-order kinetics
(D) after intramuscular administration, drug absorption follows first-order kinetics
(E) with intravenous administration, drug absorption follows first-order kinetics

8. All of the following statements about efficacy and potency are true EXCEPT that

(A) efficacy is usually a more important clinical consideration than potency
(B) efficacy is indicated by the height of the log dose–response curve
(C) the ED_{50} is a measure of a drug's efficacy
(D) drugs that produce a similar pharmacologic effect can have very different levels of efficacy
(E) on a log dose–response curve, two drugs with the same action but with different potencies usually have parallel curves

9. All of the following statements regarding the use of viral vectors for gene delivery are true EXCEPT

(A) viral replication is rendered defective by deletion of essential genes
(B) therapeutic genes are inserted into an engineered virus
(C) the vector infects the target cell, transferring the therapeutic gene
(D) the retroviral vector integrates into the host genome resulting in permanent expression
(E) adenovirus vectors integrate effectively into nuclear DNA of the recipient cell

10. All of the following statements regarding signal transduction are true EXCEPT

(A) it allows cells to communicate with each other
(B) the signal is initiated by extracellular ligands
(C) activation of G proteins occurs
(D) activation of protein kinases occurs
(E) hormones and neurotransmitters are the final products of transduction

1. The answer is B *[II F]*. The patient's dosage should be 200 mg every 8 hours to maintain the patient's total body store at 300 mg of the antibiotic. A drug accumulates in the body if the time interval between doses is less than four half-lives, in which case the total body store of the drug increases exponentially to a plateau. The average total body store of a drug at the plateau is a function of the dose, the interval between doses, and the elimination half-life of the drug. When the drug is administered at the half-life of elimination, the average total body store of the drug is approximately equal to 1.5 times the amount administered.

2. The answer is B *[III B 2 c, 6]*. E_{max} reflects the efficacy of a drug and is indicated by the height of the dose–response curve. Potency refers to the different doses of two drugs that are needed to produce the same effect. Potency is independent of efficacy, and efficacy is more important than potency in selecting drugs for a particular clinical situation. The quantal response of a drug relates to the all-or-none relationship seen in a population with a given dose of a drug. The therapeutic index (TI) is defined as the LD_{50}/ED_{50} and is independent of the E_{max}.

3. The answer is A *[II B 1 a (3) (d)]*. After oral administration, a drug is absorbed through the gastrointestinal mucosa and then passes through the liver. Some drugs (e.g., propranolol) undergo extensive hepatic metabolism (first-pass effect) before reaching the site of action. With most other routes of administration, the first-pass effect does not occur because extensive hepatic passage immediately after drug absorption is avoided.

4. The answer is E *[III A 1]*. A drug receptor is a specific drug-binding site in a cell or on its surface that mediates the action of the drug. Some drugs bind to various plasma proteins, such as gamma globulin, but these molecules do not serve as drug receptors. Most drugs combine reversibly with their receptors to form a drug–receptor complex, and it is this complex that exerts a biologic effect (e.g., a decrease in blood pressure). However, some drugs are believed not to have specific receptors and act by some other mechanism. If a drug has no inherent pharmacologic activity but binds to a receptor, it acts as an antagonist.

5. The answer is B *[II A 1 a]*. Fick's law is expressed as:

$$dQ/dt = (-D)(A)(dc/dx)$$

where dQ/dt is the rate of drug flux, D is the temperature-dependent diffusion constant of the molecule, A is the area of the absorbing surface, and dc/dx is the concentration gradient. Thus, the larger the surface area, the greater the drug flux. All of the other statements in the question are true.

6. The answer is E *[II B 1]*. Inhalation provides rapid access to the general circulation (e.g., gaseous anesthetics). The rapid response gained by intravenous administration can be critical in an emergency. All forms of parenteral administration (i.e., administration by injection) require the use of sterile technique, and all can cause local irritation, depending on the drug being given. For a drug to be administered orally, the patient must be conscious and alert to avoid the risk of aspiration.

7. The answer is E *[II B 1, 2]*. The route of administration is an important determinant of the rate and efficiency of absorption of a drug. Delivery of the drug into the circulation is relatively slow after oral administration, and the rate of absorption is variable. Parenteral routes of administration bypass the alimentary tract and usually result in rapid, direct drug absorption. After intravenous administration, the absorption of a drug follows zero-order kinetics; thus, a constant **amount** (i.e., 100%) of the drug is absorbed. After any other route of administration, the absorption of most drugs follows first-order (exponential) kinetics; thus, a constant **fraction** of the drug is absorbed.

8. The answer is C *[III B 2 c, 3]*. The ED_{50} is a measure of a drug's potency, not its efficacy. The smaller the ED_{50}, the greater the potency of the drug. Efficacy is usually a more important clinical consideration than potency. Drugs that produce a similar pharmacologic effect can have very different levels of efficacy. Efficacy is indicated by the height of the log dose–response curve; two drugs with the same action but with different potencies usually have parallel curves.

9. The answer is E *[III A 2]*. Replication-defective adenoviruses do not integrate effectively into the nuclear DNA of the recipient cell, resulting in the transient expression of therapeutic genes. Detrimental effects of the virus are mitigated by rendering viral replication defective by depleting essential genes. Therapeutic genes are inserted into the engineered virus, whereby the viral vector infects the target cell and transfers the therapeutic gene. Integration into the host genome then occurs.

10. The answer is E *[III A 1 c]*. Cellular communication is initiated by extracellular ligands such as hormones and neurotransmitters. These molecules bind to membrane-sparing receptors, resulting in activation of G proteins. Signaling cascades can activate protein kinases, ultimately leading to diverse physiologic responses.

Chapter 2
Drugs Affecting Peripheral Neurohumoral Transmission

I. **PERIPHERAL EFFERENT NERVOUS SYSTEM.** The peripheral efferent nervous system consists of the **somatic** and the **autonomic nervous systems**.

A. The **somatic nervous system** innervates and controls the motor function of the body. Axons from the spinal cord innervate skeletal muscle; the neurotransmitter (see I C) is acetylcholine.

B. **Autonomic nervous system.** Axons from preganglionic neurons within the spinal cord connect to neurons in ganglia outside the spinal cord. Postganglionic axons from the ganglia innervate smooth and cardiac muscle and exocrine glands. The autonomic nervous system has two parts: the **parasympathetic** and **sympathetic nervous systems**. These two divisions control homeostatic functions that are primarily involuntary.

1. **Parasympathetic nervous system**
   a. **Location of preganglionic neurons.** In the parasympathetic (craniosacral) nervous system, preganglionic neurons are located in cranial and sacral portions of the spinal cord.
   b. **Location of ganglia.** In the parasympathetic nervous system, the ganglia are close to the innervated organ, so that the preganglionic axons are long and the postganglionic axons are short.
   c. **Innervation of organs**
      (1) The parasympathetic nervous system innervates the heart, bronchial smooth muscle, iris, salivary glands, and urinary bladder.
      (2) Under normal conditions, the heart, eye, gastrointestinal tract, urinary bladder, bronchi, and salivary glands are under parasympathetic control.

2. **Sympathetic nervous system**
   a. **Location of preganglionic neurons.** In the sympathetic (thoracolumbar) nervous system, the neurons are located in lumbar and thoracic portions of the spinal cord.
   b. **Location of ganglia.** In the sympathetic nervous system, the ganglia are close to the spinal cord, so that the preganglionic axons are short and the postganglionic axons are long.

C. **Neurotransmitters** are chemical mediators that transmit nerve impulses across junctions such as synapses (see Chapter 3 I A).

1. At the **ganglionic synapse** in both the sympathetic and the parasympathetic nervous systems, the neurotransmitter is **acetylcholine** (see IV A).

2. At the **postganglionic synapse,** the two systems differ.
   a. The **parasympathetic** neurotransmitter is **acetylcholine**.
   b. The **sympathetic** transmitter is usually **norepinephrine** (see II A), but at sweat glands and at some blood vessels, it is **acetylcholine**.

D. **Receptors of the nervous system.** More than one type of receptor exists for each neurotransmitter. The receptors are distinguished in part on the basis of their affinity for various agonists and antagonists.

1. **Cholinergic receptors** (for acetylcholine) are broadly subdivided into **muscarinic** and **nicotinic receptors**.
   a. **Muscarinic receptors**
      (1) Muscarinic receptors are further subdivided into M_1 and M_2 receptors. Muscarinic receptors of both types are found in the central nervous system (CNS). In addition, M_1 receptors are found at autonomic ganglia; M_2 receptors are found at end-organ effector sites.
      (2) Muscarine is the classic agonist for muscarinic receptors, and atropine is an antagonist.
   b. **Nicotinic receptors** are found in the CNS, in autonomic ganglia, and in striated muscle.
      (1) Nicotine, the classic agonist, first stimulates and then blocks autonomic ganglia and skeletal muscle end-plates.
      (2) *d*-Tubocurarine blocks nicotinic receptors, particularly in striated muscle and in autonomic ganglia, whereas hexamethonium preferentially blocks ganglionic nicotinic receptors.
   c. The various cholinergic receptors and their sites are summarized in Table 2-1.

2. **Adrenergic receptors** [for norepinephrine (noradrenaline) and epinephrine (adrenaline)] are also of several types.
   a. **α-Adrenergic receptors.** Agonists, in decreasing order of potency, are epinephrine > norepinephrine > isoproterenol. Antagonists are phentolamine and phenoxybenzamine. Some α-adrenergic receptors precede the synapse between nerve terminal and effector organ; others are postsynaptic.
      (1) **α_1-Adrenergic receptors** are **postsynaptic** receptors. They are found on blood vessels, on the radial muscle of the eye, in the gastrointestinal tract, and on the splenic capsule.
      (2) **α_2-Adrenergic receptors** are **presynaptic** or **postsynaptic;** all seem to serve an inhibitory function. Isoproterenol is ineffective on α_2-receptors.
         (a) **Presynaptic α_2-receptors** are found at adrenergic and cholinergic nerve terminals. Presynaptic α_2-receptors, when activated, inhibit the release of further neurotransmitter.
         (b) **Postsynaptic α_2-receptors** are found in blood vessels and in the CNS.
   b. **β-Adrenergic receptors.** Agonists for β-receptors are isoproterenol, epinephrine, and norepinephrine. Propranolol is an antagonist. The β-receptors are also subdivided on the basis of their relative response to agonists and antagonists.
      (1) **β_1-Adrenergic receptors** are found predominantly on cells in the heart and intestine. The relative potency of agonists is isoproterenol > epinephrine and norepinephrine.
      (2) **β_2-Adrenergic receptors** are found at other sites, most importantly, on bronchial and vascular smooth muscle. The relative potency of agonists is isoproterenol > epinephrine >> norepinephrine.

TABLE 2-1. Sites of Cholinergic Receptors

	Receptors		
	Muscarinic		
Site	M_1	M_2	**Nicotinic**
Skeletal muscle	–	–	+
Autonomic ganglia	+	–	+
Central nervous system	+	+	+
End-organ innervation	–	+	–

E. **Direct effects of autonomic stimulation on various organs.** Stimulation of effector organs may be either direct or indirect. A **direct** effect occurs when the nerve innervating an organ is stimulated. **Indirect** responses are mediated by changes caused in other organs.

1. **Direct effects of parasympathetic and sympathetic stimulation on various organs**
    a. **Heart**
        (1) **Sympathetic stimulation** increases the heart rate (**chronotropic effect**) and the contractile force (**inotropic effect**).
        (2) **Parasympathetic stimulation** decreases the heart rate but has little effect on contractile force because there is no parasympathetic innervation of the ventricles.
    b. **Blood vessels**
        (1) **Sympathetic stimulation**
            (a) Stimulation of α-receptors causes constriction of the arteries, arterioles, and veins.
            (b) Stimulation of β-receptors causes dilation of skeletal muscle arteries.
        (2) **Parasympathetic stimulation** has no effect on blood vessels because most have no parasympathetic innervation.
    c. **Gastrointestinal tract. Sympathetic stimulation** decreases the activity of the gastrointestinal tract, whereas **parasympathetic stimulation** increases it.
    d. **Eye**
        (1) **Sympathetic stimulation** contracts the radial muscle, causing dilation of the pupil.
        (2) **Parasympathetic stimulation** produces contraction of the circular and ciliary muscles, causing pupillary constriction and changes in accommodation.
    e. **Bronchial smooth muscle** is relaxed by sympathetic stimulation and contracted by parasympathetic stimulation.
    f. **Glycogenolysis** is increased in liver and muscle by sympathetic stimulation.

2. Table 2-2 summarizes the effects of autonomic stimulation on various end-organs, depending on the type of receptor stimulated.

TABLE 2-2. Receptor–End-Organ Response

Organ	Receptor Type	End-Organ Effect
Heart	β_1	Increased inotropism and chronotropism
	M_2	Decreased inotropism and chronotropism
Coronary and pulmonary arterioles, blood vessels to skeletal muscle	β_2 (predominant type)	Dilation
	α	Constriction
	M_2	Dilation
Other arterioles	α	Constriction
	β	Dilation
	M_2	Dilation
Veins	α	Constriction
	β_2	Dilation
Bronchi	β_2	Relaxation
	M_2	Constriction
Gastrointestinal tract	α, β	Decreased motility and secretion
	M_2	Increased motility and secretion
Bladder	α, β	Retention
	M_2	Evacuation
Eye	α_1	Mydriasis
	β	Relaxation of ciliary muscle
	M_2	Miosis, constriction of ciliary muscle

Adapted from Lefkowitz RJ, Hoffman BB, Taylor P: Drugs acting at synaptic and neuroeffector junctional sites. In *Goodman and Gillman's The Pharmacological Basis of Therapeutics*, 8th ed. Edited by Gilman AG, et al. New York, Pergamon Press, 1990, p 89.

TABLE 2-3. Sites of Action of Drugs Affecting the Sympathetic Nervous System*

Site*	Process*	Inhibitor
1	Tyrosine uptake	None
2	Tyrosine hydroxylase (TH)	α-Methyl-p-tyrosine, dopamine (DA), norepinephrine (NE)
3	Dopa decarboxylase (DD)	α-Methyldopa
4	Movement of DA into vesicles	Reserpine
4A	Movement of NE back into vesicles	
5	Dopamine β-hydroxylase (DBH)	Disulfiram
6	Depolarization of adrenergic terminals	Bretylium, guanethidine
7	Exocytotic release of NE	See site 6
8	Release by indirect-acting sympathomimetics	Cocaine (blocks uptake), reserpine (eliminates stores)
9	α_1-Adrenergic receptors (postsynaptic)	Phentolamine, tolazoline, phenoxybenzamine, ergotamine, prazosin
10	β_1-Adrenergic receptors	Propranolol (also β_2), atenolol, metoprolol
11	β_2-Adrenergic receptors	Propranolol (also β_1)
12	α_2-Adrenergic receptors (presynaptic)	See site 9 (not prazosin)
13	Norepinephrine uptake (U-1)	Cocaine, imipramine, ouabain, bretylium, guanethidine, phenoxybenzamine
14	Extraneuronal uptake (U-2)	Phenoxybenzamine, corticosterone, normetanephrine
15	Catechol O-methyltransferase	Pyrogallol
16	Monoamine oxidase	Phenelzine (a hydrazine), tranylcypromine (derivative of amphetamine)

*Site numbers and processes are as in Figure 2-1.
Adapted from Molinoff PB: Drugs affecting the sympathetic nervous system. In lecture notes for course in medical pharmacology. University of Pennsylvania School of Medicine, August, 1985.

F. Drug effects on neurohumoral transmission

1. **Drugs** can affect neurohumoral transmission at various steps. They can affect the following:
   a. Synthesis, storage, or release of a neurotransmitter
   b. Interaction between transmitter and receptor
   c. Enzymatic destruction of a neurotransmitter
   d. Transport of a transmitter into cells
   e. Recovery of a cell membrane after the transmitter–receptor interaction

2. Figure 2-1 and Table 2-3 show the mechanisms and sites of drug effects on the sympathetic nervous system.

II. SYMPATHOMIMETIC (ADRENERGIC) AGENTS are drugs that mimic the actions of the sympathetic nervous system.

A. Catecholamines: norepinephrine and epinephrine (Figure 2-2)

1. **Chemistry**
   a. Tyrosine is hydroxylated on the aromatic ring by tyrosine hydroxylase, yielding **dopa** (dihydroxyphenylalanine); this step is the rate-limiting step in the biosynthesis of adrenergic transmitters.
   b. Dopa is decarboxylated to give **dopamine**.

FIGURE 2-1. Site of action of drugs affecting the sympathetic nervous system. The figure depicts the events taking place at the junction of a sympathetic nerve terminal and an end-organ cell.

Tyrosine from the circulation enters the nerve terminal (1) and is converted, first (2) via tyrosine hydroxylase (*TH*) into dopa and then (3) via dopa decarboxylase (*DD*) into dopamine (*DA*). Dopamine enters the vesicles of the nerve terminal (4), where it is converted (5), via dopamine β-hydroxylase (*DBH*) into norepinephrine (*NE*), which is stored in the vesicles. Free NE in the axoplasm also enters and leaves the vesicles (4A).

In the process of nerve impulse transmission across the neuroeffector junction, the nerve terminal is depolarized (6) by an action potential. The storage vesicle fuses with the plasma membrane, and the neurotransmitter NE is released into the junction (7) by exocytosis. Indirect-acting sympathomimetics can also cause NE to leave the vesicles and enter the neuroeffector junction (8).

Once released from the nerve cell, NE activates the postsynaptic α_1-, β_1-, and β_2-receptors (9, 10, 11) on the effector cell, thereby producing the effector response. NE also activates the presynaptic α_2-receptors (12) on the nerve terminal itself.

Several mechanisms terminate the action of NE. Most important is the reentry of NE into the nerve terminal (a process known as uptake-1) (13). Some of the NE enters the effector cell (uptake-2) (14), and some enters the circulation.

Two enzymes play a role in the metabolism of NE. The NE that enters the effector cell is methylated (15) by catechol *O*-methyltransferase (*COMT*) to the normetanephrine. The NE in the axoplasm of the nerve terminal is converted (16) by monoamine oxidase (*MAO*) in the nerve cell's mitochondria, first to the aldehyde, and then to the glycol or to 3-methoxy-4-hydroxymandelic acid (vanillylmandelic acid, or VMA). The glycol and the acid are the major metabolites excreted in the urine.

Drugs that affect the sympathetic nervous system act at specific steps in the process. Such drugs, and the processes they inhibit, are listed in Table 2-3. (Adapted from Molinoff PB: The regulation of the noradrenergic neuron. *J Psychiatr Res* 11:339–345, 1974.)

FIGURE 2-2. Structures of norepinephrine (*A*) and epinephrine (*B*).

    c. Dopamine is hydroxylated on the β-carbon to give **norepinephrine**.
    d. Epinephrine is formed in the adrenal medulla by the methylation of norepinephrine. The medulla releases 85% epinephrine and 15% norepinephrine.

  2. Pharmacokinetics of epinephrine and norepinephrine
    a. Absorption is poor with oral administration because the drugs are rapidly conjugated and oxidized.
    b. Absorption is slow with subcutaneous administration because the drugs cause local vasoconstriction.
    c. Nebulized and inhaled solutions are usually used for their actions on the respiratory tract.
    d. The drugs can be given intravenously, but this route must be used with caution so that the heart does not fibrillate.
    e. The liver is important in the degradation of epinephrine and norepinephrine. The majority of the dose is metabolized by catechol *O*-methyltransferase (COMT) and monoamine oxidase (MAO), and the metabolites are excreted in the urine.

  3. Pharmacologic effects of epinephrine. Epinephrine interacts strongly with both β- and α-receptors. Its effects on some body systems depend on the concentration of epinephrine as well as the type of receptor. At low concentrations, β effects predominate, and, at high concentrations, α effects predominate.
    a. Effects on blood pressure
      (1) A large dose of epinephrine administered intravenously causes an increase in blood pressure, with the systolic pressure increasing more than the diastolic. Subsequently, the mean pressure decreases to below normal before returning to the control value. The rise in pressure is due to:
        (a) Vasoconstriction through activation of α-receptors
        (b) Increased ventricular contraction through activation of β-receptors
        (c) An initial increase in heart rate, which, at the height of the vasopressor response, is slowed by a compensatory vagal discharge
      (2) Low doses cause a decrease in blood pressure because the β_2 (vasodilator)-receptors are more sensitive to epinephrine than are the α (vasoconstrictor)-receptors.
    b. Vascular effects. Epinephrine exerts its action on small arterioles and precapillary sphincters. Its vascular effects include:
      (1) Decreased cutaneous blood flow
      (2) Increased blood flow to skeletal muscle at low concentrations and decreased flow at higher concentrations

(3) Increased hepatic blood flow with increased splanchnic vascular resistance

(4) Increased renal vascular resistance, producing decreased renal blood flow

(5) Increased arterial and venous pulmonary pressure

(6) Increased coronary blood flow, caused indirectly by an increase in the work of the heart, and mediated by local effectors

c. **Effects on the heart** produced by epinephrine include:

(1) A direct effect on β_1-receptors, producing a slight initial increase in heart rate, which is slowed by a compensatory vagal discharge

(2) Increased stroke volume

(3) Increased cardiac output

(4) A propensity toward arrhythmias

d. **Effects on smooth muscle** depend on the predominant type of adrenergic receptor in the muscle.

(1) Epinephrine relaxes gastrointestinal smooth muscle (α_2- and β-receptor stimulation), whereas it usually increases sphincter contraction (α stimulation).

(2) Uterine contractions may be inhibited (β) or stimulated (α), depending on menstrual phase or state of gestation.

(3) In the bladder, the detrusor muscle relaxes (β), while the trigone and sphincter contract (α).

(4) Bronchiolar smooth muscle relaxes (β_2).

e. **Metabolic effects** of epinephrine also depend on the type of adrenergic receptor. These effects include:

(1) An increase in glucose and lactate production via liver and muscle glycogenolysis (β_2)

(2) Inhibition of insulin secretion (α)

(3) An increase in free fatty acids, mediated by cyclic adenosine 3',5'-monophosphate (cAMP) (β_1)

(4) An increase in oxygen consumption

4. **Pharmacologic effects of norepinephrine.** Norepinephrine is equipotent to epinephrine in its reaction on β_1-receptors, and slightly less potent on α-receptors. It has very little effect on β_2-receptors.

a. An intravenous infusion raises both systolic and diastolic pressure by constriction of vascular smooth muscle (α-receptors).

b. The increased peripheral vascular resistance produces a compensatory vagal reflex that slows the heart rate. Cardiac output may actually decrease, although coronary blood flow is increased.

5. **Termination of action**

a. **Transport, or uptake into the cells,** is an important mechanism for terminating the action of many neurotransmitters. There are two active **amine transport systems:**

(1) A system in the plasma membrane transports amines from the extracellular fluid to the cytosol.

(2) A system in the secretory granular membrane transports amines into granules.

b. **Deactivation by conversion to inactive metabolites** is also a way of terminating action. Two enzymes are involved:

(1) COMT adds a methyl group to the hydroxyl of the catechol ring.

(2) MAO removes the amine group. When metabolic breakdown or transport is prevented (as in patients taking MAO inhibitors or tricyclic antidepressants), then the dosage of sympathomimetic agents must be reduced.

6. **Therapeutic uses**

a. Epinephrine is used:

(1) To treat bronchospasm

(2) For relief of hypersensitivity reactions; it is the primary treatment for anaphylactic shock

(3) To prolong the duration of infiltrative anesthesia

(4) To restore cardiac activity in cardiac arrest

(5) To facilitate aqueous drainage in chronic open-angle glaucoma

b. Norepinephrine is used for treating hypotension during anesthesia when tissue perfusion is good.

7. Adverse effects. Both epinephrine and norepinephrine can cause:
   a. Anxiety
   b. Headache
   c. Cerebral hemorrhage from the vasopressor effects
   d. Cardiac arrhythmias, especially in the presence of digitalis and certain anesthetic agents
   e. Pulmonary edema from pulmonary hypertension

B. Isoproterenol

1. Pharmacokinetics
   a. Absorption of orally administered isoproterenol is unreliable.
   b. It is readily absorbed when given parenterally or as an inhaled aerosol.
   c. It is principally metabolized by COMT; MAO plays a smaller role than in epinephrine or norepinephrine metabolism.

2. Pharmacologic effects
   a. Isoproterenol has an *N*-alkyl substitution, which makes it act almost entirely on β-receptors and have little effect on α-receptors.
   b. Intravenous infusion produces a reduction of peripheral vascular resistance in skeletal muscles and in renal and mesenteric vascular beds.
   c. Diastolic blood pressure falls, but because there are increased venous return and positive inotropic and chronotropic effects, cardiac output is increased.
   d. Systolic blood pressure may increase, but mean pressure decreases.
   e. Renal blood flow decreases in normotensive individuals, but it increases in patients with nonhemorrhagic shock.
   f. Relaxation of both bronchial and gastrointestinal smooth muscle occurs.
   g. A release of free fatty acids occurs; hyperglycemia is less than with epinephrine.
   h. Pancreatic islet cells are activated, stimulating insulin secretion.

3. Therapeutic uses. Isoproterenol is used as a bronchodilator and as a cardiac stimulant.

4. Adverse effects
   a. These are similar to the adverse effects of epinephrine.
   b. Overdosage by inhalation can induce fatal ventricular arrhythmias.
   c. Tolerance to the desired effects occurs with overuse in the asthmatic.

C. Dopamine

1. Chemistry. Dopamine is an intermediate in the synthesis of norepinephrine (see II A 1).

2. Pharmacokinetics. Dopamine resembles epinephrine and norepinephrine in its pharmacokinetics.

3. Central dopamine receptors (D_1, D_2, D_3)
   a. The central D_1 receptor site is excitatory and directly activates the adenylate cyclase system.
   b. The D_2 receptor site is inhibitory in some brain tissues and uses cAMP as its intracellular messenger. Pituitary-related side effects of neuroleptics are thought to be mediated through D_2 receptors in the pituitary.
   c. The D_3 receptor is localized in the limbic system and is not found in the pituitary. It is principally associated with emotional and cognitive behavior.

4. Pharmacologic effects
   a. Dopamine is an important neurotransmitter in the CNS. It is a direct agonist, acting on β_1-receptors and releasing norepinephrine from nerve terminals. The result is a positive inotropic effect on the myocardium.

b. Low or intermediate doses of dopamine reduce arterial resistance in the mesentery and kidney; this raises the glomerular filtration rate. The effect is mediated by a receptor for dopamine.

c. Dopamine increases systolic pressure but has little effect on diastolic pressure.

d. At higher doses, it acts on α-receptors and causes vasoconstriction with a consequent reduction in renal function.

5. **Therapeutic uses.** Dopamine is used in the treatment of cardiogenic and septic shock and in chronic refractory congestive heart failure.

6. **Adverse effects**

a. Overdosage results in excessive sympathomimetic activity.

b. Anginal pain, arrhythmias, nausea, and hypertension can occur, but these effects are short-lived because dopamine has rapid metabolism.

D. Dobutamine

1. **Pharmacokinetics**

a. Dobutamine is not absorbed when given orally.

b. It has a half-life of 2 minutes when given by intravenous injection.

2. **Pharmacologic effects**

a. Although dobutamine resembles dopamine chemically, it is a direct β_1-receptor agonist. It has a greater inotropic than chronotropic effect.

b. Dobutamine does not act on dopaminergic receptors.

3. **Therapeutic uses.** Dobutamine is used to improve myocardial function in congestive heart failure. Oxygen demands are less than with other sympathetic agonists because dobutamine causes minimal changes in heart rate and systolic pressure.

4. **Adverse effects**

a. Dobutamine increases atrioventricular conduction and must, therefore, be used with caution in atrial fibrillation.

b. Other adverse effects are similar to those of other catecholamines.

E. Phenylephrine

1. **Pharmacologic effects**

a. Phenylephrine is a direct-acting sympathomimetic agent. Its effects are similar to those of norepinephrine, but it is less potent and has a longer duration of action.

b. Vasoconstriction, increased atrial pressure, and reflex bradycardia occur with parenteral administration.

2. **Therapeutic uses.** Phenylephrine is used:

a. As a nasal decongestant

b. As a pressor agent

c. To provide local vasoconstriction as:

(1) A 10% ophthalmic solution

(2) An adjunct for use with local anesthetics

d. For relief of paroxysmal atrial tachycardia

3. **Adverse effects**

a. Large doses cause cardiac irregularities.

b. Ophthalmic solutions, like intranasal solutions, can be systemically absorbed. Their use in patients taking β-blockers increases the risk of cardiac irregularities, myocardial infarction, and intracranial hemorrhage.

c. Rebound nasal congestion can occur with chronic use as a nasal decongestant.

F. Ephedrine

1. **Pharmacokinetics**

a. Ephedrine is absorbed when taken orally.

b. It is resistant to COMT and MAO, so that its action is prolonged.

2. Pharmacologic effects

a. Ephedrine is a **mixed-acting** sympathomimetic agent; that is, it has both direct and indirect actions.

(1) Its **primary action** is **indirect.** It causes the release of norepinephrine from storage in nerve terminals, apparently by competing with norepinephrine for transport into the granules.

(2) It also produces direct stimulation of adrenergic receptors.

b. When administered intravenously, its action is similar to that of epinephrine. However,

(1) Its pressor response occurs more slowly and lasts 10 times longer.

(2) Its potency is 1/250 that of epinephrine in producing an equivalent pressor response.

c. Ephedrine increases arterial pressure by causing peripheral vasoconstriction and cardiac stimulation.

d. Its effects on the bronchi and other smooth muscle are qualitatively similar to those of epinephrine.

e. It causes CNS stimulation, which can result in effects such as insomnia, nervousness, nausea, and agitation.

f. Tachyphylaxis occurs with repeated administration.

3. Therapeutic uses. Ephedrine is used:

a. In the treatment of bronchial asthma

b. As a nasal decongestant

c. As a pressor agent in spinal anesthesia

d. As a mydriatic

4. Adverse effects

a. These are similar to the adverse effects seen with epinephrine.

b. In addition, CNS effects may occur.

c. Ephedrine must be used with caution in patients with cardiovascular disease or hyperthyroidism because it is a powerful heart stimulator.

G. Amphetamine

1. Pharmacologic effects

a. Amphetamine acts indirectly by releasing norepinephrine.

b. Amphetamine is also a CNS stimulant (see Chapter 3 VIII A).

c. The dextrorotatory (*d*-) form is more active in the CNS than the levorotatory (*l*-) form.

d. Amphetamine depresses the appetite, decreasing food intake, by affecting the feeding center in the lateral hypothalamus.

e. It increases metabolism to a small extent.

2. Therapeutic uses

a. Amphetamine is used in the treatment of narcolepsy and the hyperkinetic syndrome in children (see Chapter 3 VIII A 2).

b. The control of obesity is not a recommended use because abuse of amphetamine is not rare and because tolerance to the anorexic effects develops within a few weeks.

3. Adverse effects

a. Tolerance to amphetamine can occur within several weeks.

b. Psychic and physical dependence can occur.

c. Toxic psychosis can result from large doses.

d. Prolonged use can lead to mental depression and fatigue.

e. Reactions attributable to CNS stimulation occur, such as restlessness or insomnia.

f. Cardiovascular stimulation can result in tachycardia and hypertension.

g. Mydriasis and dry mouth can occur.

h. Amphetamine is contraindicated in patients with cardiovascular disease because it stimulates the heart and in those receiving MAO inhibitors or guanethidine because these compounds increase norepinephrine concentrations outside the cells, as amphetamine does.

i. Treatment of acute intoxication involves:
  (1) Acidification of the urine by ammonium chloride administration
  (2) Administration of chlorpromazine, which is effective for treating both the CNS symptoms and the elevated blood pressure because of its α-blocking activity

H. **Methamphetamine and hydroxyamphetamine**

1. **Methamphetamine** is related chemically to both amphetamine and ephedrine.
   a. A mixed-acting sympathomimetic agent, it is equal to amphetamine in central stimulant activity and is more potent than ephedrine in pressor activity.
   b. Therapeutic indications are limited to those that make use of its CNS effects, such as narcolepsy.

2. **Hydroxyamphetamine** has an action resembling that of ephedrine but without CNS effects. It is used as a mydriatic, decongestant, and pressor agent.

I. **Mephentermine**

1. Mephentermine is a mixed-acting sympathomimetic. Its peripheral vasopressor actions are similar to those of methamphetamine; it lacks significant central actions.

2. Its major therapeutic use is in the treatment of hypotension.

J. **Methoxamine**

1. Methoxamine is a direct-acting stimulator of α-adrenergic receptors with pharmacologic properties similar to those of phenylephrine.

2. It produces little CNS stimulation.

3. Its large pressor effect results from an increase in total peripheral resistance.

4. It causes a reflex bradycardia.

5. Methoxamine is used therapeutically in hypotensive states and to end attacks of paroxysmal atrial tachycardia.

K. **Metaraminol**

1. Metaraminol is a mixed-acting sympathomimetic that is similar to norepinephrine in its actions, although it is less potent.

2. Metaraminol increases systolic and diastolic blood pressure via vasoconstriction, and produces a marked reflex bradycardia.

3. It has little stimulant effect on the CNS.

4. Its major therapeutic use is in the treatment of hypotensive states.

L. **β_2-Stimulating bronchodilators**

1. **Pharmacologic effects.** The adrenergic agents that are primarily β_2-agonists have a relaxing effect on bronchial smooth muscle and show little effect on cardiac β_1-receptors.

2. **Therapeutic uses.** These agents are used therapeutically for the treatment of bronchial asthma or bronchospasm, where their lack of cardiac stimulation is a decided advantage. Experts recommend regular use of inhaled corticosteroids to decrease inflammation and as-needed use of β_2-agonists to control acute symptoms.

3. **Administration.** β_2-Stimulating bronchodilators are used chiefly as aerosol inhalants; oral and injectable forms are also available.

4. **Adverse effects** of the β_2-agonists are similar to those seen with the sympathomimetic drugs listed previously.
   a. Regular use of a short-acting β_2-agonist can be associated with increased bronchial hyperresponsiveness to methacholine challenge.

   b. Overuse of β_2-agonists by patients with asthma has been associated with increased mortality.
   c. Even though their effects are primarily bronchial, β_2-agonists should be used with caution in patients with cardiovascular disease or hyperthyroidism because they can have minimal effects on the β_1-receptors of the heart.

5. **Specific agents**
   a. Metaproterenol has a more rapid onset of bronchodilating action in asthma than either albuterol or terbutaline.
   b. Albuterol is somewhat more bronchoselective than isoproterenol when given as an inhalant. In asthma, the effects of albuterol are apparent within 15 minutes, are maximal at about 60–90 minutes, and last about 3–4 hours.
   c. Salmeterol is a long-acting β_2-selective adrenergic agonist inhalant used for the maintenance treatment of asthma, with or without inhaled corticosteroids. It also appears to inhibit the release of inflammatory mediators from human lung tissue.
      (1) Salmeterol is not recommended for acute treatment of bronchospasm; bronchodilation begins in 15 minutes but can last up to 12 hours.
      (2) Because salmeterol is long-acting, a short-acting β_2-agonist can be administered as needed to control acute symptoms.
   d. Terbutaline, when used in the treatment of bronchial asthma, has a longer duration of action than metaproterenol. It may have more side effects than other sympathomimetic agents.
   e. Bitolterol is a prodrug that is converted in the lung to **colterol,** an active catecholamine. It may have a longer duration of action than terbutaline, metaproterenol, or albuterol. It may cause tremor due to stimulation of skeletal muscle, in addition to the adverse effects seen with all sympathomimetic agents.

III. SYMPATHETIC ANTAGONISTS.
Synonyms for this class of drugs are **sympatholytics, antiadrenergic agents,** and **adrenergic blocking agents.**

A. α-Adrenergic blocking agents (α-blockers)

1. **Phenoxybenzamine**
   a. Mechanism of action
      (1) Phenoxybenzamine is a haloalkylamine and is closely related to the nitrogen mustards.
      (2) It binds covalently to the α-receptor, producing an irreversible blockade.
      (3) Phenoxybenzamine is somewhat more potent in blocking α_1 (postsynaptic)-receptors than in blocking α_2 (presynaptic)-receptors.
   b. Pharmacologic effects. Phenoxybenzamine antagonizes sympathetic responses mediated by α-adrenergic receptors.
      (1) Cardiovascular effects. Phenoxybenzamine induces postural hypotension caused by a lack of compensatory sympathetic vasoconstriction. In addition, it increases cardiac output and decreases total peripheral resistance.
      (2) Most **metabolic effects** produced by catecholamines are the result of their effects on β-receptors; thus, α-adrenergic blocking agents do not have significant metabolic actions.
      (3) CNS effects. Phenoxybenzamine stimulates the CNS, producing nausea, hyperventilation, and loss of time perception.
   c. Therapeutic uses. Phenoxybenzamine is used:
      (1) For acute hypertensive episodes caused by use of sympathomimetics or MAO inhibitors, or by pheochromocytomas
      (2) To reverse vasoconstriction in shock (if use is attempted in shock, the patient must have an elevated central venous pressure)
      (3) To relieve vasospasm in Raynaud's phenomenon
      (4) For control of autonomic hyperreflexia resulting from spinal cord transection

d. Adverse effects
   (1) Postural hypotension and reflex tachycardia may occur, especially in patients who are hypovolemic.
   (2) Ejaculation may be inhibited.
   (3) Miosis and nasal stuffiness may occur.
   (4) Nausea and vomiting may occur with oral administration.
   (5) Injections cause local tissue irritation.

2. **Phentolamine** and **tolazoline** act by a reversible α-adrenergic blockade.
   a. Pharmacologic effects
      (1) These agents produce vasodilation and reflex cardiac stimulation.
      (2) They decrease peripheral resistance and increase venous capacity.
      (3) Both stimulate salivary, lacrimal, pancreatic, and respiratory tract secretions.
      (4) They cause a gastric secretion that induces effects similar to those of histamine.
      (5) Phentolamine is more potent than tolazoline.
      (6) Tolazoline is absorbed when given orally and is rapidly excreted by the kidneys; phentolamine is excreted more slowly. Both can be given parenterally.
   b. Therapeutic uses
      (1) Phentolamine has been used to control acute hypertensive episodes caused by use of sympathomimetics.
      (2) In the past, phentolamine was used as a diagnostic test for pheochromocytoma, but it has been replaced by assays for urinary catecholamines.
      (3) Tolazoline can be used in the treatment of neonates with persistent pulmonary hypertension, despite use of oxygen therapy and mechanical ventilation.
      (4) Tolazoline has been used experimentally to relieve vasospasm and in the treatment of Raynaud's phenomenon.
   c. Adverse effects
      (1) Both drugs can cause cardiac stimulation, leading to arrhythmias and anginal pain, especially after parenteral administration; they must be used with caution in patients with coronary artery disease.
      (2) Tolazoline can produce a paradoxical hypertension.
      (3) Because they induce gastrointestinal stimulation, both drugs must be used with caution in patients with peptic ulcer disease.

3. **Prazosin** is a selective blocker of postsynaptic α_1-receptors, producing vasodilation.
   a. Pharmacologic effects
      (1) Prazosin reduces vascular tone in both resistance and capacitance vessels.
      (2) Because prazosin has no effect on α_2-receptors, neurotransmitter feedback inhibition is maintained, so that prazosin causes only a small degree of tachycardia.
      (3) It decreases arterial pressure with little change in cardiac output, heart rate, and right atrial pressure.
   b. Prazosin is discussed further in Chapter 5 IV F 2.

4. **Ergot alkaloids**
   a. Mechanism of action
      (1) These agents are weak α-adrenergic blockers and are serotonin antagonists (see Chapter 8 V B).
      (2) They are also partial agonists at α-adrenergic receptors and agonists at tryptaminergic and dopaminergic receptors.
   b. Pharmacologic effects
      (1) Ergot alkaloids are CNS stimulants and, therefore, may cause effects such as confusion, irregular respiration, and anxiety.
      (2) They directly stimulate smooth muscle.
      (3) They cause a significant elevation of blood pressure via peripheral vasoconstriction.
   c. Therapeutic uses
      (1) Ergotamine tartrate, by virtue of its vasoconstricting effects, is used in the treatment of migraine headaches.

      (2) Ergonovine maleate is a powerful oxytocic but lacks the adrenergic blocking activity of ergotamine. It causes direct contraction of uterine smooth muscle and is used to decrease postpartum bleeding.

      (3) Methylergonovine maleate is also used to decrease postpartum uterine bleeding.

      (4) Methysergide (see Chapter 8 V B 1) is used for prophylaxis of migraine attacks.

  d. Adverse effects

      (1) Ergot preparations often cause nausea and vomiting.

      (2) Their vasoconstricting effects can cause vascular insufficiency, leading to gangrene.

B. **β-Adrenergic blocking agents (β-blockers)** (Table 2-4)

  1. Propranolol is a nonselective β-antagonist. It competes for both β_1- and β_2-receptors.

    a. Pharmacokinetics

      (1) Although propranolol is completely absorbed from the gastrointestinal tract, a large portion of the drug is extracted by the liver before it enters the systemic circulation.

      (2) Wide variation in the hepatic metabolism of the drug among individuals causes significant differences in the plasma concentrations attained.

      (3) Propranolol is approximately 90% bound to plasma proteins.

      (4) The elimination half-life is approximately 3 hours for a small dose, but it is prolonged with larger doses and is significantly prolonged in the presence of cirrhosis.

      (5) A metabolic product, 4-hydroxypropranolol, is active but has a short half-life.

    b. Pharmacologic effects

      (1) Propranolol decreases the heart rate and cardiac output and prolongs systole.

      (2) It decreases total coronary blood flow and oxygen consumption.

      (3) It reduces blood flow to most tissues, except to the brain.

      (4) Propranolol's antihypertensive effect is slow to develop, and the mechanisms that cause the effect are not clear. However, propranolol inhibits the renal secretion of renin, which may play a part.

      (5) It depresses sodium (Na^+) excretion because it alters renal hemodynamics, an effect that is secondary to the decrease in cardiac output.

      (6) Propranolol increases airway resistance by β_2 blockade.

      (7) Because most of the effects of catecholamines on carbohydrate and fat metabolism are mediated by β-receptors, propranolol interferes with these events.

    c. Therapeutic uses. Propranolol is used for:

      (1) Treatment of hypertension, often in combination with a diuretic

      (2) Prophylaxis of angina pectoris (see Chapter 5 III B)

      (3) Prophylaxis of supraventricular and ventricular arrhythmias (see Chapter 5 II E 1)

      (4) Long-term prophylaxis in patients who have had a myocardial infarction and are at high risk for infarction or sudden death

TABLE 2-4. β-Blockers for Hypertension

Drug	β-Blocking Selectivity
Carteolol	Nonselective, intrinsic sympathomimetic
Labetalol	Nonselective β- and selective α_1-blocking activity
Nadolol	Nonselective
Penbutolol	Nonselective, intrinsic sympathomimetic
Pindolol	Nonselective, intrinsic sympathomimetic
Propranolol	Nonselective
Timolol	Nonselective
Sotalol	Nonselective
Acebutolol	β_1-selective, intrinsic sympathomimetic
Atenolol	β_1-selective
Betaxolol	β_1-selective
Metoprolol	β_1-selective

(5) Management of hypertrophic obstructive cardiomyopathies to reduce the force of myocardial contractions

(6) Management of hyperthyroidism and anxiety states to decrease the heart rate

(7) Prophylaxis of migraine headaches

d. Adverse effects and precautions

(1) Propranolol can induce heart failure, especially in patients with compromised myocardial function.

(2) Rapid withdrawal can lead to "supersensitivity" of β-adrenergic receptors, which can provoke anginal attacks, arrhythmias, or myocardial infarction.

(3) Because propranolol increases airway resistance, it must be used with caution in asthmatics.

(4) Because of its effects on carbohydrate metabolism, the hypoglycemic action of insulin may be augmented. Therefore, diabetics being treated with insulin and persons prone to hypoglycemia must use propranolol with caution.

(5) Rash, fever, and purpura are characteristic of an allergic response and require discontinuation of the drug.

(6) Prolonged use may cause fatigue, depression, nightmares, sexual dysfunction, and peripheral arterial insufficiency.

(7) Because of its effects on peripheral blood flow, propranolol is contraindicated in patients with Raynaud's phenomenon.

2. **Timolol** is a nonselective β-adrenergic antagonist that is 5–10 times more potent than propranolol.

a. **Therapeutic uses.** Timolol is used for the **same applications as propranolol**. In addition, timolol is used for:

(1) Glaucoma. Timolol lowers intraocular pressure by reducing the production of aqueous humor; the mechanism is not clear. It does not change the size of the pupil, and vision is not affected. For this use, timolol is available as eyedrops.

(2) Migraines. Timolol decreases the frequency of migraine attacks, but not their duration or severity.

b. **Adverse effects.** Systemic absorption can occur with ocular use, but the amount absorbed is usually not enough to affect patients with asthma or heart failure.

3. **Nadolol** is a nonselective β-adrenergic blocking agent that is not metabolized and is excreted unchanged in the urine. Its effect and adverse reactions are similar to those of propranolol.

4. **Sotalol** is a nonselective β-blocker without intrinsic sympathomimetic or local anesthetic activity (see Chapter 5 II F). It is approved for the treatment of life-threatening ventricular arrhythmias.

5. **Labetalol** is a nonselective β-blocker, which also has α_1-blocking activity. It is used in the treatment of mild to severe hypertension.

a. Labetalol reduces peripheral vascular resistance while preventing reflex tachycardia.

b. When combined with either prazosin or hydralazine, labetalol is faster acting than other β-blockers.

c. It can be given intravenously in hypertensive emergencies.

d. **Adverse effects.** Labetalol may cause postural hypotension and jaundice in addition to the adverse effects seen with other β-blockers.

6. **Pindolol** is a nonselective β-blocker, which also has some degree of intrinsic sympathomimetic (α-adrenergic) activity. Unlike the case with propranolol, no rebound tachycardia occurs upon abrupt withdrawal of pindolol.

7. **Acebutolol** is a β-blocker with mild intrinsic sympathomimetic activity (ISA).

a. Its β_1-blocking effects exceed its β_2-blocking effects.

b. Because of its ISA, it may not cause as slow a bradycardia as propranolol does.

c. **Adverse effects,** in addition to those seen with other β-blockers, include arthritis, myalgia and arthralgia, and the presence of antinuclear antibodies.

8. **Metoprolol** is a selective β_1-adrenergic antagonist.
   a. **Pharmacologic effects**
      (1) Metoprolol inhibits the inotropic and chronotropic cardiac responses to isoproterenol.
      (2) It is 1/50th as potent as propranolol in inhibiting the vasodilator response to isoproterenol; however, it is long-acting.
      (3) It is absorbed well when given orally.
   b. **Therapeutic uses.** Metoprolol is used chiefly in the treatment of hypertension.
   c. **Adverse effects**
      (1) Metoprolol produces fewer deleterious effects in asthmatic patients because of its selective β_1-adrenergic antagonism, but its use in asthmatics still requires caution.
      (2) Other adverse effects are similar to those of propranolol.

9. **Atenolol** is a selective β_1-adrenergic antagonist that is administered once daily.

10. **Betaxolol** is a selective β_1-adrenergic antagonist that is administered once daily. It is more lipophilic than atenolol. It is also available as a topical formulation for the treatment of glaucoma.

C. **Agents that inhibit the action of adrenergic nerves**

1. **Reserpine**
   a. **Mechanism of action.** Reserpine, a rauwolfia alkaloid, acts via catecholamine depletion. It inhibits the uptake of norepinephrine into vesicles, and intraneuronal degradation of norepinephrine by MAO then occurs. This action takes place both centrally and peripherally.
   b. **Pharmacologic effects**
      (1) Large doses given parenterally may cause a transient sympathomimetic effect as stored catecholamines are released from the cell, because uptake into vesicles is inhibited.
      (2) Blood pressure decreases, which usually triggers reflex tachycardia in normal people through sympathetic stimulation. However, because sympathetic stores are depleted, bradycardia may ensue in people taking reserpine.
      (3) Sedation often results because there are depleted stores of catecholamines and serotonin (5-hydroxytryptamine, 5-HT) in the brain.
   c. **Therapeutic uses.** The major therapeutic use of reserpine is in the treatment of hypertension (see Chapter 5 IV H 1).
   d. **Adverse effects** include:
      (1) Sedation
      (2) Psychic depression that may result in suicide
      (3) Abdominal cramps and diarrhea
      (4) Gastrointestinal ulceration
      (5) Possible increased incidence of breast carcinoma

2. **Guanethidine**
   a. **Mechanism of action**
      (1) Guanethidine acts presynaptically. It impairs the response to sympathetic stimulation by inhibiting the release of neurotransmitters from peripheral adrenergic neurons.
      (2) Guanethidine is taken up by adrenergic nerves and displaces norepinephrine from intraneuronal storage granules. This action does not inhibit the release of granule contents; that occurs through another, unknown, mechanism.
      (3) Much of the norepinephrine released from the adrenergic nerve terminals is deaminated by intraneuronal MAO. Some norepinephrine does leak from the cell.
   b. **Pharmacokinetics**
      (1) With oral administration, absorption varies and the onset of action is slow.
      (2) The drug is rapidly cleared by the kidney.
   c. **Pharmacologic effects**
      (1) A large intravenous dose causes a transient increase in blood pressure.

      (2) This is followed by a fall in systemic and pulmonary arterial pressures that is much more intense in the erect than in the supine individual.

    d. Therapeutic uses. The major therapeutic indication is a potent, long-acting antihypertensive agent (see Chapter 5 IV H 2).

    e. Adverse effects include:

      (1) Postural hypotension

      (2) Syncope, especially with strenuous exercise

      (3) Diarrhea

      (4) Edema

    f. Guanethidine is contraindicated in patients taking MAO inhibitors.

    g. The antihypertensive effects of guanethidine may be reversed by tricyclic antidepressants or indirect-acting sympathomimetic amines, such as ephedrine or phenylpropanolamine.

3. Guanadrel is similar to guanethidine in its mode of action and indications, but it has a shorter duration of action.

    a. Guanadrel causes less morning hypotension and less diarrhea than guanethidine does.

    b. Like guanethidine, guanadrel is contraindicated in patients taking MAO inhibitors, and its effects may be reversed by the same types of drugs as for guanethidine.

    c. Guanadrel causes water retention and should, therefore, be given in combination with a diuretic.

4. Bretylium

    a. Pharmacologic effects

      (1) Bretylium is taken up by adrenergic nerve terminals and produces a block in the release of norepinephrine.

      (2) It also inhibits the re-uptake of norepinephrine into nerve terminals.

      (3) Initially, bretylium produces a sympathomimetic effect, before it blocks the action of the nerves.

    b. Therapeutic uses. Bretylium is no longer used for hypertension but is used mainly as an antiarrhythmic agent (see Chapter 5 II G 1). It is poorly absorbed when given orally.

    c. Adverse effects include cardiac stimulation caused by the sympathomimetic effects of bretylium and strong hypotension.

IV. PARASYMPATHETIC (CHOLINERGIC) AGONISTS

A. Acetylcholine

1. Chemistry. Acetylcholine is a quaternary ammonium ester (Figure 2-3) that is rapidly hydrolyzed by acetylcholinesterase and plasma cholinesterase.

2. Pharmacologic effects

    a. Cardiovascular effects

      (1) Acetylcholine produces:

        (a) A negative inotropic effect

        (b) A negative chronotropic effect

        (c) Vasodilation

      (2) Its actions on the heart are the same as the effects of vagal stimulation.

      (3) Large intravenous doses cause an increase in blood pressure because there is release of catecholamines from the adrenal medulla and activation of sympathetic ganglia.

$$(CH_3)_3 - \overset{+}{N} - CH_2 - CH_2 - O - \overset{\displaystyle O}{\overset{\|}{C}} - CH_3$$

FIGURE 2-3. Acetylcholine.

b. Effects on other systems

    (1) Acetylcholine increases gastrointestinal motility and secretory activity.

    (2) It contracts smooth muscle in the uterus, ureters, bladder, and bronchioles, and the constrictor muscles of the iris.

    (3) It stimulates the salivary, sweat, and lacrimal glands.

3. Therapeutic uses. Acetylcholine is used as a miotic in cataract surgery.

B. **Methacholine (acetyl-β-methylcholine)**

1. Chemistry. Methacholine differs chemically from acetylcholine by the addition of a methyl group to the β position of choline. As a result:

    a. Methacholine is hydrolyzed only by acetylcholinesterase and, therefore, has a longer duration of action than acetylcholine.

    b. It becomes virtually a pure muscarinic-acting agent.

2. Pharmacologic effects. The effects of methacholine on the cardiovascular system and other systems are similar to those of acetylcholine.

C. **Carbachol (carbamylcholine)**

1. Carbachol has a carbamic acid–ester link, which is not readily susceptible to hydrolysis by cholinesterases.

2. Carbachol has all the pharmacologic properties of acetylcholine. It exerts both nicotinic and muscarinic effects.

3. Carbachol is used ophthalmically as a miotic agent.

D. **Bethanechol**

1. Chemically, bethanechol has the structural features of both methacholine and carbachol. It is resistant to hydrolysis by cholinesterases and is mainly muscarinic in action.

2. Bethanechol shows no negative inotropic or chronotropic cardiovascular effects.

3. It is used therapeutically for abdominal distention, esophageal reflux, and urinary bladder distention.

E. **Pilocarpine**

1. Pilocarpine is a tertiary amine alkaloid.

2. Its actions are similar to those of methacholine. When applied locally to the eye, it causes miosis and an eventual decrease in intraocular pressure.

3. Its major therapeutic indication is in the treatment of glaucoma.

F. **Metoclopramide**

1. Metoclopramide stimulates the motility of the upper gastrointestinal tract.

2. It is useful for the treatment of diabetic gastroparesis (delayed gastric emptying) and gastroesophageal reflux disease.

3. It is also an antiemetic and is used for this purpose during cancer chemotherapy.

4. Adverse effects include possibly irreversible tardive dyskinesia [see Chapter 3 V B 5 a (3)], acute dystonia, and prolactin secretion, which can cause loss of libido, galactorrhea, and menstrual disorders.

G. **Adverse effects and precautions for parasympathetic agonists**

1. Atropine often blocks serious adverse effects, such as the increase in gastrointestinal motility, muscle paralysis, and stimulation of glandular secretion, that can occur with use of these drugs.

2. Use of these drugs is contraindicated in patients with coronary insufficiency, hyperthyroidism, peptic ulcer, or asthma. In addition, **metoclopramide** is contraindicated in patients taking phenothiazines, butyrophenones, or thioxanthenes and in patients with pheochromocytoma or acute porphyria.

V. ANTICHOLINESTERASE AGENTS

A. Physostigmine

1. **Mechanism of action.** This alkaloid forms a reversible complex at the site of acetylcholinesterase where acetylcholine is broken down.

2. **Pharmacokinetics**
   a. Physostigmine is well absorbed from the gastrointestinal tract, subcutaneous tissues, and mucous membranes.
   b. Its metabolism is at the ester linkage by hydrolytic cleavage.

3. **Pharmacologic effects.** The pharmacologic properties of physostigmine mimic those of acetylcholine.
   a. It produces miosis and, thus, can antagonize the mydriasis induced by atropine.
   b. When given in large doses, it causes fasciculation, then paralysis, of skeletal muscle because of the accumulation of acetylcholine at the neuromuscular junction that results when acetylcholine is not broken down.

4. **Therapeutic uses**
   a. Treatment of atropine, phenothiazine, and tricyclic antidepressant intoxication
   b. Treatment of glaucoma, especially simple and secondary glaucoma
   c. Treatment of early stages of Alzheimer's disease, because degeneration of cortical cholinergic axons has been seen at autopsy in some patients with this disorder

B. Neostigmine

1. **Chemistry.** Neostigmine is a synthetic reversible anticholinesterase that contains a quaternary nitrogen.

2. **Pharmacokinetics**
   a. Neostigmine is not well absorbed orally.
   b. It does not penetrate the blood–brain barrier, which minimizes the toxicity due to inhibition of acetylcholinesterase that is in the brain.
   c. It is destroyed by plasma esterases and is excreted in the urine.

3. **Pharmacologic effects**
   a. The pharmacologic properties of neostigmine mimic those of acetylcholine.
   b. It also has a direct action on nicotinic receptors, in addition to blocking acetylcholinesterase.
   c. It reverses the neuromuscular blockade produced by curare and its derivatives; the mechanism of action involves the release of increased amounts of acetylcholine from nerve endings, cholinesterase inhibition, and a direct action on skeletal muscle cholinergic receptors.

4. **Therapeutic uses**
   a. Neostigmine is used to reverse the effects of competitive neuromuscular blocking agents (see VIII).
   b. It is used in the management of paralytic ileus and atony of the urinary bladder.
   c. It is also used in the symptomatic treatment of myasthenia gravis.

C. Edrophonium

1. **Pharmacokinetics.** Edrophonium is more rapidly absorbed and has a shorter duration of action than neostigmine. It is administered parenterally.

2. Pharmacologic effects. In its actions, edrophonium is similar to neostigmine, except that with high doses it can stimulate the neuromuscular junction without affecting muscarinic effector organs.

3. Therapeutic uses include:
   a. Diagnosis of myasthenia gravis
   b. Antagonism of curare-like agents

D. **Other physostigmine-like anticholinesterases**

1. Pyridostigmine and **ambenonium** are used in the symptomatic treatment of myasthenia gravis.

2. Demecarium is used as an ophthalmic solution for the treatment of chronic glaucoma.

E. **Organophosphate cholinesterase inhibitors**

1. Preparations
   a. Diisopropyl fluorophosphate (DFP) is an organophosphate compound, which forms a covalent bond between its phosphorus atom and the esteratic site of cholinesterase. The enzyme-inhibitor complex thus formed is irreversible. Its use is limited to the treatment of certain types of glaucoma.
   b. Echothiophate is a long-acting organophosphate cholinesterase inhibitor with pharmacologic properties similar to those of DFP. Spontaneous regeneration of the phosphorylated enzyme can occur. Its major use is in the treatment of glaucoma.
   c. Parathion is an organophosphate anticholinesterase agent used as an insecticide. Its active form is **paraoxon,** a metabolite. Pharmacologic and adverse effects are similar to those of DFP.

2. Adverse effects of DFP and other organophosphate cholinesterase inhibitors include:
   a. Miosis
   b. Increased bronchial secretions, profuse sweating, and increased lacrimation
   c. Anorexia, vomiting, and involuntary diarrhea
   d. Bradycardia
   e. Weakness of all skeletal muscles, but especially those of respiration, after twitching and fasciculations
   f. Anxiety, confusion, and convulsions, followed by vasomotor depression

3. Reversal of cholinesterase inhibition. Pyridine-2-aldoxime methyl chloride (PAM, pralidoxime) reverses the effects of the organophosphate anticholinesterase agents.
   a. It combines with and splits off the phosphorus from the esteratic site on cholinesterase in such a way that the enzyme is restored.
   b. With reactivation of the enzyme, the effects of acetylcholine begin to disappear.
   c. Treatment must be within hours, because the phosphorylated enzyme slowly changes to a form that cannot be reversed.

VI. **PARASYMPATHETIC ANTAGONISTS**

A. **Atropine** is an alkaloid derived from the plant *Atropa belladonna* (deadly nightshade). The active component is the racemic mixture *dl*-hyoscyamine, an ester compound of tropic acid and the organic base tropine.

1. Mechanism of action
   a. Atropine competes reversibly with acetylcholine at muscarinic receptors.
   b. At very high concentrations, it blocks acetylcholine at ganglionic synapses and motor nerve endings.
   c. Atropine antagonizes the action of acetylcholine in the CNS.

2. Pharmacokinetics
   a. Atropine is rapidly but poorly absorbed when given orally.
   b. It disappears rapidly from the blood and is excreted in the urine.

3. Pharmacologic effects
   a. Effects on the heart
      (1) The heart rate slows initially because there is medullary stimulation of the cardio-inhibitory center.
      (2) Tachycardia then follows with increased cardiac output and shortening of the P–R interval. Higher doses cause only tachycardia.
   b. Effects on blood pressure
      (1) Oral or intramuscular doses have little effect on blood pressure.
      (2) With intravenous injection, total peripheral resistance increases.
      (3) The increase in heart rate and cardiac output causes arterial pressure to increase.
      (4) Atropine has a direct vasodilating effect on small blood vessels.
   c. Effects on the CNS
      (1) Large doses can produce hallucinations and, ultimately, coma, but therapeutic doses exert little effect.
      (2) Atropine possesses antitremor activity via a central antimuscarinic mechanism.
   d. Effects on involuntary muscles
      (1) Atropine decreases the amplitude and frequency of peristaltic contractions and reduces the tone of the stomach, small intestine, and colon.
      (2) It also relaxes the smooth muscle of the biliary tract.
      (3) Urinary bladder and ureter tone are decreased, whereas vesical sphincter tone is increased.
   e. Effects on the eye. Atropine blocks the acetylcholine response of the ciliary muscle of the lens and of the circular smooth muscles of the iris, producing cycloplegia and mydriasis.
   f. Effects on secretions
      (1) Sweat gland secretions are greatly reduced.
      (2) Bronchial and salivary secretions are decreased.
      (3) There is a reduction in gastric secretion during both the psychic and gastric phases, and a reduction in total acid content, especially at doses greater than 1 mg.
   g. Effects on the bronchi. Atropine produces slight bronchodilation.

4. Therapeutic uses
   a. Ophthalmic administration is used for producing cycloplegia and mydriasis.
   b. Its ability to reduce secretions in the upper and lower respiratory tract makes it useful as a preanesthetic agent.
   c. It is used in myocardial infarction to treat sinus node bradycardia or a high-grade arteriovenous block.
   d. It is effective for prophylaxis of motion sickness.
   e. Combined with an opioid, it is used for the treatment of renal and biliary colic.
   f. Because it antagonizes the actions of acetylcholine, it may be used in large doses for the treatment of poisoning by anticholinesterase agents and for the rapid type of mushroom poisoning.

5. Adverse effects include:
   a. Rapid pulse
   b. Dilated pupils, resulting in photophobia
   c. Dry mouth
   d. Flushed skin
   e. An increase in body temperature, especially in children
   f. Restlessness, confusion, and disorientation

6. The **antidote** in atropine poisoning is **physostigmine**.

B. **Scopolamine** (hyoscine), like atropine, is an alkaloid and is an ester of tropic acid but with the organic base scopine.

   1. Pharmacologic effects. Like atropine, scopolamine has antimuscarinic actions.
      a. It is more potent than atropine in producing mydriasis and cycloplegia, in decreasing bronchial, salivary, and sweat gland secretions, and in its sedative effect.
      b. It is less potent than atropine in its effects on the heart, bronchial muscles, and intestines.
      c. Atropine has a longer duration of action, and, in therapeutic doses, it does not depress the CNS.

   2. Therapeutic uses and adverse effects are generally similar to those of atropine. Scopolamine is excellent for treatment of motion sickness.

C. **Propantheline** is a synthetic antimuscarinic agent. High doses produce skeletal neuromuscular blockade. It is useful in the treatment of urinary bladder spasm and enuresis.

D. **Dicyclomine** is another synthetic antimuscarinic drug.

   1. At normal therapeutic doses, it decreases spasm in most smooth muscles without producing atropine-like effects on the heart, eye, or salivary and sweat glands.

   2. It is thought to act by direct relaxation of muscle rather than by competitive antagonism of acetylcholine at muscarinic receptors.

E. **Homatropine and eucatropine** are used in ophthalmology.

   1. Homatropine is a rapidly acting muscarinic blocking agent used to produce cycloplegia and mydriasis for ophthalmic refractions.

   2. Eucatropine is used as a mydriatic.

VII. GANGLIONIC STIMULATORS AND BLOCKERS

A. Nicotine

   1. Mechanism of action
      a. Nicotine interacts with the acetylcholine receptor on the postsynaptic membrane of autonomic ganglia.
      b. It causes an initial stimulation of the ganglion similar to the effect of acetylcholine.
      c. Large amounts produce a prolonged blockade following the initial stimulation.
      d. In small doses, it causes the release of catecholamines from the adrenal medulla, whereas larger doses prevent their release.
      e. Nicotine affects chemoreceptors in the carotid and aortic bodies and centers in the medulla oblongata.

   2. Pharmacokinetics
      a. Nicotine is readily absorbed through the skin, respiratory tract, and buccal membranes.
      b. It is metabolized in the liver, kidney, and lung and is eliminated via the kidney.
      c. It is excreted in the breast milk of lactating women who are heavy smokers.

   3. Pharmacologic effects
      a. Nicotine is a CNS stimulant.
         (1) Via motor cortex excitation, it produces tremors, which, with larger doses, can be followed by convulsions.
         (2) Small doses stimulate respiration, whereas toxic doses depress it.
         (3) Nicotine stimulates the release of antidiuretic hormone (ADH).

    b. Tachycardia, increased blood pressure, and increased total peripheral resistance result from stimulation of sympathetic ganglia and the adrenal medulla.

    c. Increased bowel motility results predominantly from parasympathetic ganglionic stimulation.

    d. Salivary and bronchial secretions are first stimulated, then blocked.

4. No therapeutic uses for nicotine exist. Its inherent toxicity has been applied in the control of insects. Its presence in tobacco is of major medical importance.

B. Hexamethonium

1. Chemistry. Hexamethonium $[(CH_3)_3—N^+—(CH_2)_6—{}^+N—(CH_3)_3]$ has a bridge of six methylene groups between two quaternary nitrogen atoms. The addition of more intervening carbon groups decreases the activity at the ganglionic receptor and increases activity at the skeletal muscle receptor. Ten carbons (as in **decamethonium**) produce maximal activity at the skeletal muscle receptor.

2. Mechanism of action. Hexamethonium produces competitive ganglionic blockade by occupying ganglionic cholinergic receptors.

3. Pharmacologic effects

    a. Hexamethonium reduces systemic vascular resistance, venous return, and cardiac output.

    b. Gastric secretions are reduced in volume and acidity, and gastric motility is reduced.

    c. Salivary secretions are decreased, and some bronchodilation occurs.

    d. The glomerular filtration rate is decreased and renal vascular resistance is increased.

    e. Urinary excretion may be impaired because of reduced urinary bladder contractions.

    f. Partial mydriasis and loss of accommodation may occur.

    g. Dryness of the skin and flushing occur.

4. Therapeutic uses. Hexamethonium is not used therapeutically.

C. **Trimethaphan** is a sulfonium ganglionic blocking agent with a very short duration of action.

1. It is used therapeutically in treating hypertensive crises, in the management of autonomic hyperreflexia, and to provide controlled hypotension to reduce bleeding in the operative field during surgery.

2. It may reduce pulmonary edema associated with congestive heart failure by decreasing the return of blood to the right heart.

D. **Mecamylamine,** a ganglionic blocking agent, can be taken orally for the treatment of hypertension.

VIII. NEUROMUSCULAR BLOCKING AGENTS (Table 2-5). These agents, which act by blocking transmission at the neuromuscular junction, can be divided into two classes on the basis of their mechanism of action: **depolarizing agents** and **competitive,** or **stabilizing, blocking agents.**

A. Mechanism of action

1. Depolarizing agents (succinylcholine, decamethonium)

    a. Like acetylcholine, depolarizing agents react with receptors at the muscle end-plate leading to depolarization of the excitable membrane. This **phase I block** is seen clinically as fasciculation.

    b. With prolonged exposure, a reduction in receptor sensitivity occurs, leading to a **phase II,** or **desensitization, block** manifested by flaccid paralysis. This phase II block is not competitive in nature.

TABLE 2-5. Neuromuscular Blocking Agents

Neuromuscular Blocker	Type	Onset/ Duration	Principal Metabolism/ Excretion	Histamine Release	Cardiovascular Effects
SUX	Depolarizing	R/S	PCE	0	Bradycardia
Tubocurarine	Nondepolarizing	S/L	Kidney	+3	Hypotension (histamine/ ganglionic blockade)
Pancuronium	Nondepolarizing	S/L	Kidney/lung	0	Tachycardia (vagolytic)
Gallamine	Nondepolarizing	S/L	Kidney	0	Tachycardia (vagolytic)
Atracurium	Nondepolarizing	I	Blood	+2	0
Vecuronium	Nondepolarizing	I	Kidney/lung	0	0
Doxacurium	Nondepolarizing	S/L	Kidney	0	0
Pipercuronium	Nondepolarizing	S/L	Kidney	0	0
Mivacurium	Nondepolarizing	R/S	AChE	+1	0
Rocuronium	Nondepolarizing	R/S	Lung	0	0

AChE = acetylcholinesterase; I = intermediate; L = long; P = pseudocholinesterase; R = rapid; S = short; 0 = none; +1 = slight; +2 = mild; +3 = moderate.

    2. Competitive blocking agents (tubocurarine, gallamine, pancuronium, atracurium, vecuronium, metocurine, pipercuronium, rocuronium)
        a. Competitive blocking agents combine with acetylcholine receptors at the muscle end-plate but do not activate them.
        b. By decreasing the number of available acetylcholine receptors, these agents reduce the height of the end-plate potential; thus, the threshold for excitation is not reached.

B. **Pharmacokinetics**

    1. Distribution. After injection, neuromuscular blocking agents are found in high concentration in venous blood flowing to the heart and ultimately in the extracellular space around the muscle end-plate.

    2. Onset and duration of action. Nondepolarizing (competitive) blockers are safer, but slower in onset and dose-dependent (i.e., the larger the dose, the more rapid the onset and the longer the duration of action).
        a. Depolarizing agents. Succinylcholine has a rapid onset of action, which facilitates rapid endotracheal intubation.
        b. Nondepolarizing agents
            (1) Rocuronium has the fastest onset of action of any nondepolarizing agent.
            (2) Atracurium has a longer onset of action than succinylcholine, and spontaneous recovery occurs after 30–60 minutes.

    3. Metabolism
        a. Metabolism of gallamine, tubocurarine, and decamethonium is negligible.
        b. Pancuronium is deacetylated, and its metabolites show some activity.
        c. Succinylcholine is rapidly metabolized to succinylmonocholine and choline, which accounts for its brief duration of action.
        d. Atracurium is inactivated in the plasma by enzymatic ester hydrolysis and by a nonenzymatic process known as Hofmann elimination.

C. Therapeutic uses

1. Neuromuscular blocking agents are used:
   a. As surgical adjuvants to anesthesia
      (1) For promoting skeletal muscle relaxation
      (2) For facilitating endotracheal intubation
   b. With electroconvulsant shock therapy to prevent trauma
   c. In the diagnosis of myasthenia gravis (tubocurarine), although provocative tests of this sort are potentially hazardous

2. Atracurium may be useful in patients with renal failure because it does not rely on the kidney for excretion.

3. **Pipercuronium** does not have vagolytic activity nor does it cause histamine release.

D. Adverse effects

1. **All neuromuscular blocking agents**
   a. These agents do not affect the sensorium, so that, despite the paralysis, individuals remain conscious and are able to feel pain.
   b. Prolonged apnea may occur.

2. **Depolarizing agents**
   a. The fasciculations can cause muscle pain; this occurs most frequently in young patients.
   b. Fasciculation of the abdominal muscles can result in increased intragastric pressure. This is important in patients at risk of aspirating gastric contents.
   c. Contraction of extraocular muscles can lead to an increase in intraocular pressure.
   d. The muscle fasciculations and the increased intraocular and intragastric pressure may be diminished by the prior administration of a small dose of a competitive blocking agent.
   e. Succinylcholine may exert some action at other acetylcholine receptors, such as stimulation of autonomic ganglia and muscarinic receptors.
   f. The resulting effects, such as bradycardia and increased bronchial secretions, are seen more commonly with repeated intravenous administration in children; cardiac arrest has occurred.
   g. In some genetically predisposed individuals, the combination of succinylcholine and halothane results in a rapid and potentially fatal increase in temperature (malignant hyperthermia).

3. **Tubocurarine**
   a. A dose-related decrease in arterial pressure, the most common side effect, is the result of both ganglionic blockade and histamine release.
   b. Histamine release can also result in bronchospasm.

4. **Metocurine** causes histamine release less often than tubocurarine does, and **atracurium** is a less potent histamine releaser than either tubocurarine or metocurine.

5. **Vecuronium** causes no histamine release; thus, the risk of histamine-induced hypotension or bronchoconstriction is reduced.

6. **Gallamine** causes tachycardia and increased arterial pressure, the results of both vagolytic and tyramine-like effects.

7. **Pancuronium** also causes an increase in the heart rate and in arterial pressure, but to a lesser extent than gallamine does; the mechanism is not understood.

8. **Pipercuronium** can have a prolonged duration of action in patients with renal failure.

E. Factors influencing the action of neuromuscular blocking agents

1. Serum cholinesterase is determined genetically; the normally transient effects of succinylcholine are greatly prolonged in an individual with deficient serum cholinesterase.

2. Because serum cholinesterase is synthesized in the liver, hepatic disease can double the duration of action of succinylcholine.

3. Echothiophate, an irreversible cholinesterase inhibitor used in the treatment of glaucoma, can significantly decrease cholinesterase activity and thereby increase the duration of action of succinylcholine.

4. Patients with myasthenia gravis are highly sensitive to competitive neuromuscular blocking agents, and phase II block occurs sooner than in normal individuals when depolarizing blockers are given.

5. Patients with Eaton-Lambert syndrome (small cell, or oat cell, carcinoma of the lung) have increased sensitivity to both competitive and depolarizing neuromuscular blockers.

6. Depolarizing neuromuscular blockers increase serum potassium; this is exacerbated in conditions that are associated with hyperkalemia, such as burns.

7. Aminoglycoside antibiotics and lincomycin exert a synergistic neuromuscular blockade when given with either competitive or depolarizing neuromuscular blocking agents; the mechanism is presynaptic.

8. All inhalation anesthetics increase the effects of neuromuscular blocking agents.

F. | **Reversal of neuromuscular blockade**

1. Competitive neuromuscular blockers can be antagonized by cholinesterase inhibitors, such as edrophonium, neostigmine, or pyridostigmine.

2. No antagonists exist for depolarizing blockers.
   a. Controlled ventilation is used until spontaneous recovery occurs.
   b. If an anticholinesterase is given, phase I block increases, but an anticholinesterase may reverse phase II block.

DIRECTIONS: Each of the numbered items or incomplete statements in this section is followed by answers or by completions of the statement. Select the ONE lettered answer or completion that is BEST in each case.

1. A patient who is using a direct-acting sympathomimetic agent as a decongestant is most likely to be taking

(A) ephedrine
(B) amphetamine
(C) phenylephrine
(D) metaraminol
(E) mephentermine

2. A patient is taking a mixed-acting sympathomimetic as a nasal decongestant. This agent, which causes tachyphylaxis and qualitatively resembles epinephrine in its cardiovascular effects, most likely is

(A) ephedrine
(B) phenylephrine
(C) metaproterenol
(D) terbutaline
(E) amphetamine

3. Which of the following agents would bring a rapid heart rate (120 beats/minute) back to normal?

(A) Isoproterenol
(B) Phentolamine
(C) Propranolol
(D) Phenoxybenzamine
(E) Edrophonium

4. A 29-year-old woman says that her eyes will not stay open despite the fact that she is not tired. On physical examination, her facial musculature weakens as she continues to talk. Which of the following drugs would be most useful in helping to make a diagnosis in this patient?

(A) Physostigmine
(B) Neostigmine
(C) Pyridostigmine
(D) Edrophonium
(E) Demecarium

5. Atropine is useful in treating poisoning produced by organophosphate insecticides because it

(A) reactivates inhibited acetylcholinesterase
(B) stimulates α-receptors directly
(C) stimulates β-receptors directly
(D) inhibits normal ganglionic transmission
(E) blocks the action of acetylcholine at both central and peripheral sites

6. Which neuromuscular blocking agent has the potential to cause the greatest release of histamine?

(A) Succinylcholine
(B) Pancuronium
(C) Tubocurarine
(D) Mivacurium
(E) Rocuronium

7. A 15-year-old girl presents with complaints of frequent migraine headaches. Which of the following drugs might help to prevent them?

(A) Aspirin
(B) Propranolol
(C) Ibuprofen
(D) Ephedrine
(E) Phenylephrine

8. Dopamine can be used to treat which of the following?

(A) Parkinson's disease
(B) Angina
(C) Side effects of phenothiazines
(D) Atrioventricular (AV) conduction disturbances
(E) Cardiogenic shock

9. Which nondepolarizing neuromuscular blocking agent has the most rapid onset of action?

(A) Succinylcholine
(B) Pancuronium
(C) Tubocurarine
(D) Rocuronium
(E) Doxacurium

DIRECTIONS: Each of the numbered items or incomplete statements in this section is negatively phrased, as indicated by a capitalized word such as NOT, LEAST, or EXCEPT. Select the ONE lettered answer or completion that is BEST in each case.

10. All of the following agents are β-adrenergic agonists EXCEPT

(A) epinephrine
(B) isoproterenol
(C) norepinephrine
(D) phentolamine
(E) dobutamine

11. All of the following neuromuscular blockers would be contraindicated in patients with renal failure EXCEPT

(A) atracurium
(B) doxacurium
(C) pipercuronium
(D) gallamine
(E) tubocurarine

12. Characteristics of carbachol include all of the following EXCEPT

(A) it is a parasympathetic agent
(B) it exerts both nicotinic and muscarinic effects
(C) it is resistant to acetylcholinesterase
(D) it causes mydriasis
(E) it has a carbonic acid–ester link

13. Characteristics of pancuronium include all of the following EXCEPT

(A) it can increase heart rate
(B) it acts by the same mechanism as tubocurarine
(C) it produces analgesia
(D) it can increase arterial pressure
(E) it can be antagonized by cholinesterase inhibitors

DIRECTIONS: The set of matching questions in this section consists of a list of four to twenty-six lettered options (some of which may be figures) followed by several numbered items. For each numbered item, select the ONE lettered option that is most closely associated with it. To avoid spending too much time on matching sets with large numbers of options, it is generally advisable to begin each set by reading the list of options. Then, for each item in the set, try to generate the correct answer and locate it in the option list, rather than evaluating each option individually. Each lettered option may be selected once, more than once, or not at all.

Questions 14–18

Match each description to the most appropriate β-adrenergic blocking agent.

(A) Acebutolol
(B) Labetalol
(C) Sotalol
(D) Pindolol
(E) Timolol

14. Nonselective β-blocker used to treat glaucoma

15. Nonselective β-blocker with α_1-blocking activity

16. Nonselective β-blocker with α-adrenergic activity

17. β-blocker with a stronger β_1-blocking effect than β_2-blocking effect

18. Nonselective β-blocker that lacks intrinsic sympathomimetic and local anesthetic activity

Questions 19–22

Match each effect with the correct receptor type.

(A) β_1
(B) β_2
(C) α
(D) α, β
(E) M_2

19. Bronchial relaxation

20. Increased gastrointestinal motility and secretion

21. Increased myocardial contraction strength

22. Constriction of veins

ANSWERS AND EXPLANATIONS

1. The answer is C *[II E 1 a, 2 a]*. All of the substances listed in the question are sympathomimetic agents. Phenylephrine is direct-acting and is used clinically as a decongestant. Ephedrine, amphetamine, mephentermine, and metaraminol are all mixed-acting agents.

2. The answer is A *[II F 2, 3 b]*. Phenylephrine, metaproterenol, and terbutaline are all direct-acting sympathomimetic agents, whereas amphetamine is indirect-acting. Ephedrine is mixed-acting and is used as a nasal decongestant. While its primary action is indirect, causing release of norepinephrine from storage in nerve terminals, it also directly stimulates sympathetic receptors.

3. The answer is C *[III B 1 b (1)]*. Propranolol is an effective agent for treating an abnormal tachycardia. Its mechanism of action is β-adrenergic blockade. Propranolol decreases the heart rate, reduces cardiac output, and prolongs systole. It reduces total coronary blood flow to most tissues (except the brain) and lowers oxygen consumption.

4. The answer is D *[V C 3 a]*. If the patient's symptoms are caused by myasthenia gravis, they will be reversed by a cholinesterase inhibitor. Although neostigmine and pyridostigmine are used for the symptomatic treatment of myasthenia gravis, edrophonium is more useful for the diagnosis of this disorder because it is more rapidly absorbed and has a shorter duration of action. Demecarium and physostigmine are used in the treatment of glaucoma; the latter drug is also useful for reversing the anticholinergic effects of various drugs.

5. The answer is E *[VI A 1, 4 f]*. Atropine is both a central and a peripheral muscarinic blocker. Atropine competes reversibly with acetylcholine at muscarinic receptors, antagonizes the action of acetylcholine in the central nervous system (CNS), and, at high concentrations, blocks acetylcholine action at ganglionic synapses and motor nerve endings.

6. The answer is C *[VIII D; Table 2-5]*. Tubocurarine can cause histamine release, which may result in bronchospasm and a dose-related fall in arterial pressure. The latter is also a result of ganglionic blockade. Succinylcholine, pancuronium, and rocuronium do not cause histamine release. Mivacurium only has a slight potential to cause histamine release.

7. The answer is B *[III B 1 c (7)]*. Propranolol, a β-adrenergic receptor blocker, is used for the prophylaxis of migraine headaches. Aspirin and ibuprofen are both analgesics and can be used for the treatment of migraine headaches, but not for the prevention of acute attacks. Ephedrine and phenylephrine are used as nasal decongestants and pressor agents.

8. The answer is E *[II C 5]*. Dopamine, an intermediate in the biosynthesis of norepinephrine, is an important neurotransmitter in the central nervous system (CNS). Dopamine, a β_1-adrenergic agonist with positive inotropic effects on the myocardium, is used in the treatment of cardiogenic and septic shock and in chronic refractory congestive heart failure (CHF). In Parkinson's disease, a dopamine deficiency in the stratum appears to cause the neurologic symptoms. However, the drug dopamine does not cross the blood–brain barrier, and, therefore, levodopa (L-dopa), the precursor of dopamine, is administered instead. The neurologic side effects of antipsychotic agents, such as the phenothiazines, resemble the symptoms of Parkinson's disease, but again dopamine would be ineffective as therapy. Dopamine could exacerbate arrhythmias and anginal pain.

9. The answer is D *[Table 2-5]*. Rocuronium has the fastest onset of action of any nondepolarizing agent. Although succinylcholine has a rapid onset of action, it is a depolarizing agent. Tubocurarine, pancuronium, and doxacurium have slow onsets of action.

10. The answer is D *[II A 3, B 2 a, D 2 a; III A 2]*. Phentolamine is an α-adrenergic antagonist. Isoproterenol, epinephrine, and norepinephrine are agonists for all adrenergic receptors, α and β. Dobutamine, though resembling dopamine chemically, is a direct β_1-receptor agonist. The relative potency at β_1-receptors is isoproterenol > dobutamine > epinephrine and norepinephrine.

11. The answer is A *[VIII C 2; Table 2-5]*. Doxacurium, pipercuronium, gallamine, and tubocurarine are all excreted via the kidney and therefore would be contraindicated in patients with renal failure. Atracurium is inactivated in the plasma by enzymatic ester hydrolysis and by a nonenzymatic process known as Hofmann elimination.

12. The answer is D *[IV C]*. Carbachol (carba-mylcholine) is a parasympathetic agent that is resistant to cholinesterase because of its car-bamic acid–ester link. It exerts both muscarinic and nicotinic effects. Because it is a parasympa-thetic agonist, it causes miosis, not mydriasis.

13. The answer is C *[VIII D 1 a, 7]*. Pancuro-nium is, like tubocurarine, a competitive mus-cular blocker. Unlike tubocurarine, it can cause an increase in arterial pressure, whereas tubo-curarine causes histamine-induced hypoten-sion. Unlike succinylcholine, pancuronium can increase the heart rate. None of the neuromus-cular blocking agents affect awareness of pain. Reversal of neuromuscular blockade is via cholinesterase inhibitors such as neostigmine.

14–18. The answers are: 14-E *[III B 2]*, **15-B** *[III B 5]*, **16-D** *[III B 6]*, **17-A** *[III B 7]*, **18-C** *[III B 4]*. Timolol is a nonselective β-adrenergic blocking agent (i.e., it competes for both β_1- and β_2-receptors). Timolol lowers intraocular pressure by reducing the produc-tion of aqueous humor and is therefore useful for the treatment of glaucoma; it is available as eye drops for this purpose.

Labetalol is another nonselective β-blocker; it also has α_1-blocking activity. Labetalol is a potent antihypertensive agent.

Pindolol is a nonselective β-blocker that also has some degree of intrinsic sympatho-mimetic (α-adrenergic) activity.

Acebutolol is primarily a β_1-blocking agent but has some β_2-blocking activity. It can cause arthralgia and myalgia as well as the usual untoward effects seen with β-blockers.

Sotalol is a nonselective β-blocker without intrinsic sympathomimetic or local anesthetic activity. It is approved for the oral treatment of life-threatening ventricular arrhythmias.

19–22. The answers are: 19-B, 20-E, 21-A, 22-C *[Table 2-2]*. β_2-Agonists (e.g., metapro-terenol, albuterol, salmeterol) have relaxing effects on bronchial smooth muscle and are used therapeutically for the treatment of bronchial asthma.

M_2 agonists (e.g., bethanechol) can increase gastrointestinal motility and secretion and have been used therapeutically to treat abdominal distention.

β_1-Agonists, such as dobutamine, are occa-sionally used to improve myocardial function in patients with congestive heart failure (CHF).

α-Agonists, such as phenylephrine, act on vascular smooth muscle and produce constric-tion of veins.

Chapter 3
Agents Acting on the Central Nervous System

I. INTRODUCTION

A. **Transmission of nerve impulses** (see Figure 2-1).

   1. **Information transfer.** The brain and spinal cord are involved in information transfer via electrical signals passing along axons (**action potentials**).

   2. **Synaptic transmission**
      a. The **locus of communication** between neurons is the **synapse**.
         (1) In general, a chemical **neurotransmitter** is released from a presynaptic neuron, diffuses across the synaptic cleft, and interacts with a special cell-surface receptor located on a second, postsynaptic neuron.
         (2) The neurotransmitter–receptor complex initiates a sequence of events (e.g., the opening of channels for particular ions), which can excite, inhibit, or otherwise modulate the electrical activity of the postsynaptic neuron.
      b. Synaptic transmission between neurons can be affected by altering the levels of neurotransmitter in the presynaptic neuron. This can be accomplished by various agents, which:
         (1) Block or enhance the biosynthesis of the neurotransmitter
         (2) Block or enhance the metabolic degradation of the neurotransmitter
         (3) Alter the reuptake and reutilization of the neurotransmitter in presynaptic terminals
      c. It is possible to alter the amount of neurotransmitter that is released by activating **presynaptic receptors (autoreceptors)** that are located at some synapses.
      d. Many drugs are believed to bind to receptors and, bypassing the normal neurotransmitter, either to activate or block the response of the postsynaptic neuron, serving as agonists or antagonists, respectively.
      e. Some drugs may act directly on ion channels, bypassing the neurotransmitter–receptor interaction entirely.

   3. **Mechanism of action.** Although the basic mechanisms underlying many of the agents that act on the central nervous system (CNS) are only partially understood, most are believed to alter either the basic cellular functioning of neurons or the communication between neurons.
      a. Any agent that slows or blocks the axonal electrical conduction (e.g., a local anesthetic) will affect behavior.
      b. At therapeutic doses, most of the pharmacologically useful agents that affect the CNS are believed to act at various specific synaptic sites.

B. **Blood–brain barrier.** The ability of an agent to affect CNS function depends on its ability to cross or mediate an effect across the **blood–brain barrier**.

   1. The blood–brain barrier restricts the passage of polar compounds and macromolecules from the blood into the brain interstitium.
      a. Agents that are lipid-soluble, are un-ionized to physiologic pH, and bind poorly to plasma proteins are better able to diffuse across the blood–brain barrier.
      b. Some metabolically important compounds (e.g., nutrients) apparently are actively transported across this barrier.

2. The morphologic basis for the blood–brain barrier appears to be the structure of the endothelial cell layer lining the brain capillaries. Transendothelial vesicular transport (pinocytosis) is a primary cellular mechanism by which plasma protein constituents and macromolecules pass through the cerebrovascular endothelium.

II. SEDATIVE–HYPNOTICS

A. Barbiturates (Table 3-1)

1. **Chemistry**
   a. The parent compound, **barbituric acid,** is derived from a dehydration of urea and malonic acid. Barbituric acid itself has no depressant effect on the CNS.
   b. Changes in structure that favor increased lipid solubility speed up the onset of action, shorten the duration of action, and increase the hypnotic potency.
   c. When the oxygen at C-2 of oxybarbiturates is replaced with a sulfur, it becomes a thiobarbiturate, a compound with enhanced lipid solubility.

2. **Classification.** Barbiturates are classified on the basis of their onset and duration of action.
   a. **Ultra–short-acting** barbiturates (e.g., **thiopental**) act within seconds, and their duration of action is 30 minutes. Their principal use is as intravenous adjuvants to anesthesia.
   b. **Short-acting** barbiturates (e.g., **pentobarbital**) have a duration of action of about 2 hours; their principal use is as sleep-inducing hypnotics.
   c. **Intermediate-acting** barbiturates (e.g., **amobarbital**) have an effect lasting 3–5 hours. Their principal use is as hypnotics; however, they have a "hangover" liability, the result of residual depression of the CNS.
   d. **Long-acting** barbiturates (e.g., **phenobarbital**) have a duration of action greater than 6 hours. They are effective hypnotics and sedatives and at low doses are used as antiepileptic agents, but they are likely to cause hangover.

3. **Mechanism of action**
   a. At low doses, barbiturates either have a γ-aminobutyric acid (GABA)-like action or enhance the effects of GABA, an inhibitory neurotransmitter.
   b. When GABA receptors are activated, chloride channels open. Chloride enters the cell, hyperpolarizes it, and produces decreased excitation.
   c. There is also a picrotoxin site associated with the GABA receptor to which barbiturates bind. The greater the affinity of a barbiturate for the picrotoxin binding site, the greater is its potency.
   d. Barbiturates are less selective than benzodiazepines, which also have GABA-like actions, because elevating the dose of barbiturates produces a generalized CNS depression in addition to selective depression at synaptic sites.

TABLE 3-1. Common Barbiturates: Duration of Action

Drug	Duration of Action
Thiopental	Ultra-short
Hexobarbital	Short
Pentobarbital	Short
Secobarbital	Short
Amobarbital	Intermediate
Butabarbital	Intermediate
Barbital	Long
Phenobarbital	Long

4. Pharmacokinetics
   a. The duration of action of a barbiturate depends on:
      (1) Its rate of metabolic (hepatic) degradation
      (2) Its degree of lipid solubility
      (3) The extent to which it binds to serum proteins, which reduces renal excretion
   b. Long-acting barbiturates are metabolized principally in the liver by a slow oxidation of the radicals at C-5, which produces more polar derivatives with low lipid solubility.
   c. Ultra–short-acting barbiturates are highly lipid-soluble and, thus, have a short onset and duration of action.
      (1) High lipid solubility allows rapid transport across the blood–brain barrier.
      (2) Removal of the ultra–short-acting barbiturates from the brain occurs via redistribution to other tissues (e.g., muscle).
   d. Barbiturates are absorbed from the stomach, small intestine, rectum, and intramuscular sites.
   e. They readily cross the placental barrier, and concentrations in the fetal blood approach those in maternal blood.
   f. Barbiturates and their metabolites are principally excreted via the renal route. Alkalinization of the urine profoundly expedites the excretion of barbiturates with lower lipid solubility, such as phenobarbital.

5. Pharmacologic effects
   a. Barbiturates depress the CNS at all levels in a dose-dependent fashion. A barbiturate plus another CNS depressant (e.g., a phenothiazine, ethanol, or an antihistamine) can result in marked depression.
   b. As hypnotics, barbiturates decrease the amount of time spent in rapid eye movement (REM) sleep.
   c. Barbiturates are not analgesic and, at low doses, are thought to be hyperalgesic.
   d. All barbiturates suppress convulsant activity if given in sufficient doses.
   e. Respiration is depressed at multiple levels. As CNS depression develops and the neurogenic respiratory drive is eliminated, the respiratory drive shifts to the carotid and aortic bodies.
   f. At sedative doses, barbiturates have little effect on the cardiovascular system. Toxic dose levels can cause circulatory collapse, due, in part, to medullary vasomotor depression.
   g. Most barbiturates, but especially phenobarbital, can induce hepatic microsomal drug-metabolizing enzymes.
      (1) This results in increased degradation of the barbiturate, ultimately leading to barbiturate tolerance.
      (2) It also causes increased inactivation of other compounds, such as the anticoagulants, phenytoin, digitoxin, theophylline, and glucocorticoids, leading to potentially serious problems with drug interactions.
   h. Barbiturate-induced porphyria can occur as a result of more rapid hemoglobin degradation.

6. Therapeutic uses
   a. Although still used as sedative–hypnotic agents, barbiturates are being replaced for this purpose by the benzodiazepines (see II B 3; VI C) because of the following disadvantages:
      (1) They have a narrow therapeutic-to-toxic dosage range.
      (2) They suppress REM sleep.
      (3) Tolerance develops relatively quickly.
      (4) They have a high potential for physical dependence and abuse.
      (5) Drug interactions secondary to microsomal enzyme induction are frequent.
   b. Due to their rapid onset of action, barbiturates (i.e., phenobarbital, pentobarbital, amobarbital, thiopental) are used in the emergency treatment of convulsions as in status epilepticus (see III A). In adults, however, the benzodiazepines are the drugs of choice.

   c. The ultra–short-acting thiobarbiturates are useful as intravenous adjuncts to surgical anesthetics.

   d. Barbiturates, especially in anesthetic doses, significantly decrease oxygen utilization by the brain, which may be of value in lessening cerebral edema caused by surgery or trauma and in protecting against cerebral infarction during cerebral ischemia.

   e. The ability of barbiturates to stimulate liver glucuronyl transferase has been applied successfully in the treatment of hyperbilirubinemia and kernicterus in the neonate.

7. Adverse effects

   a. Depressant effects include oversedation and a decrease in REM sleep.

   b. Skin eruptions and porphyria can occur.

   c. Barbiturate dependence

     (1) Physiologic as well as psychological dependence can occur.

     (2) Withdrawal of a barbiturate may result in grand mal seizures, severe tremors, vivid hallucinations, and psychoses. Abrupt withdrawal should be avoided.

   d. Acute barbiturate overdosage

     (1) An overdose can result in coma, diminished reflexes (although deep tendon reflexes are usually intact), severe respiratory depression, hypotension leading to cardiovascular collapse, and renal failure.

     (2) Treatment of acute overdosage

       (a) Primary treatment consists of supporting respiration and circulation.

       (b) Excretion of the drug is fostered by alkalinizing the urine and promoting diuresis. These measures are most effective with the long-acting barbiturates.

       (c) Hemodialysis or peritoneal dialysis is useful and often needed.

B. **Nonbarbiturate sedative–hypnotics**

1. Chloral hydrate

   a. Pharmacokinetics

     (1) Chloral hydrate is metabolized in the liver by alcohol dehydrogenase to trichloroethanol, which is thought to be the active metabolite producing the CNS effects.

     (2) Trichloroethanol and, to a lesser extent, chloral hydrate are oxidized to trichloro-acetic acid, which is excreted in the kidney, as the glucuronide conjugate.

   b. Therapeutic uses

     (1) Chloral hydrate is a relatively safe hypnotic drug, inducing sleep in a half hour and lasting about 6 hours. It causes a relatively small reduction in REM sleep.

     (2) It is used mainly in children and the elderly and is most effective when used for 1–3 nights to treat transient insomnia.

   c. Adverse effects

     (1) Chloral hydrate is bad-tasting and irritating to the gastrointestinal tract.

     (2) The CNS depressant effects are potentiated by alcohol (the combination being dubbed a "Mickey Finn").

     (3) Addiction can occur.

2. Paraldehyde

   a. Chemistry. Paraldehyde is a trimer of acetaldehyde.

   b. Mechanism of action

     (1) Paraldehyde produces hypnosis in about 15 minutes, and its effects last 4–8 hours.

     (2) Its CNS depressant activity resembles that of alcohol, chloral hydrate, and the barbiturates.

   c. Route of administration. Paraldehyde can be administered orally, parenterally, or rectally.

   d. Therapeutic uses

     (1) Paraldehyde is used exclusively for patients undergoing withdrawal from alcohol.

     (2) It is used for patients with hepatic or renal failure because it is mainly eliminated via the lungs.

e. Adverse effects

(1) Its strong odor and disagreeable taste limit its use mainly to hospitals.

(2) It is a gastrointestinal irritant.

(3) It should not be used with disulfiram.

3. Benzodiazepine derivatives (see VI C). The benzodiazepines are generally considered to be the preferred drugs for sedation–hypnosis. In contrast to the various other sedative–hypnotics, the benzodiazepines are not general neuronal depressants. They act on the allosteric site of the GABA receptor, facilitating chloride entry into the neuron, which produces an inhibitory effect on neuronal conduction. Whether the antianxiety properties of the benzodiazepines are distinct from their sedative–hypnotic effects is presently unclear.

a. Flurazepam

(1) **Pharmacologic effects.** Flurazepam produces hypnotic effects within 20–40 minutes after an oral dose, which may last for 6–8 hours. The major metabolite has a long half-life and may cause daytime sedation and motor impairment.

(2) **Adverse effects**

(a) Flurazepam causes less suppression of REM sleep than other benzodiazepines.

(b) Overdosage can occur and is treated as for other benzodiazepines (see VI C 4 b).

(c) At moderate dosage, addiction potential is low, as is withdrawal (rebound) insomnia, which is often seen with many of the other hypnotics.

b. Triazolam

(1) **Pharmacokinetics.** Triazolam has the shortest latency period before sleep, but because of its short duration of action, its effects may not persist through the night.

(2) **Therapeutic uses.** Triazolam is used for the short-term treatment of insomnia.

(3) **Adverse effects**

(a) It is least likely to cause residual drowsiness but may cause daytime anxiety.

(b) Rebound insomnia may occur.

(c) Profound anterograde amnesia and toxic psychosis have been reported.

c. Temazepam

(1) **Pharmacokinetics**

(a) Temazepam is conjugated with glucuronic acid and is excreted in the urine; therefore, hepatic dysfunction has little effect on its elimination.

(b) While it has a short elimination half-life, temazepam has an intermediate-to-slow onset and may accumulate with repeated use.

(2) **Pharmacologic effects.** Temazepam decreases awakenings and increases sleep time. It does not affect sleep latency.

III. AGENTS USED IN THE TREATMENT OF SEIZURES

A. Barbiturates (see II A)

1. Pharmacologic effects

a. As antiseizure agents, barbiturates have a narrow margin of safety. However, phenobarbital possesses more selectivity in its anticonvulsant action than in its sedative effect.

b. If a barbiturate is used as an anticonvulsant during pregnancy, the neonate can experience withdrawal symptoms.

2. Therapeutic uses

a. Barbiturates are the drugs of choice for status epilepticus in infants and children.

b. They are no longer a preferred treatment for the prophylactic control of general seizure states (generalized tonic–clonic seizures, simple and complex partial seizures).

e. Adverse effects
- **(1)** Diplopia, ataxia, and nausea
- **(2)** Bone marrow depression, including aplastic anemia
- **(3)** Congestive heart failure
- **(4)** Atropine-like symptoms
- **(5)** Kidney and liver toxicity

2. Valproic acid (dipropylacetic acid) was used as a solvent in the screening of certain compounds for antiepileptic activity. It was itself found to possess antiseizure activity.
- **a.** Valproate is most effective in seizure states with a subcortical focus (e.g., absence seizures). It is somewhat effective in grand mal seizures and less effective in partial seizures.
- **b.** Valproate is rapidly absorbed from the gastrointestinal tract. Its mechanism of anticonvulsant action is unclear but is thought to involve inhibition of GABA transaminase, the enzyme responsible for the breakdown of GABA; valproate also inhibits succinic aldehyde dehydrogenase. Valproate antagonizes pentylenetetrazol-induced convulsions, suggesting an additional postsynaptic site of action.
- **c. Adverse effects**
  - **(1)** Teratogenicity
  - **(2)** Pancreatitis and hepatic failure, especially when the drug is used in combination with other antiseizure medication
  - **(3)** Anorexia and nausea
  - **(4)** Menstrual disturbances
  - **(5)** Sedation and ataxia
  - **(6)** Alopecia
  - **(7)** Drug interactions, including a 40% rise in plasma phenobarbital concentration with concurrent administration

3. Felbamate is a phenyldicarbamate structurally similar to meprobamate.
- **a. Mechanism of action.** Felbamate blocks sustained repetitive neuronal firing through an effect on sodium channels.
- **b. Therapeutic uses.** Felbamate is orally absorbed. It has been used in the treatment of refractory partial seizures or various types of seizures associated with Lennox–Gastaut syndrome.
- **c. Adverse effects**
  - **(1)** Because of a much higher than expected incidence of aplastic anemia, the use of felbamate has been suspended, except in cases where, in the physician's opinion, the patient's well-being is dependent on continued treatment. Specific risk factors have not yet been identified.
  - **(2)** When taken with other antiepileptic drugs, drug interactions can occur.

G. Dantrolene

1. Mechanism of action. Dantrolene is an antispasticity drug, which works peripherally in the muscle by decreasing Ca^{2+} release from the sarcoplasmic reticulum.

2. Therapeutic uses. It is used in the treatment of malignant hyperthermia and for controlling the manifestations of clinical spasticity, resulting from upper motor neuron disorder.

3. Adverse effects. Dantrolene may cause generalized skeletal muscle weakness. Another major potential adverse reaction is life-threatening hepatic dysfunction of an idiosyncratic or hypersensitivity type.

IV. AGENTS USED IN THE TREATMENT OF PARKINSONIAN DISORDERS

A. Levodopa (L-dopa)

1. Mechanism of action. A dopamine deficiency in the striatum needs to be corrected in the treatment of parkinsonism.

a. Dopamine does not cross the blood–brain barrier; thus, levodopa, the precursor of dopamine, is given instead.

b. Levodopa is formed from L-tyrosine and is an intermediate in the synthesis of catecholamines.

c. Levodopa itself has minimal pharmacologic activity, in contrast to its decarboxylated product, dopamine.

d. Levodopa is rapidly decarboxylated in the gastrointestinal tract. Prior to the advent of decarboxylase inhibitors (carbidopa), large oral doses of levodopa were required; thus, toxicity from dopamine was a limiting factor.

2. **Pharmacokinetics**

a. Levodopa is well absorbed from the small bowel; however, 95% is rapidly decarboxylated in the periphery.

b. Peripheral dopamine is metabolized in the liver to dihydroxyphenylacetic acid (DOPAC) and homovanillic acid (HVA), which are then excreted in the urine.

3. **Pharmacologic effects**

a. The effects on bradykinesia and rigidity are more rapid and complete than the effects on tremor. Other motor defects in Parkinson's disease improve. The psychological well-being of the patient is also improved.

b. Tolerance to both beneficial and adverse effects (see IV A 4) occurs with time. Levodopa is most effective in the first 2–5 years of treatment. After 5 years of therapy, patients have dose-related dyskinesias, inadequate response, or toxicity.

4. **Adverse effects**

a. Because the decarboxylation of levodopa increases peripheral concentrations of dopamine, prominent α- and β-adrenergic effects are seen, but these effects are significantly less severe than those seen with epinephrine, norepinephrine, or isoproterenol.

b. Principal adverse effects include:

(1) Anorexia, nausea, and vomiting upon initial administration, which often limit the initial dosage

(2) Cardiovascular effects, including tachycardia, arrhythmias, and orthostatic hypotension

(3) Mental disturbances, including vivid dreams, delusions, and hallucinations

c. Sudden discontinuation can result in fever, rigidity, and confusion. The drug should be withdrawn gradually over 4 days.

5. **Drug interactions**

a. Pyridoxine reduces the beneficial effects of levodopa by enhancing its extracerebral metabolism. The decarboxylation of levodopa to dopamine is mediated by an enzyme that is pyridoxine-dependent.

b. Phenothiazines, reserpine, and butyrophenones antagonize the effects of levodopa because they lead to a junctional blockade of dopamine action.

c. Therapy with monoamine oxidase (MAO) inhibitors must be stopped 14 days prior to the initiation of levodopa therapy.

d. Dietary amino acids can decrease effectiveness of levodopa by competing for absorption from the intestine.

B. | **Carbidopa**

1. **Pharmacokinetics.** Carbidopa is an inhibitor of dopa decarboxylase. Because it is unable to penetrate the blood–brain barrier, it acts to reduce the peripheral conversion of levodopa to dopamine. As a result, when carbidopa and levodopa are given concomitantly:

a. Levodopa blood levels are increased, and drug half-life is lengthened.

b. The dose of levodopa can be significantly reduced, also reducing toxic side effects.

c. A shorter latency period precedes the occurrence of beneficial effects.

d. If the patient has been taking levodopa alone, it should be withheld for 8 hours before starting combined carbidopa–levodopa therapy, and the dosage of levodopa should be reduced by 75%.

2. **Preparations. Sinemet** is the trade name of a preparation that combines carbidopa and levodopa in fixed proportions (1:10 and 1:4). It is considered the most effective treatment for Parkinson's disease.

3. **Adverse effects** of the combination are similar to those seen with high doses of levodopa.

C. Selegiline

1. **Mechanism of action.** Selegiline is a selective MAO type B inhibitor, also known as deprenyl.

2. **Therapeutic use.** Treatment with selegiline postpones the need for levodopa for 6–9 months.

3. **Adverse effects**
   a. Unlike MAO-A inhibitors (used for depression), selegiline does not cause hypertension after ingesting tyramine-rich foods.
   b. Fluoxetine and meperidine have been associated with toxic reactions when taken with selegiline.

D. Amantadine

1. **Therapeutic uses and mechanism of action**
   a. Amantadine is an antiviral agent used in the prophylaxis of influenza A_2 (see Chapter 12 VIII B). It was found to improve parkinsonian symptoms by stimulating the release of dopamine from dopaminergic nerve terminals in the nigrostriatum and delaying its reuptake.
   b. Amantadine may be more efficacious in parkinsonism than the anticholinergic atropine derivatives (see IV F) but is less effective than levodopa. It has been used alone to treat early Parkinson's disease and as an adjunct in later stages.

2. **Excretion.** Amantadine is well absorbed orally and is excreted unchanged in the urine.

3. **Adverse effects** are infrequent; however, long-term use can produce livedo reticularis in the lower extremities. Tolerance is observed in 6–8 weeks.

E. Bromocriptine and pergolide

1. **Therapeutic uses and mechanism of action**
   a. Bromocriptine and pergolide provide additional therapeutic benefit when added to levodopa therapy, but have less antiparkinsonian effect than levodopa.
   b. As ergot derivatives, bromocriptine and pergolide mimic the action of dopamine.

2. **Adverse effects** such as hallucinations, postural hypotension, and livedo reticularis are more common with bromocriptine than with levodopa; however, it induces less dyskinesia than levodopa.

F. Anticholinergic agents

1. **Mechanism of action**
   a. Since the deficiency of dopamine in the striatum augments the excitatory cholinergic system in the striatum, the blockade of this system by anticholinergic agents, such as trihexyphenidyl, helps to alleviate the motor dysfunction.
   b. Improvement in the parkinsonian tremor is more pronounced than improvement in bradykinesia and rigidity.

2. **Therapeutic uses.** Although not as effective as levodopa or bromocriptine, anticholinergic agents may have an additive therapeutic effect at any stage of the disease when taken concurrently.

3. **Adverse effects,** such as mental confusion and hallucinations due to central muscarinic toxicity, can occur as can peripheral atropine-like toxicity (e.g., cycloplegia, urinary retention, constipation).

G. **Antihistamines** (e.g., diphenhydramine) are less effective therapeutically but are better tolerated than anticholinergic agents.

H. **Antidepressants.** Depression commonly accompanies Parkinson's disease. A tricyclic antidepressant or trazodone is usually the drug of choice.

V. ANTIPSYCHOTIC AGENTS

A. **General considerations**

1. Antipsychotic agents are prescribed for the management of psychotic symptoms; they are sometimes referred to as **major tranquilizers**.

2. They are useful in both acute and chronic psychoses and in nonpsychotic individuals who are delusional or excited. They improve mood and behavior without producing excessive sedation.

3. As a group, these agents produce little physical dependence or habituation but, notably, are capable of causing extrapyramidal symptoms, both reversible (parkinsonian symptoms, akathisia) and irreversible (tardive dyskinesia).

B. **Phenothiazines** (Table 3-2)

1. **Chemistry.** The phenothiazines have a three-ring structure in which two benzene rings are linked by a sulfur and a nitrogen atom (Figure 3-1). Differences within this group result from substitution on the nitrogen.

2. **Pharmacokinetics**
   a. The phenothiazines are erratically absorbed from the gastrointestinal tract.
   b. They are highly protein-bound and enter the fetal circulation.
   c. Their biologic effects last 24 hours, allowing once-daily dosing.
   d. Phenothiazines are metabolized in the hepatic microsomal system by hydroxylation, followed by conjugation with glucuronic acid. In addition, the formation of sulfoxides is an important metabolic pathway.

3. **Pharmacologic effects**
   a. **CNS effects**
      (1) The psychotic patient has fewer hallucinations and delusions. Improvements in behavior are most often noted with long-term therapy.

TABLE 3-2. Common Phenothiazine Derivatives

Drug	Major Use	Orthostatic Hypotension	Extrapyramidal Symptoms
Chlorpromazine (Thorazine)	Antipsychotic Antiemetic	Moderate	Moderate
Clozapine (Clozaril)	Antipsychotic Anticholinergic Antihistaminic	Low	Low
Thioridazine (Mellaril)	Antipsychotic	Moderate	Low
Triflupromazine (Vesprin)	Antipsychotic	Moderate	High
Fluphenazine (Prolixin)	Antipsychotic	Low	High
Prochlorperazine (Compazine)	Antiemetic	Low	Low–moderate
Promethazine (Phenergan)	Antihistaminic	Moderate	Low

The columns "Orthostatic Hypotension" and "Extrapyramidal Symptoms" fall under **Frequency of Adverse Effects**.

FIGURE 3-1. Phenothiazine nucleus.

    (a) Tolerance to these effects is rarely seen.

    (b) The antipsychotic effects are believed to be due to antagonism of dopaminergic neurotransmission in the limbic, nigrostriatal, and hypothalamic systems.

(2) Extrapyramidal symptoms occur most often with chronic administration.

    (a) These effects arise, presumably, because of antidopaminergic effects in the basal ganglia. They can be treated by lowering the dose or by using an anticholinergic antiparkinsonian drug such as benztropine mesylate.

    (b) Phenothiazines having the greatest antihistaminic and anticholinergic properties will exhibit the fewest extrapyramidal effects.

(3) The **neuroleptic effects** of the antipsychotic drugs consist of emotional quieting, reduced physical movement, and a potential for neurologic side effects. The drugs have little effect on the intellectual functioning of the patient.

(4) Most phenothiazines are antiemetic. They antagonize agents, such as apomorphine, which stimulate the chemoreceptor trigger zone. In high doses, phenothiazines may directly depress the medullary vomiting center.

(5) Phenothiazines are capable of altering temperature-regulating mechanisms. Normally, they produce hypothermia; however, in a hot climate they can cause hyperthermia because of failure to lose body heat.

(6) Since phenothiazines depress the hypothalamus, endocrine alterations may occur.

    (a) This includes the release of lactogenic hormone (prolactin), inducing lactation.

    (b) Abnormal pigmentation can occur because of an increased release of melanocyte-stimulating hormone from the pituitary.

    (c) Increased levels of prolactin may lead to galactorrhea and gynecomastia.

    (d) Phenothiazines decrease corticotropin release and secretion of pituitary growth hormone.

    (e) Weight gain and increased appetite are seen with phenothiazine use.

b. Peripheral effects

    (1) An α-adrenergic blocking activity is seen, especially with the prototypic phenothiazine, chlorpromazine.

    (2) Adrenergic potentiation, especially with chronic administration, is probably a result of the ability of phenothiazines to inhibit the reuptake of norepinephrine.

    (3) Anticholinergic effects can result in blurred vision, constipation, dry mouth, decreased sweating, and, rarely, urinary retention. Miosis is seen with chlorpromazine and is probably due to α-adrenergic blockade. Other phenothiazines can produce mydriasis.

    (4) Chlorpromazine is a potent local anesthetic.

    (5) Antihistaminic activity is seen with most phenothiazine derivatives.

    (6) Inhibition of ejaculation without interference with erection can occur, especially with thioridazine.

    (7) Inhibition of antidiuretic hormone (ADH) secretion by chlorpromazine can result in a weak diuretic effect.

    (8) Orthostatic hypotension can occur as a result of both the central action of phenothiazines and inhibition of norepinephrine uptake mechanisms. In addition, chlorpromazine has an antiarrhythmic effect upon the heart.

(9) Phenothiazines are known to enhance the pharmacologic actions of barbiturates, narcotics, and ethyl alcohol.

4. **Therapeutic uses**
   a. Phenothiazines are used chiefly in the treatment of psychotic disorders, including mania, paranoid states, schizophrenia, and psychoses associated with chronic alcoholism (alcoholic hallucinosis).
   b. In addition, several phenothiazines are effective in the treatment of nausea and vomiting of certain causes, such as drug-induced nausea.
   c. Due to their H_1 antihistaminic activity, some phenothiazines are useful as antipruritics.
   d. Chlorpromazine is useful in the control of intractable hiccup.

5. **Adverse effects**
   a. **CNS effects**
      (1) A parkinsonian syndrome may occur in which patients display rigidity and tremor at rest.
      (2) Acute dystonic reactions may be seen with initial drug therapy. Patients display facial grimacing and torticollis.
      (3) Tardive dyskinesia may be seen with chronic therapy. Patients display sucking and smacking of the lips and other involuntary facial movements. The dyskinesia may persist far after discontinuation of therapy.
      (4) Lethargy and drowsiness may occur.
   b. **Cardiovascular effects** include orthostatic hypotension, which can result in syncope, and reflex tachycardia.
   c. **Allergic reactions** most often occur during the first few months of therapy.
      (1) Cholestatic jaundice can occur; it resolves with discontinuation of drug therapy.
      (2) Blood dyscrasias (e.g., agranulocytosis) and eosinophilia can occur but are rare.
      (3) Various forms of dermatitis may occur, including a photosensitivity reaction that resembles a severe sunburn.
   d. Children exhibit extrapyramidal symptoms and, less commonly, may develop jaundice, blood dyscrasias, or hyperpyrexia.
   e. Somnolence and hypotension are prominent adverse effects of acute intoxication.

C. **Thioxanthene derivatives** are similar chemically and pharmacologically to the phenothiazine derivatives. They differ chemically in that a carbon is substituted for a nitrogen in the central ring of the phenothiazine nucleus (position 10). The thioxanthenes in clinical use are **chlorprothixene** and **thiothixene**.

D. **Butyrophenones**

1. The prototype is **haloperidol,** which resembles the phenothiazine derivatives pharmacologically. It has potent antiemetic properties, antagonizing stimulation of the chemoreceptor trigger zone. Significant extrapyramidal symptoms are associated with its use.

2. Another butyrophenone, **droperidol,** is often combined with a potent narcotic analgesic, such as fentanyl, to produce neuroleptanalgesia. This combination is known by the trade name Innovar.

E. **Clozapine**

1. **Chemistry.** It is a tetracyclic N-methyl-piperazinyl-dibenzodiazepine analog.

2. **Pharmacokinetics.** At least 80% of orally administered clozapine appears in the urine or feces as metabolites. The half-life is 12 hours.

3. **Pharmacologic effects**
   a. Unlike standard neuroleptic and antipsychotic agents, clozapine lacks extrapyramidal side effects.
   b. It also differs from typical neuroleptic agents by having low affinity for D_1 and D_2 dopamine receptors.

    c. Clozapine has relatively potent anticholinergic activity.

    d. Other activities include antiadrenergic, antiserotoninergic, and possible antihistaminergic activities.

4. Therapeutic uses. Clozapine can be effective in treating some patients with psychosis who are unresponsive to standard neuroleptic drugs. It can be used safely if granulocyte counts are monitored weekly.

5. Adverse effects. Although clozapine was developed 30 years ago as an antipsychotic agent, development was slowed by the recognition that it caused agranulocytosis in 1%–2% of patients. Because of the high risk of potentially fatal agranulocytosis, risk of seizures at high doses, inconvenience of weekly white cell counts, and the high cost of the drug, it is important to consider risk–benefit and cost–benefit relations.

F. Risperidone

1. Chemistry. Risperidone is a benzisoxcizole derivative.

2. Pharmacokinetics. Risperidone is well absorbed from the gastrointestinal tract and metabolized in the liver by the cytochrome P-450 enzymes to an active metabolite.

3. Mechanism of action. Risperidone has an affinity, like clozapine, for serotonin type 2 receptors and, like haloperidol, for dopamine type 2 receptors. Risperidone also binds to α-adrenergic and histamine-1 (H_1) receptors.

4. Therapeutic uses. Risperidone is as effective as haloperidol for chronic schizophrenia with less toxicity.

5. Adverse effects include asthenia, sedation, and lack of concentration.

VI. AGENTS USED IN THE TREATMENT OF ANXIETY

A. General considerations.
Unlike the antipsychotic agents, these agents are used to treat anxiety or neurosis. They are not used in the treatment of psychosis. These drugs, therefore, are known as **antianxiety agents** or **minor tranquilizers**.

1. Antianxiety agents have sedative and hypnotic properties and possess some central skeletal muscle relaxant activity.

2. They have a habituation and physical dependence liability.

3. Generally, the antianxiety agents have a lower incidence of adverse effects than the antipsychotic agents.

B. Meprobamate
is a propyl alcohol derivative (propanediol carbamate). At one time, meprobamate was a widely used antianxiety agent; however, it has largely been replaced by the benzodiazepines.

1. Pharmacokinetics. Meprobamate is well absorbed from the gastrointestinal tract, and its peak serum concentration is reached in about 1½ hours. Metabolism occurs in the liver, and the inactive metabolites are excreted via the kidney.

2. Pharmacologic effects
    a. Meprobamate depresses the CNS in a fashion similar to that of the barbiturates, especially phenobarbital, but meprobamate is shorter acting.
    b. It is capable of promoting sleep, but, like phenobarbital, it decreases the REM phase.
    c. The skeletal muscle relaxant activity demonstrated by meprobamate is probably a combination of its sedative effect and specific central skeletal muscle relaxant activity.

3. Adverse effects
    a. Drowsiness, often seen with full therapeutic doses

   b. Blood dyscrasias, including purpura, but these are rare
   c. Habituation and physical dependence with long-term administration (withdrawal from drug therapy should, therefore, be gradual)

C. **Benzodiazepines** are considered the drugs of choice in the treatment of anxiety, partly because of their high therapeutic index. The first benzodiazepine developed was **chlordiazepoxide** (Figure 3-2). Others include **diazepam, clonazepam, lorazepam, oxazepam, clorazepate, halazepam, prazepam, alprazolam,** the anesthetic **midazolam,** and the sedative–hypnotics **flurazepam, triazolam,** and **temazepam** (see II B 3).

1. **Pharmacokinetics** (Table 3-3)
   a. Diazepam, flurazepam, and clorazepate are relatively rapidly absorbed, while oxazepam, prazepam, and temazepam are more slowly absorbed. Triazolam, midazolam, alprazolam, and clonazepam have an intermediate onset of action.
   b. All benzodiazepines are soluble in lipids and cross the blood–brain barrier. Plasma levels reflect brain levels.
   c. Benzodiazepines are metabolized primarily by microsomal oxidation and glucuronide conjugation.

2. **Pharmacologic effects**
   a. **CNS effects**
      (1) Benzodiazepines potentiate the binding of GABA to receptors. The benzodiazepine receptor that helps to potentiate the GABA binding is as yet unidentified.
      (2) Because they increase the seizure threshold, benzodiazepines are useful as anticonvulsants, especially diazepam in status epilepticus. They prevent convulsions caused by strychnine or pentylenetetrazole.
      (3) Benzodiazepines are also effective hypnotics, and flurazepam, temazepam, and triazolam are promoted as such.
   b. At therapeutic doses, the benzodiazepines have minimal effects on the cardiovascular system.
   c. Although the benzodiazepines, especially diazepam, are widely used as central skeletal muscle relaxants, their effectiveness has not been firmly established.

3. **Therapeutic uses**
   a. Treatment of anxiety
   b. Anesthetic premedication (midazolam is a parenteral benzodiazepine that will replace diazepam for perioperative use; its advantages include less tissue irritation, faster onset of action, and more rapid elimination)
   c. Use as amnestics, such as in cardioversion
   d. Use as sedative–hypnotics

FIGURE 3-2. Chlordiazepoxide.

TABLE 3-3. Pharmacokinetics of Benzodiazepines

Agent	Duration of Action	Gastrointestinal Absorption Rate	Active Metabolite	Elimination Half-life
Midazolam	Short	Intermediate	No	2.5 hours
Triazolam	Short	Intermediate	No	3 hours
Alprazolam	Intermediate	Intermediate	No	14 hours
Lorazepam	Intermediate	Intermediate	No	15 hours
Oxazepam	Intermediate	Slow	No	10 hours
Temazepam	Intermediate	Slow	No	15 hours
Chlordiazepoxide	Long	Intermediate	Yes	2–4 days
Clonazepam	Long	Intermediate	Yes	2–3 days
Clorazepate	Long	Rapid	Yes	2–4 days
Diazepam	Long	Rapid	Yes	2–4 days
Flurazepam	Long	Intermediate	Yes	2–3 days
Halazepam	Long	Slow	Yes	2–4 days
Prazepam	Long	Slow	Yes	2–4 days

  e. Management of seizure disorders
  f. Treatment of alcohol withdrawal syndromes
  g. Use as central skeletal muscle relaxants
  h. Treatment of night terrors
  i. Panic attacks (alprazolam only; physical dependence can occur)

4. Adverse effects
  a. Adverse effects are partially age- and dose-dependent. These effects include:
    (1) Ataxia, drowsiness, and sedation (additive depressant effects are seen when benzodiazepines are combined with other agents possessing CNS depressant activity)
    (2) Paradoxically increased anxiety, including psychoses, especially with high doses
    (3) Reversible confusion in the elderly
    (4) Menstrual irregularities, including anovulation
  b. Overdoses, although frequent, are seldom fatal. Treatment is supportive. Owing to the high plasma–protein-binding characteristics of benzodiazepines, the benefit from dialysis is limited.
  c. Withdrawal symptoms are influenza-like muscle aches and nausea. These symptoms are rare, except in the case of alprazolam.
  d. Agent-specific effects include:
    (1) Triazolam may cause rebound insomnia.
    (2) Lorazepam and triazolam have a greater risk of inducing anterograde amnesia.
    (3) Flurazepam at higher doses (30 mg) is associated with daytime residual sedation.

D. **Buspirone** is an antianxiety agent that is not chemically or pharmacologically related to the benzodiazepines, barbiturates, or other sedative–anxiolytic drugs.

  1. Mechanism of action. Although the exact mechanism of action is unknown, buspirone can bind to dopamine and serotonin receptors. It does not bind to benzodiazepine receptors and does not have muscle-relaxant, anticonvulsant, or hypnotic activity.

  2. Pharmacokinetics
    a. Buspirone is rapidly and completely absorbed from the gastrointestinal tract.
    b. The drug undergoes an extensive first-pass effect. One hydroxylated metabolite is pharmacologically active.
    c. Buspirone is highly protein-bound.
    d. It is partly excreted in the urine and has an elimination half-life of 4.8 hours.

  3. Therapeutic uses. Buspirone is used for the short-term treatment of generalized anxiety. It may require 1–2 weeks for a therapeutic effect to take place.

4. **Adverse effects** include restlessness and dysphoria with high doses. Buspirone is remarkably free of other adverse effects. It has little potential for abuse.

VII. MOOD-ALTERING DRUGS

A. **Lithium carbonate** is used in the treatment of mania and manic episodes of bipolar disorder (manic–depressive illness).

1. **Mechanism of action** is thought to be related to lithium's inhibition of hormone-sensitive adenylate cyclase and the greater stabilization of dopamine and β-adrenergic receptors.

2. **Pharmacokinetics.** Lithium ion is well absorbed from the gastrointestinal tract and eventually reaches equilibrium between plasma and tissues. It is eliminated by renal excretion; 80% of the lithium is reabsorbed in the proximal tubule. Lithium ion is secreted into breast milk.

3. **Route of administration.** Lithium is given orally. Because lithium has a low therapeutic index, serum concentrations must be carefully maintained between 0.8 and 1.5 mEq/L.

4. **Therapeutic uses**
   a. The major therapeutic indications are the prevention of bipolar illness and the treatment of acute mania.
   b. Lithium may also be useful in reducing the intensity of depression and increasing the duration between bouts of depression in unipolar depression.
   c. Lithium has no effect on schizophrenia and does not produce psychotropic effects in normal individuals.

5. **Adverse effects**
   a. High serum concentrations of lithium are associated with anorexia, vomiting, diarrhea, excessive thirst, and polyuria. The latter two symptoms probably involve the ability of lithium to inhibit the action of ADH on renal adenylate cyclase. This ultimately can result in diabetes insipidus; in fact, lithium is the most common cause of nephrogenic diabetes insipidus.
   b. Epileptic seizures have been reported, as well as somnolence, confusion, and psychomotor disturbances.
   c. The use of lithium during early pregnancy can result in cardiovascular anomalies in the newborn.
   d. Adverse cardiovascular effects include hypotension and cardiac arrhythmias.
   e. Chronic lithium use can result in thyroid enlargement.
   f. Lithium intoxication can usually be reversed by osmotic diuresis or, in more severe cases, by dialysis.

B. **Antidepressant agents**

1. **General considerations**
   a. Depression is an alteration of mood characterized by sadness, worry, and anxiety. The patient may suffer from losses of weight and libido.
   b. Most antidepressants are believed to improve mood by increasing catecholamine stores, although there may be a correlation between improvement in mood and a decrease in adenylate cyclase.
   c. There are various pharmacologic modalities that may be useful, and selection often depends on the patient's history and symptoms.

2. **Monoamine oxidase inhibitors**
   a. **Chemistry.** Chemically, the MAO inhibitors consist of two major groups, the hydrazides and the nonhydrazides.
      (1) The **hydrazide derivatives** include **isocarboxazid, phenelzine,** and **iproniazid.** The latter is no longer used because of its hepatotoxicity.

(2) The prototypic **nonhydrazide** is **tranylcypromine,** which structurally resembles dextroamphetamine.

b. Mechanism of action

(1) The MAO inhibitors form stable complexes with the enzyme MAO, irreversibly inactivating it, thereby preventing the oxidative deamination of biogenic amines, such as norepinephrine, epinephrine, dopamine, serotonin, and tyramine.

    (a) These biogenic amines are, thus, increased significantly in the brain, intestines, heart, and blood.

    (b) The increase of biogenic amine levels in the brain is thought to underlie the observed antidepressant effects.

(2) The two types of MAO inhibitors are distinguished by differing responses to specific inhibitors and by differing preferences for substrates.

    (a) Type A deaminates serotonin and norepinephrine but not phenylethylamine.

    (b) Type B deaminates phenylethylamine better than serotonin or norepinephrine, and it is inhibited by deprenyl. MAO-B is the type found largely in the CNS.

(3) The nonhydrazide, tranylcypromine, by way of its amphetamine-like action, releases norepinephrine centrally. This probably accounts for the relative rapidity of action with tranylcypromine (action can occur in 48 hours) in contrast to the other MAO inhibitors, which have latency periods of 2–3 weeks.

c. Pharmacokinetics

(1) All MAO inhibitors are rapidly absorbed from the gastrointestinal tract, but, inexplicably, the observed therapeutic response does not occur for 2–3 weeks.

(2) The hydrazide derivatives are cleaved, resulting in biologically active products. Inactivation occurs by acetylation, and, in patients who are genetically slow acetylators, conventional doses of agents, such as phenelzine, may produce exaggerated effects.

(3) Enzyme regeneration terminates the drug effect, but this frequently takes weeks after use of the drug is stopped.

(4) When switching antidepressant therapy, a minimum of 2 weeks' delay is required after termination of MAO-inhibitor therapy [see VII B 3 g (3)].

d. Pharmacologic effects

(1) **CNS effects**

    (a) Besides their effect on depression, MAO inhibitors are effective in sleep disorders, including narcolepsy. They suppress REM sleep.

    (b) Except for tranylcypromine, which has a stimulant effect on the electroencephalogram (EEG), other MAO inhibitors have minimal EEG effects.

(2) **Cardiovascular effects**

    (a) Hypotension, especially postural, can result from the ability of MAO inhibitors to affect ganglionic transmission and reduce the release of norepinephrine in certain organ systems. This effect is believed to be due to the uptake and release of "false transmitters," such as tyramine.

    (b) MAO inhibitors can **interact with foods containing a high tyramine content,** such as cheese, beer, and chicken liver.

        (i) The high concentrations of tyramine absorbed from these foods cannot undergo oxidative deamination.

        (ii) The tyramine can, therefore, induce the release of large amounts of stored catecholamines from nerve terminals. This can precipitate a **hypertensive crisis,** which is the most serious adverse effect of MAO inhibitors.

(3) **Hepatic effects**

    (a) MAO inhibitors interfere with the detoxification of many drugs.

    (b) They enhance the action of general anesthetics, sedatives, atropine-like agents, narcotics (especially meperidine, which can result in hyperpyrexia), and tricyclic antidepressants.

e. Therapeutic uses. MAO-A inhibitors are especially effective in the treatment of atypical depression, characterized by symptoms such as hypersomnolence, hyperphagia, and hyperanxiety. Deprenyl (see IV C) is an MAO-B inhibitor, which may be useful in the treatment of Parkinson's disease.

f. Adverse effects
 (1) The most serious effect is marked hypertension from an interaction between an MAO-A inhibitor and certain amines or their precursors (see VII B 2 b).
 (2) Hydrazide-derived MAO inhibitors can cause hepatocellular damage.
 (3) Excessive CNS stimulation has occurred, resulting in insomnia and convulsions.
 (4) Overdosage can result in agitation, headache, hallucinations, convulsions, and hypotension or hypertension. Treatment of overdosage is usually supportive. Since the effects of MAO inhibitors are lengthy, patients should be observed in the hospital for at least 1 week.

3. Tricyclic antidepressants
 a. Chemistry. Chemically, the tricyclic antidepressants and their desmethyl derivatives are similar to the phenothiazines. The basic structure is shown in Figure 3-3.
 b. Specific agents
  (1) Imipramine is closely related to the phenothiazines.
  (2) Amitriptyline is thought to be better tolerated than imipramine in older psychotic or depressed patients. Amitriptyline is effective in multiple sclerosis patients with **pseudobulbar palsy,** the syndrome of pathologic laughing and weeping.
  (3) Desipramine, the monodesmethyl derivative of imipramine, is less sedating than its parent compound.
  (4) Nortriptyline, like desipramine, produces less sedation than its parent compound amitriptyline.
  (5) Doxepin is also effective in treating depression when anxiety is present.
  (6) Protriptyline has a 3- to 5-day half-life and causes little sedation.
 c. Mechanism of action
  (1) Tricyclic antidepressants potentiate the action of biogenic amines, presumably by blocking the inactivating reuptake of the amines after release from the presynaptic neuron. It is thought that the demethylated antidepressants (secondary amines) are more selective in blocking the uptake of norepinephrine.
  (2) Tricyclic antidepressants have both antihistaminic (H_1-receptor–blocking) and α-adrenergic properties.
  (3) In addition, the tricyclic antidepressants possess antimuscarinic action and block the reuptake of serotonin. Tertiary amines (imipramine, amitriptyline) are more effective at blocking serotonin uptake.
 d. Pharmacokinetics
  (1) The tricyclic antidepressants are well absorbed from the gastrointestinal tract.
  (2) Because of their lipophilic nature, these agents become widely distributed and have relatively long half-lives. They are metabolized in the microsomal metabolizing system. Hydroxylation, N-demethylation, and conjugation with glucuronic acid are the major metabolic pathways.
  (3) The demethylated metabolites of both amitriptyline and imipramine have antidepressant activity.
  (4) Excretion of metabolites is via the kidney.

FIGURE 3-3. Basic structure of tricyclic antidepressants.

e. Pharmacologic effects

(1) CNS effects

(a) A nondepressed person experiences sleepiness when a tricyclic antidepressant is administered. In addition, anxiety and toxic anticholinergic effects may be experienced.

(b) In the depressed patient, an elevation of mood occurs 2–3 weeks after administration begins. The latency period can be as long as 4 weeks.

(c) Tricyclic antidepressants can cause extrapyramidal symptoms and ataxia.

(d) High doses of tricyclic antidepressants are capable of producing seizures and coma.

(2) Cardiovascular effects

(a) Orthostatic hypotension and arrhythmias are two common effects.

(b) Tachycardia in response to the hypotension and interference with atrioventricular conduction similar to that produced by quinidine can occur.

(3) The most common **autonomic nervous system effect** is anticholinergic. Amitriptyline possesses the most potent antimuscarinic effects.

f. Therapeutic uses

(1) These agents are considered the treatment of choice for severe endogenous depression (characterized by regression and inactivity). In terms of overall efficacy, the various tricyclic antidepressants are equivalent at appropriate dosages.

(2) Enuresis has been successfully treated with imipramine.

(3) Obsessive–compulsive neurosis accompanied by depression, and phobic–anxiety syndromes, chronic pain, and neuralgia may respond to tricyclic agents; it should be noted that these indications are investigational.

g. Adverse effects

(1) The adverse effects of tricyclic antidepressants often resemble those seen with phenothiazines, owing to the common structural features of the two groups of drugs.

(a) Anticholinergic effects can be prominent and occur both peripherally and centrally. Amitriptyline produces the highest incidence of antimuscarinic effects. Because of these actions, caution is required in treating patients with prostatic hypertrophy and glaucoma. Tolerance often develops to these effects.

(b) Sweating is common, although its mechanism is unknown.

(c) The elderly may suffer from dizziness and muscle tremor.

(d) As with phenothiazines, cardiac arrhythmias can occur. In addition, hypotension is frequent and results from a down-regulation of adrenergic receptors.

(e) Manic excitement and delirium can occur in patients with bipolar illness.

(2) Acute poisoning is often treated with activated charcoal, although gastric lavage and physostigmine have been used successfully as adjuncts. Vital functions need to be supported and constantly monitored, because seizures, ventricular arrhythmias, and death can result from overdoses.

(3) The combination of an MAO inhibitor with a tricyclic antidepressant should be avoided, because hyperpyrexia, convulsions, and coma can result.

4. Serotonin (5-hydroxytryptamine, 5-HT) reuptake inhibitors

a. Fluoxetine

(1) Chemistry. Chemically, fluoxetine is a phenyltolylpropylamine that inhibits the uptake of serotonin.

(2) Mechanism of action

(a) It is a selective inhibitor of serotonin uptake in the CNS.

(b) It has little effect on central norepinephrine or dopamine function.

(c) It has less adverse effects because of minimal binding to cholinergic, histaminic, and α-adrenergic receptors.

(3) Pharmacokinetics

(a) Fluoxetine is well absorbed after oral ingestion.

(b) It undergoes extensive hepatic biotransformation to the active metabolite norfluoxetine. The inactive metabolites are excreted in the urine.

(c) The elimination half-life is 1–3 days for fluoxetine and 7–15 days for nor-fluoxetine.

(d) The onset of action is within 1–3 weeks after beginning treatment.

(4) Therapeutic uses

(a) Fluoxetine is used for treatment of mild to moderate endogenous depression.

(b) It may be useful in treating obsessive–compulsive disorder, obesity, and alcoholism.

(5) Adverse effects

(a) Fluoxetine has caused anorexia and, unlike the tricyclics, does not cause weight gain.

(b) It may precipitate mania or hypomania.

(c) Nausea, nervousness, headache, and insomnia occur more frequently with fluoxetine than with tricyclics.

(d) Urticaria or some other rash develops in 4% of patients.

b. **Sertraline** and **paroxetine** are similar to fluoxetine in mechanism of action and therapeutic use. Sertraline is less likely than fluoxetine or paroxetine to interact adversely with other drugs.

c. **Bupropion**

(1) Chemistry. Chemically, bupropion is a trimethylated monocyclic phenyl-aminoketone.

(2) Mechanism of action. Although the exact mechanism of action is unknown, the drug does weakly block dopamine reuptake.

(3) Pharmacokinetics

(a) Bupropion is rapidly absorbed from the gastrointestinal tract and undergoes extensive first-pass metabolism.

(b) It is eliminated primarily in the urine.

(4) Therapeutic uses. Bupropion is used for the treatment of major depression. Significant improvement is often seen within 1 week of treatment. Bupropion is sometimes effective in depressed patients who do not respond to tricyclics.

(5) Adverse effects. Bupropion does not produce sedation, orthostatic hypotension, weight gain, or the sexual dysfunction associated with other antidepressants; however, it is contraindicated in patients with eating disorders, seizures, or major head trauma because it may produce or exacerbate grand mal seizures.

d. **Venlafaxine** is chemically related to bupropion and inhibits norepinephrine and serotonin reuptake. It also weakly inhibits dopamine reuptake. High dosages may cause a sustained diastolic hypertension.

VIII. CNS STIMULANTS

A. **Amphetamine** (β-phenylisopropylamine)

1. CNS effects

a. In addition to its peripheral sympathomimetic action (see Chapter 2 II G), amphetamine is a powerful CNS stimulant, presumably acting by releasing biogenic amines from storage sites in the nerve terminals.

b. Amphetamine stimulates the medullary respiratory center and has analeptic action, counteracting the central depression produced by other drugs (e.g., barbiturates).

c. Increased alertness, decreased sense of fatigue, increased motor and speech activity, and elevation of mood are often produced.

2. Therapeutic uses

a. Amphetamine is an anorectic and has been used in weight control of obese individuals. Because tolerance develops rapidly, psychologically driven food intake is not affected, and abuse potential is significant, this therapeutic use is of questionable merit.

b. The stimulant effect of amphetamine is useful in the treatment of narcolepsy.

c. A paradoxical calming effect is produced with long-term therapy in many abnormally hyperactive children (i.e., those with hyperkinetic syndrome).

3. Adverse effects
   a. Some individuals experience dysphoria, headache, confusion, dizziness, fatigue, or delirium.
   b. Blood pressure is usually raised, and cardiac arrhythmias may occur.
   c. Larger doses or prolonged usage are usually followed by fatigue and mental depression.
   d. The toxic dose of amphetamine shows wide variation.
      (1) Overdosage results in psychotic reactions, marked cardiovascular effects, such as hypertension or hypotension and circulatory collapse, and, eventually, convulsions and coma.
      (2) Treatment of acute intoxication is facilitated by acidification of the urine to increase excretion.

B. **Dextroamphetamine and methamphetamine** are preferred to amphetamine because of their increased CNS action and reduced peripheral effects.

C. **Cocaine**

   1. Chemistry. Cocaine is benzoylmethylecgonine; its sole clinical use is as a local anesthetic (see Chapter 4 II C 1).

   2. Pharmacokinetics
      a. Cocaine is well absorbed across mucous membranes and the mucosa of the gastrointestinal tract.
      b. Cocaine is degraded by plasma esterases and, in some animals, by hepatic enzymes.
      c. The half-life of cocaine is approximately 1 hour.

   3. Pharmacologic effects
      a. Cocaine is a CNS stimulant that blocks neuronal uptake of norepinephrine. Initially, there is an intense euphoric experience followed in minutes by dysphoria.
         (1) Alkaloidal cocaine (free base) is a form of the drug that is suitable for smoking. When the cocaine crystals are heated, a cracking sound is produced, thus, the moniker "crack." "Freebasing" or smoking delivers cocaine to the vascular bed of the lung, producing an effect comparable to that achieved by intravenous injection.
         (2) Intranasal use of cocaine hydrochloride does not provide the "rush" generally associated with freebasing. Vasoconstriction of the nasal mucous membranes limits the absorption of the drug when it is snorted.
      b. Blocking neuronal uptake of norepinephrine increases heart rate and blood pressure.
      c. At higher doses, central depression occurs, followed by respiratory failure.

   4. Adverse effects
      a. Increased heart rate and blood pressure occur, which may produce or exacerbate angina pectoris, myocardial infarction, and ventricular arrhythmias.
      b. High doses may cause hyperpyrexia, seizures, and cardiac arrhythmias.
      c. Cocaine crosses the placenta and may accumulate in the fetus. Exposure to cocaine during pregnancy increases the incidence of spontaneous abortion, fetal growth retardation, and possibly congenital anomalies.
      d. Cocaine intoxication can occur in breast-fed babies via maternal use.

IX. **NARCOTIC ANALGESICS** (Table 3-4)

A. **General considerations**

   1. Definitions
      a. Analgesia is the relief of pain without loss of consciousness, as opposed to anesthesia. The chief action of opiates and similar compounds is to impair the normal sensory awareness and response to tissue injury.
      b. Opiates are derived from the poppy plant. The exudate of the seed capsule contains morphine, codeine, thebaine, and papaverine. The term **opioid** refers to both naturally occurring opiates and synthetic drugs with similar actions.

TABLE 3-4. Narcotic Analgesics

Morphine-like agonists
    Hydromorphone
    Oxymorphone
    Heroin
 	
Codeine-like agonists
    Dihydrocodeine
    Hydrocodeine
    Oxycodone
 	
Synthetic narcotic (opioid) agonists
    Meperidine
    Fentanyl
    Methadone
    Propoxyphene
    Levorphanol
	Partial agonists and mixed
	        agonists/antagonists
	    Buprenorphine (partial agonist)
	    Pentazocine (mixed agonist/
	        antagonist)
	    Butorphanol (mixed agonist/
	        antagonist)
	    Nalbuphine (mixed agonist/
	        antagonist)
	
	Full antagonists
	    Naloxone
	    Naltrexone

2. **Mechanism of action**
   a. Through the use of ligand-binding techniques, **opiate receptors** of several types have been identified and quantitated within the CNS (Table 3-5). These receptors are found in the following sites:
      (1) The limbic system, including the amygdaloid nucleus and the hypothalamus
      (2) The medial and lateral thalamus and the area postrema, which is the site of the chemoreceptor trigger zone governing nausea and emesis
      (3) The nucleus of the solitary tract, which is the location of the cough center
      (4) The substantia gelatinosa and, to a lesser degree, other areas of the spinal cord
   b. Endogenous ligands known as **enkephalins** are pentapeptides that are localized in some nerve endings. Their distribution closely parallels the distribution of opioid receptors. It is thought that the enkephalins may be involved in the modulation of the pain response.
   c. In addition, longer polypeptides called **endorphins** possess potent analgesic activity and are found in the anterior pituitary and hypothalamus.
   d. Analgesia produced at opioid receptors requires binding by a molecule that has a terminal quaternary nitrogen that is capable of being charged at physiologic pH and resides four or five atoms from an aromatic group.
   e. The interruption of pain impulses may be mediated by calcium gating via endorphin receptors, enkephalin receptors, or both.

3. **Administration**
   a. Patient-controlled intravenous administration of analgesics may offer advantages over intramuscular injections for some patients.
   b. Intraspinal opioids have been used to control postoperative and cancer pain with few adverse effects.

TABLE 3-5. Classification of Opiate Receptors

Receptor Type	Action
Mu (μ)	Supraspinal analgesia, respiratory depression, euphoria, physical dependence
μ_1	Analgesia
μ_2	Respiratory depression
Kappa (κ)	Spinal analgesia, miosis, sedation
Sigma (σ)	Dysphoria, hallucinations, respiratory and vasomotor stimulation

FIGURE 3-4. Morphine.

B. | **Morphine and related opioids**

1. **Morphine** (Figure 3-4) is a member of the phenanthrene series of alkaloids.
   a. **Pharmacokinetics**
      (1) Morphine is well absorbed from the gastrointestinal tract. However, the analgesic effect is greater when the drug is administered intramuscularly or intravenously, rather than orally.
      (2) Morphine is metabolized in the liver, where it is transformed into inactive metabolites by conjugation with glucuronide. It undergoes a significant first-pass effect.
      (3) Ninety percent of a given dose is excreted in the urine; the remaining 10% is excreted in the feces. This latter component is derived from bile as conjugated morphine.
   b. **Pharmacologic effects**
      (1) **CNS effects**
         (a) Dose-related analgesia and increased tolerance of pain are the most prominent effects of morphine. Consciousness is not lost, and the patient can usually still locate the source of pain. Some patients become euphoric. If morphine is given to a person who is pain-free, dysphoria, anxiety, or mental clouding may be produced.
         (b) Morphine stimulates the chemoreceptor trigger zone, producing nausea and vomiting. In most cases, after the first therapeutic dose, subsequent doses of morphine do not produce vomiting.
         (c) Morphine produces miosis by stimulating the Edinger-Westphal nucleus, and pinpoint pupils are indicative of toxic dosage prior to asphyxia. The miosis can be blocked with atropine.
         (d) Morphine is a powerful respiratory depressant, which acts by reducing the responsiveness of the respiratory centers in the brain stem to blood levels of carbon dioxide.
            (i) Both alveolar and serum carbon dioxide tension (Pco_2) are increased because of the depression of medullary responsiveness.
            (ii) Due to the depressed respiration and increased arterial carbon dioxide retention, cerebral vasodilation can occur, causing an increase in intracranial pressure.
         (e) Morphine is believed to stimulate the release of ADH, producing oliguria.
         (f) Morphine is a potent cough suppressant.
         (g) Morphine has a biphasic, dose-dependent effect on body temperature. Low doses of morphine cause a decrease in body temperature; higher doses cause an increase.
      (2) **Cardiovascular effects.** Orthostatic hypotension can occur due to vasomotor medullary depression and histamine release.
      (3) **Gastrointestinal effects**
         (a) Constipation results from reduced peristalsis and stomach motility. In addition, spasmodic nonpropulsive contractions of gastrointestinal smooth muscle are produced.
         (b) Both biliary and pancreatic secretions are decreased.
         (c) Constriction at the sphincter of Oddi causes an increase in biliary pressure.

(4) Other systemic effects

(a) Morphine increases detrusor muscle tone in the urinary bladder, producing a feeling of urinary urgency. Vesical sphincter tone is also increased, making voiding difficult.

(b) Prolongation of labor can occur by an undefined uterine mechanism.

(c) Bronchoconstriction can occur because morphine causes the release of histamine and causes vagal stimulation.

(d) Cutaneous vasodilation secondary to histamine release can result in pruritus and sweating.

c. Therapeutic uses

(1) Analgesia, such as the relief of pain from myocardial infarction, terminal illness, surgery, and obstetrical procedures, is the major use of morphine.

(2) It is also used for the acute treatment of dyspnea due to pulmonary edema, in which morphine produces decreased peripheral resistance and increased capacity of peripheral and splanchnic vascular compartments.

(3) Because of their constipating effects, the morphine-like drugs can be useful in treating severe diarrhea.

d. Adverse effects

(1) Respiratory depression is the most important effect and is dose-dependent.

(2) Nausea and sometimes dysphoria can occur.

(3) Increased biliary tract pressure can occur, and caution should be exercised in giving opiates to patients with gallbladder disease.

(4) Long-term chronic administration can result in physical dependence. Pinpoint pupils are a consistent finding in addiction.

(5) Allergic reactions can occur, and skin rashes are a common manifestation.

(6) Due to morphine's bronchoconstrictive action, the drug is contraindicated for asthmatic patients.

(7) Some phenothiazines are capable of producing antianalgesia when combined with an opiate such as morphine, whereas other phenothiazines can enhance the analgesic action of morphine. However, phenothiazines are likely to increase the sedative and respiratory depressant effects of opioids.

e. Tolerance and dependence

(1) Tolerance may develop to the analgesia, the euphoria, and the respiratory depression.

(2) Tolerance to the miosis and to the delayed gastric emptying and constipation also develops, but to a much lesser extent.

(3) Physical addiction occurs, although the morphine withdrawal syndrome is not as severe as barbiturate withdrawal.

2. Codeine

a. Codeine is the 3-methyl ether of morphine. It can be obtained from opium or synthesized by methylation of morphine.

b. Although the pharmacologic effects of codeine are similar to those of morphine, it has about one-twelfth the analgesic potency of morphine, and it is generally used for somewhat milder pain.

c. Codeine has a high oral–parenteral potency ratio so that when it is administered orally, it is 60% as potent as when injected intramuscularly.

d. An oral dose of 30 mg of codeine is equivalent in analgesia to 600 mg of aspirin.

e. Codeine is also very useful as a cough suppressant.

f. Codeine produces less sedation or respiratory depression than morphine and fewer gastrointestinal effects.

g. Addiction liability is lower than with morphine, and withdrawal is less severe.

3. Hydrocodone and oxycodone

a. Although these agents are codeine derivatives, they possess an analgesic potency closer to that of morphine.

b. Their potential for causing respiratory depression is also greater than that of codeine; this is especially true of oxycodone.

c. They possess a significant addiction liability.

4. Heroin
   a. Heroin is diacetylated morphine.
   b. Heroin has a more rapid onset and shorter duration of action than morphine.
   c. It has an analgesic potency greater than that of morphine: 3 mg of heroin is equivalent to 10 mg of morphine.
   d. Heroin is not used clinically in the United States.

5. Hydromorphone
   a. Hydromorphone is 10 times more potent than morphine in producing analgesia with correspondingly more respiratory depressant activity.
   b. Hydromorphone is less nauseating and less constipating than morphine.
   c. It is highly physically addicting.
   d. Hydromorphone can be administered orally, parenterally, or rectally.

6. Levorphanol produces effects similar to those of morphine but with a lower incidence of nausea and vomiting.

C. Meperidine and congeners

1. Meperidine, a phenylpiperidine derivative, is an entirely synthetic analgesic.
   a. It is about one-eighth as potent as morphine, 100 mg of meperidine being equivalent to 15 mg of morphine.
   b. Meperidine is well absorbed by all routes of administration and is better absorbed orally than is morphine. Excretion is mainly in the urine.
   c. Meperidine causes respiratory depression and possesses addiction liability, although withdrawal effects are less severe than with morphine.
   d. Meperidine causes histamine release and smooth muscle spasm, including bronchospasm.
   e. It possesses weak, atropine-like activity and tends to cause mydriasis. In toxic doses, the pharmacologic effects are, in part, atropine-like.
   f. With intravenous administration, the incidence of adverse effects is increased. Repeated intramuscular administration can produce tissue irritation.
   g. Meperidine has no gastrointestinal or antitussive action.

2. Diphenoxylate, a derivative of meperidine, is available in combination with atropine (e.g., Lomotil).
   a. Its principal use is to control diarrhea.
   b. In the recommended dosage, it causes few morphine-like subjective effects and has low addiction liability.
   c. Due to the atropine in the combination, adverse effects, such as dry mouth and blurred vision, curtail abuse.

3. Fentanyl, like diphenoxylate, is a congener of meperidine.
   a. It has 80 times the analgesic potency and respiratory depressant properties of morphine, and is more effective than morphine in maintaining hemodynamic stability.
   b. When combined with droperidol, it produces dissociative analgesia or neuroleptanalgesia (see Chapter 4 I B 2).
   c. Its principal use is in anesthesia, where it is administered parenterally. It has a rapid onset and short duration of action. Fentanyl is also available in a controlled-release transdermal formulation. Therapeutic concentrations are not reached for 8–12 hours after application of the first dose. It is useful for the treatment of chronic cancer pain.
   d. High doses of fentanyl are capable of producing muscular rigidity.

4. Sufentanil is used as a short-acting anesthetic adjunct; it has a shorter onset of action than fentanyl.

5. Alfentanil is a synthetic opioid analgesic related to fentanyl and sufentanil.
   a. It has a more rapid onset of action and shorter duration of narcotic effect than fentanyl.
   b. It is used as an adjunct to general anesthetics and as an anesthetic induction agent.

D. **Methadone and congeners**

1. **Methadone** is a modified diphenylheptane (Figure 3-5).
   a. This synthetic analgesic has pharmacologic properties similar to those of morphine, but it is more effective orally than morphine.
   b. The duration of analgesia with methadone is equal to that of morphine, although the half-life of methadone is longer. This can result in cumulative toxicity.
   c. Methadone is well absorbed from the gastrointestinal tract, undergoes extensive bio-transformation in the liver, and is excreted in both the urine and bile.
   d. Its principal uses are in analgesia, in the suppression of withdrawal symptoms due to opiate addiction, and in treatment of heroin users.
      (1) In methadone maintenance, opiate addicts receive periodic oral doses of methadone.
      (2) In appropriate doses, methadone satisfies the craving for heroin without producing euphoria or somnolence.
      (3) Because of cross-tolerance, the effects of other self-administered opiates are blocked.
   e. Adverse effects are similar to those caused by morphine (see IX B 1 d).
   f. Both tolerance and physical dependence can occur with methadone administration. Methadone withdrawal is less severe than the withdrawal from other opiates.

2. **Propoxyphene** is a structural analog of methadone with a spectrum of pharmacologic activity similar to that of codeine.
   a. Propoxyphene is not an anti-inflammatory agent; therefore, it is less effective in treating pain associated with inflammation. In analgesic potency, it closely resembles codeine. When combined with aspirin, propoxyphene produces more analgesia than either drug alone; however, the combination of aspirin and codeine is less costly than that of aspirin and propoxyphene.
   b. The water-soluble hydrochloride is absorbed more rapidly than the water-insoluble napsylate.
   c. The N-demethylated metabolites are slowly excreted in the urine.
   d. Propoxyphene depresses respiration about one-third as much as codeine.
   e. The incidence of abuse is comparable to that seen with codeine.
   f. Physical dependence and tolerance can occur but usually are seen only after chronic high-dose administration.

E. **Opioid receptor antagonists and partial antagonists**

1. **Nalorphine** was originally used as an opioid antagonist.
   a. When it became recognized that it possessed analgesic properties with less respiratory depression than morphine, nalorphine became classified as a partial antagonist.

FIGURE 3-5. Methadone.

b. Nalorphine can lead to withdrawal symptoms when it is given to narcotic-dependent patients.

2. Pentazocine is a benzomorphan derivative with moderate agonistic and weak antagonistic activity.

    a. Due to its antagonistic activity, pentazocine can precipitate withdrawal in addicts.

    b. Although pentazocine is similar to morphine in pharmacologic properties, it has one-fifth the analgesic potency. A dose of 50 mg, given parenterally, produces analgesia equivalent to 10 mg of morphine; given orally, 50 mg is equivalent to 60 mg of codeine.

    c. Pentazocine is well absorbed from the gastrointestinal tract as well as from subcutaneous and intramuscular sites. Pentazocine is biotransformed in the liver and excreted via the kidney.

    d. Adverse effects

        (1) Pentazocine can produce psychotomimetic effects, such as anxiety and hallucinations.

        (2) There may be nausea, but less so than that associated with other opioids.

        (3) Analgesic doses are capable of increasing the pulmonary artery pressure and cardiac work.

        (4) Respiratory depression with higher doses is less pronounced than with comparable doses of morphine.

        (5) Tolerance to the analgesia can develop.

        (6) Pentazocine possesses both physical dependence potential and abuse potential.

3. Butorphanol has actions similar to those of pentazocine.

    a. As with pentazocine, but in contrast to morphine, as the analgesic dose is increased, respiratory depression is not increased proportionately.

    b. Pulmonary artery pressure and myocardial work are increased at analgesic doses.

    c. Unlike pentazocine, butorphanol does not precipitate a withdrawal syndrome in opioid addicts.

4. Nalbuphine, although structurally similar to naloxone, is equivalent (on a weight basis) to morphine in producing analgesia.

    a. It is considered to be a partial antagonist. Although its antagonistic properties are weak, it precipitates withdrawal in the opioid addict.

    b. Nalbuphine produces respiratory depression, but doses beyond 30 mg produce no further depression.

    c. Unlike pentazocine and butorphanol, nalbuphine does not cause adverse cardiac effects.

    d. Nalbuphine possesses abuse potential, and physical dependence has been reported.

5. Naloxone, an *N*-allyl derivative of oxymorphone, is a full **antagonist**.

    a. Naloxone, like other competitive receptor antagonists, blocks the opioid receptor.

    b. The sedative effects, respiratory depression, and adverse cardiovascular effects of opioid agonists are reversed within 1–2 minutes after parenteral administration of naloxone. There may be an "overshoot," producing increased respiration for a short period of time.

    c. The duration of the antagonistic effect is dose-dependent and usually lasts 1–4 hours.

    d. If naloxone is administered to opioid-addicted patients, a withdrawal syndrome is easily precipitated.

    e. Tolerance to the antagonistic effects does not develop.

    f. Naloxone is usually administered parenterally. It is metabolized in the liver via glucuronide conjugation.

    g. In obstetrics, mothers who have received opioids during labor may be given a dose of naloxone just prior to delivery to minimize neonatal respiratory depression. Alternatively, naloxone can be administered to the neonate via the umbilical vein.

6. Naltrexone

    a. Naltrexone, another full antagonist, is now the treatment of choice for patients addicted to heroin or other opioids.

   b. It can be administered orally.
   c. It has twice the potency of naloxone and three times the duration of action.
   d. An opioid abstinence syndrome can result if naltrexone is administered too vigorously.
   e. Naltrexone may cause insomnia, anxiety, abdominal cramping, nausea, and joint pain.
   f. It is **contraindicated** in patients with acute hepatitis or hepatic failure.

7. Buprenorphine is a partial antagonist with low potential for abuse (it is a schedule V drug).
   a. Its onset of action is within 15 minutes when given parenterally.
   b. It is metabolized in the liver and excreted in the feces and urine.
   c. The respiratory depression caused by buprenorphine is quantitatively similar to that caused by morphine.
   d. Buprenorphine can precipitate withdrawal symptoms in narcotic-addicted patients.
   e. Buprenorphine's pharmacologic activity is not easily reversed, even with high doses of naloxone.

F. **Nonopioid antitussives (dextromethorphan)**

1. Dextromethorphan is the *d* isomer of the codeine analog of levorphanol.

2. In contrast to the *l* isomer, dextromethorphan does not possess analgesic or addictive properties, and its principal use is as a cough suppressant.

3. Although it is as effective as codeine in cough suppression, it is not beset with codeine's adverse effects, although at high doses, CNS depression may occur.

4. It is commonly found in over-the-counter formulations.

X. **AGENTS USED IN THE TREATMENT AND PREVENTION OF MIGRAINE** (Table 3-6)

A. **General considerations**

1. **Definition.** A migraine is an episodic headache that can be unilateral or bilateral, and may be pulsatile. It is exacerbated by physical activity.

2. **Accompanying symptoms** include photophobia, phonophobia, nausea, and vomiting.

3. **Classification**
   a. Classic migraine has a premonitory aura.
   b. Common migraine does not have an aura.

4. The **male-to-female ratio** for migraine is 1 to 3.

TABLE 3-6. Drugs Used to Treat and Prevent Migraine Attacks

Treatment	Analgesics	NSAIDs	Serotonin Agonists	Dopamine Agonists
	Aspirin	Naproxen	Ergotamine	Metoclopramide
	Acetaminophen	Ibuprofen	Sumatriptan	Chlorpromazine
	Codeine	Ketorolac		
Prevention	**β-Adrenergic Antagonists**	**NSAIDs**	**Calcium-Channel Blockers**	**Serotonin-Influencing Drugs**
	Propranolol	Ketoprofen	Nifedipine	Methysergide
	Atenolol	Tolfenamic acid	Nimodipine	Amitriptyline

NSAIDs = nonsteroidal anti-inflammatory drugs.

B. **Nonsteroidal anti-inflammatory drugs** (NSAIDs; see Table 3-6) are the treatment of choice for mild to moderate migraine attacks.

1. By inhibiting prostaglandin synthesis, NSAIDs prevent neurogenically mediated inflammation in the trigeminovascular system.

2. NSAIDs are less effective when treatment is delayed.

C. **Ergot preparations** (see Table 3-6) effectively abort migraines in approximately 50% of patients.

1. Ergot preparations have a high affinity but low selectivity for serotonin ($5\text{-}HT_1$) receptors. The potent venoconstrictor and vasoconstrictor properties of serotonin help alleviate headache.

2. Ergotamine is contraindicated in patients with coronary artery or peripheral vascular disease.

D. **Sumatriptan**

1. Sumatriptan is a highly selective agonist of the D subtype $5\text{-}HT_1$ receptor. It is effective when administered subcutaneously during an attack of migraine.

2. Oral sumatriptan relieves headache, but the rate of recurrence in 48 hours is high compared with that of subcutaneously administered sumatriptan.

3. It is not used for migraine prophylaxis.

4. **Contraindications**
   a. Sumatriptan is well tolerated; however, because sumatriptan constricts coronary arteries, it is contraindicated in patients with a history of ischemic heart disease or hypertension.
   b. Because of potential "serotonin syndromes" (characterized by restlessness, hyperreflexia, and diaphoresis), sumatriptan should not be given to patients receiving MAO inhibitors, selective serotonin reuptake inhibitors, or lithium carbonate.

E. **β-Adrenergic antagonists** (see Table 3-6)

1. In patients whose migraine attacks are stress-related, β-adrenergic antagonists are the treatment of choice for prevention. Calcium-channel blockers and NSAIDs have been used for prevention with less success.

2. The mechanisms of action of these drugs in preventing migraine is not understood.

XI. **THERAPY OF ALZHEIMER'S DISEASE. Tacrine** improves or slows the decline in test scores in some patients with mild to moderate Alzheimer's disease. Function improvement is equivocal.

1. **Mechanism of action.** This acridinamine derivative is a centrally acting, noncompetitive, reversible cholinesterase inhibitor. It also:
   a. Acts as a partial agonist at muscarinic receptors
   b. Blocks reuptake of dopamine, serotonin, norepinephrine
   c. Inhibits MAO
   d. Blocks sodium and potassium channels

2. **Pharmacokinetics.** Tacrine is orally administered but has a highly variable bioavailability. It is lipid-soluble; therefore, it penetrates the blood–brain barrier and accumulates in the brain.

3. **Adverse effects.** Elevated liver enzyme levels occur in nearly 50% of patients within 4–12 weeks of first dose and return to normal 6 weeks after discontinuation. Tacrine inhibits the metabolism of theophylline and other drugs by the cytochrome P-450 pathway.

STUDY QUESTIONS

1. Granulocytopenia, gastrointestinal irritation, gingival hyperplasia, and facial hirsutism are all possible side effects of which one of the following anticonvulsant drugs?

(A) Phenobarbital
(B) Carbamazepine
(C) Dantrolene
(D) Phenytoin
(E) Valproate

2. Which of the following drugs could be prescribed for a child who suffers from night terrors?

(A) Meprobamate
(B) Clonazepam
(C) Droperidol
(D) Lithium
(E) Amphetamine

3. Type A monoamine oxidase (MAO) inhibitors and tricyclic antidepressants have which of the following features in common?

(A) Both are useful for the manic phase of bipolar disorder
(B) Both are useful for enuresis
(C) Both can precipitate hypotensive crises if certain foods are ingested
(D) Both act postsynaptically to produce their effect
(E) Both drugs increase levels of biogenic amines

4. A patient has returned from a skiing holiday with a painful sprained ankle as well as a bad cough. Which of the following agents would relieve both the pain and the cough?

(A) Meperidine
(B) Naloxone
(C) Dextromethorphan
(D) Codeine
(E) Buspirone

5. Barbiturates are being replaced by benzodiazepines for use as sedative–hypnotic agents because of the shortcomings of barbiturate therapy, which include all of the following EXCEPT

(A) a narrow therapeutic index
(B) suppression of rapid eye movement (REM) sleep
(C) induction of seizures
(D) high potential for physical dependence

6. The antianxiety agents, such as diazepam and lorazepam, differ from antipsychotic agents, such as triflupromazine, in all of the following ways EXCEPT

(A) they do not cause parkinsonian tremor
(B) they are better skeletal muscle relaxants
(C) they are good anticonvulsant agents
(D) they are ineffective in treating psychotic symptoms
(E) their adverse effects are not dose- and age-dependent

7. A physician prescribes buspirone for short-term treatment for a patient with generalized anxiety. All of the following statements about this therapy are true EXCEPT

(A) it is chemically related to the benzodiazepines
(B) it is rapidly absorbed from the gastrointestinal tract
(C) it undergoes extensive first-pass metabolism
(D) it has little abuse potential
(E) dysphoria has been reported with high doses

8. All of the following opiate receptors are correctly matched with their physiologic effect EXCEPT

(A) μ_1—analgesia
(B) μ_2—respiratory stimulation
(C) κ—spinal analgesia
(D) σ—dysphoria
(E) κ—miosis

9. A 27-year-old woman is diagnosed with chronic mild endogenous depression. Her psychiatrist suggests a combination of psychotherapy and pharmacologic therapy. Which of the following drugs is LEAST likely to be prescribed?

(A) Fluoxetine
(B) Amitriptyline
(C) Sertraline
(D) Paroxetine
(E) Bupropion

10. An otherwise healthy 37-year-old dentist is diagnosed with chronic classic migraine. These headaches occur at least twice per month. All of the following statements are true EXCEPT

(A) an ergot preparation would be effective in this patient approximately 50% of the time
(B) sumatriptan would be contraindicated in this patient
(C) sumatriptan should be prescribed prophylactically
(D) β-adrenergic antagonists are the agent of choice for prevention of migraine
(E) oral sumatriptan would relieve the headache, but the rate of recurrence within 48 hours is high

---

DIRECTIONS: Each set of matching questions in this section consists of a list of four to twenty-six lettered options (some of which may be in figures) followed by several numbered items. For each numbered item, select the ONE lettered option that is most closely associated with it. To avoid spending too much time on matching sets with large numbers of options, it is generally advisable to begin each set by reading the list of options. Then, for each item in the set, try to generate the correct answer and locate it in the option list, rather than evaluating each option individually. Each lettered option may be selected once, more than once, or not at all.

Questions 11–13

Match each clinical indication with the appropriate barbiturate.

(A) Thiopental
(B) Pentobarbital
(C) Phenobarbital
(D) Amobarbital
(E) Barbital

11. An effective antiepileptic agent at low doses

12. Used as an intravenous adjunct to anesthesia

13. Has "hangover" liability when used as a hypnotic

Questions 14–17

Match each with the agent it best describes.

(A) Phenytoin
(B) Ethosuximide
(C) Carbamazepine
(D) Dantrolene
(E) Felbamate

14. Effective for the treatment of Lennox–Gastaut syndrome

15. Drug of choice for a 9-year-old boy diagnosed with petit mal epilepsy

16. Works peripherally in the muscle by decreasing Ca^{2+} release from the sarcoplasmic reticulum

17. Effective in relieving the pain of recurring trigeminal neuralgia

ANSWERS AND EXPLANATIONS

1. The answer is D *[III C 1 c]*. Phenytoin can induce blood dyscrasias. Other adverse effects include gastrointestinal irritation, ataxia and diplopia, gingival hyperplasia, hypersensitivity reactions, hirsutism, hepatitis, and drug interactions.

2. The answer is B *[III E 3]*. Clonazepam is a benzodiazepine. Besides being useful for seizure disorders, including petit mal, it is an antianxiety agent and helps to relieve night terrors. Meprobamate, one of the earliest antianxiety agents, has been largely replaced by the benzodiazepines. Droperidol, a butyrophenone, is used in anesthesiology. Lithium is used for the treatment of bipolar disease. Amphetamine can produce a calming effect with long-term therapy in hyperkinetic syndrome.

3. The answer is E *[VII B 2 b, e, 3 c, f]*. Monoamine oxidase (MAO) inhibitors are classified as follows: Type A deaminates serotonin and norepinephrine but not phenylethylamine, and type B deaminates phenylethylamine better than serotonin or norepinephrine. They are not useful in the manic phase of bipolar illness and can precipitate a hypertensive crisis if certain foods (e.g., cheese, beer, chicken livers) are ingested. Tricyclic antidepressants act presynaptically by preventing the reuptake of biogenic amines. Only the tricyclic imipramine is used to treat enuresis. Both groups of antidepressants produce an absolute increase in biogenic amine levels. In addition, they have considerable lag time prior to the onset of clinically useful effects. This latency period is usually 2 weeks or more, although it may be as short as 48 hours with the nonhydrazide MAO inhibitor tranylcypromine.

4. The answer is D *[IX B 2 b, e]*. Of the drugs listed in the question, only codeine has both antitussive and analgesic effects. The analgesic meperidine has no antitussive activity; the cough suppressant dextromethorphan has no analgesic activity. Naloxone has neither effect: It is a pure opioid antagonist and is used to reverse the unwanted effects of opioids (e.g., in neonates whose mothers received morphine during labor). Buspirone is an antianxiety agent, which is remarkably free of adverse effects.

5. The answer is C *[II A 7 a–c]*. Barbiturates do not induce seizures. Although still used as sedative–hypnotic agents, barbiturates are being replaced by benzodiazepines because they have a narrow therapeutic index, they suppress rapid eye movement (REM) sleep, and they have a high potential for physical dependence. Certain barbiturates, because of their rapid onset of action, can be used in the emergency treatment of convulsions.

6. The answer is E *[V; VI]*. Adverse effects of therapy with benzodiazepine antianxiety agents (e.g., diazepam, lorazepam) are partially dose- and age-dependent. The benzodiazepine antianxiety agents do not produce parkinsonian tremor, are better skeletal muscle relaxants, and are good anticonvulsant agents compared to antipsychotic agents, such as the phenothiazines. Antianxiety agents are not used in the treatment of psychosis.

7. The answer is A *[VI D]*. Buspirone is an antianxiety agent that is not chemically or pharmacologically related to the benzodiazepines, barbiturates, or other sedative–anxiolytic drugs. It is rapidly and completely absorbed from the gastrointestinal tract and undergoes an extensive first-pass metabolism. Buspirone is used for the short-term treatment of generalized anxiety. Although there are few adverse effects, dysphoria has been reported with high doses. It has little potential for abuse.

8. The answer is B *[IX A 2; Table 3-5]*. Mu (μ) receptors are associated with supraspinal analgesia (μ_1), respiratory depression (μ_2), as well as euphoria and physical dependence. Kappa receptors are associated with spinal analgesia, miosis, and sedation. Sigma receptors, when stimulated, cause dysphoria, hallucinations, and respiratory and vasomotor stimulation.

9. The answer is B *[VII B 4]*. Standard therapy for chronic mild endogenous depression comprises psychotherapy and a serotonin reuptake inhibitor. Amitriptyline is a tricyclic antidepressant. Fluoxetine, sertraline, paroxetine, and bupropion are all serotonin reuptake inhibitors, which have little effect on norepinephrine or dopamine function. Compared with amitriptyline, these agents have minimal adverse effects because of minimal binding to cholinergic, histaminic, and α-adrenergic receptors.

10. The answer is B *[X C–E]*. Sumatriptan is highly selective for the D subtype 5-hydroxytriptamine (5-HT$_1$) receptor and would not be contraindicated in this patient for active treatment. Oral sumatriptan relieves headache but the rate of recurrence within 48 hours is high. When sumatriptan is administered subcutaneously, the rate of recurrence is somewhat lower. Sumatriptan is not used for migraine prophylaxis. β-Adrenergic antagonists are the treatment of choice for migraine prophylaxis. Ergot preparations effectively abort migraines in approximately 50% of patients.

11–13. The answers are: 11-C *[II A 2 d]*, **12-A** *[II A 2 a]*, **13-D** *[II A 2 c]*. Phenobarbital, a long-acting barbiturate, is an effective antiepileptic when administered in low doses.

Thiopental is an ultra–short-acting barbiturate. Its principal use is as an intravenous adjuvant to anesthesia.

Amobarbital is an intermediate-acting barbiturate. When used as a hypnotic, amobarbital has a "hangover" liability, the result of residual depression of the central nervous system (CNS).

14–17. The answers are: 14-E *[III F 3]*, **15-B** *[III D 1 c]*, **16-D** *[III G 1]*, **17-C** *[III F 1]*. Felbamate is useful in the treatment of refractory partial seizures and various types of seizures associated with Lennox-Gastaut syndrome.

Ethosuximide is considered the drug of choice in the treatment of petit mal epilepsy.

Dantrolene is an antispasticity drug that works peripherally in the muscle by decreasing Ca^{2+} release from the sarcoplasmic reticulum. It is useful in the treatment of malignant hyperthermia as well.

Carbamazepine is used in the treatment of grand mal epilepsy as an adjunct to phenytoin therapy. Other uses include the treatment of trigeminal neuralgia.

Chapter 4
Anesthetic Agents

I. INTRODUCTION

A. Local anesthetics

1. Local anesthetic agents act by blocking both sensory and motor nerve conduction to produce a temporary loss of sensation without a loss of consciousness.

2. Unlike general anesthetics, they normally do not cause central nervous system (CNS) depression.

B. General anesthetics act on the CNS or autonomic nervous system to produce analgesia, amnesia, or hypnosis. Used alone or in combination with other agents (e.g., preanesthetic medication), general anesthetics can produce an optimum depth of anesthesia for a variety of surgical procedures.

1. **Inhalation anesthetics,** notably ether and nitrous oxide, revolutionized surgery after 1846 when their anesthetic properties were accepted by the medical community.

2. **Intravenous anesthetics** (e.g., thiopental) are mostly used for induction of anesthesia before administration of more potent anesthetic agents; however, they can be used for some procedures of shorter duration.
   a. **Neuroleptanesthesia** is induced by combining a powerful narcotic analgesic with a neuroleptic agent, and administering the combination in conjunction with the inhalation of nitrous oxide and oxygen.
   b. **Dissociative anesthesia,** such as that caused by ketamine, produces rapid analgesia and amnesia while maintaining laryngeal reflexes.
   c. **Preanesthetic medication** may include sedatives, opioids, tranquilizers, and anti-cholinergic agents.

II. LOCAL ANESTHETICS

A. Chemistry

1. Structurally, all local anesthetics consist of a hydrophilic amino group linked through a connecting group to a lipophilic aromatic residue (Figure 4-1). The greater the length of the connecting and amino groups, the greater the potency and the toxicity of the local anesthetic.

2. Local anesthetics are weak bases and, thus, are usually water-insoluble. The drug may be dispensed as a crystal but usually is prepared as an acidic salt solution, which is highly water-soluble and stable.

3. At tissue pH, depending on the pK_a of the agent, the drug exists as either an uncharged tertiary or secondary amine or a positively charged ammonium cation. The former state is lipophilic and crosses connective tissue and enters nerve cells; the cation is thought to block the generation of action potentials via a membrane–receptor complex.

FIGURE 4-1. Structural comparison of the ester and amide local anesthetics. (*A*) Procaine. If the connecting link between the intermediate group and the aromatic residue is an ester group, the site of metabolism is hydrolysis by plasma pseudocholinesterase. (*B*) Lidocaine. If the link is an amide bond, hydrolysis occurs in the liver.

B. **Mechanism of action**

1. Local anesthetics slow the propagation of nerve impulses by **reducing the rate of rise of the action potential and the rate of repolarization**.
   a. The increased threshold for electrical excitability results in a complete block of conduction.
   b. Local anesthetics specifically block nerve conduction by interfering with cell membrane permeability to sodium, particularly voltage-dependent Na^+ channels. Two theories may explain the mechanism of interference with membrane permeability.
      (1) The **specific receptor theory** postulates that the local anesthetic displaces Ca^{2+} from a site near the Na^+ channel and then blocks the adjacent Na^+ channel.
      (2) The **membrane expansion theory** hypothesizes that local anesthetics, because of their lipophilic properties, incorporate into the cell membrane, preventing the opening of pores and, thus, interfering with the passage of electrolytes.

2. A **differential sensitivity of nerve fibers to local anesthetics** has been identified and characterized.
   a. The smallest unmyelinated fibers, which conduct impulses for pain, temperature, and autonomic activity, conduct slowly and are the first to be blocked by local anesthetics.
   b. **Critical length** is the exposure time required by an anesthetic in order for it to exert its action; smaller nerve fibers have a proportionally smaller critical length.

C. **Agents** (Table 4-1)

1. **Cocaine** (see Chapter 3 VIII C)
   a. **Chemistry.** Cocaine is an ester of benzoic acid.
   b. **Pharmacokinetics**
      (1) Cocaine is quickly degraded by plasma esterases and has a half-life of approximately 1 hour.
      (2) Cocaine is metabolized in the blood by ester hydrolysis using pseudocholinesterase.

TABLE 4-1. Local Anesthetics—Preparations and Therapeutic Uses

Agent	Preparation	Therapeutic Use
Cocaine	4%–10% concentration, crystals	Topical anesthesia of nose, pharynx, and tracheobronchial tree; use limited by abuse potential
Procaine	1%–2% solution	Nerve block, infiltrative anesthesia
	5%–20% solution	Spinal anesthesia
Tetracaine	10% dextrose solution	Spinal anesthesia
	2% solution	Topical anesthesia of mucous membranes
Lidocaine	1%–2% solution, ointment, jelly, or cream	Topical anesthesia of mucous membranes; nerve block anesthesia
	0.5% solution	Infiltrative anesthesia
	< 5% solution	Spinal anesthesia
Prilocaine	1%–3% solution	Infiltrative, regional, and spinal anesthesia
Etidocaine	0.5%–1.5% solution	Infiltrative, regional, and epidural anesthesia
Mepivacaine	1%–4% solution	Infiltrative and regional nerve block anesthesia
Bupivacaine	0.25%–0.75% solution	Regional nerve block anesthesia
Dibucaine	0.2% solution	Topical anesthesia of mucous membranes

    c. Pharmacologic effects. In addition to local anesthetic activity, the spectrum of activity of cocaine includes the following:

      (1) CNS effects

        (a) Cocaine initially produces euphoria and sometimes dysphoria.

        (b) The initial effect is followed by poststimulatory depression.

      (2) Cardiovascular effects

        (a) Cocaine blocks the uptake of catecholamines at adrenergic nerve terminals.

        (b) This causes sympathetically mediated tachycardia and vasoconstriction, leading to hypertension. (The vasoconstriction also decreases intraoperative mucous membrane bleeding.)

    d. Preparations and therapeutic uses (see Table 4-1)

    e. Adverse effects

      (1) Tolerance, abuse, and poisoning can occur with cocaine overuse.

      (2) Hyperpyrexia

      (3) Anorexia

2. Procaine

    a. Chemistry. Procaine (see Figure 4-1A) is an ester of diethylaminoethanol and para-aminobenzoic acid (PABA).

    b. Pharmacokinetics

      (1) Procaine is well absorbed following parenteral administration and is rapidly metabolized by pseudocholinesterase. It has a short duration of action.

      (2) The metabolic product of procaine hydrolysis is PABA, which inhibits the action of sulfonamides.

      (3) The drug lacks topical activity.

      (4) Procaine administration causes minimal systemic toxicity and no local irritation.

    c. Preparations and therapeutic uses (see Table 4-1). Procaine hydrochloride is available with and without epinephrine. **Epinephrine,** a vasoconstrictor, decreases the rate of anesthetic absorption in the bloodstream and so approximately doubles the duration of anesthesia produced by a given dose.

3. Tetracaine

    a. Chemistry. Tetracaine is an ester and derivative of PABA.

    b. Pharmacokinetics
        (1) Tetracaine is approximately 10 times more potent (and more toxic) than procaine.
        (2) Its onset of action is approximately 5 minutes, and its duration of action is between 2 and 3 hours.
    c. Preparations and therapeutic uses (see Table 4-1)
        (1) Tetracaine hydrochloride is a commonly used local anesthetic for spinal anesthesia and, in this context, usually is combined with 10% dextrose to increase the specific gravity so that the solution is heavier than cerebrospinal fluid.
        (2) A 2% solution is used topically on mucous membranes.

4. Lidocaine
    a. Chemistry. Lidocaine (see Figure 4-1B) is an amide local anesthetic and an acetanilid derivative.
    b. Pharmacokinetics. Lidocaine is rapidly absorbed after parenteral administration and is metabolized in the liver by microsomal mixed-function oxidases.
    c. Pharmacologic effects include:
        (1) Rapid onset of anesthesia
        (2) Minimal local irritation
        (3) A greater potency and longer duration of action than procaine
        (4) Moderate topical activity
    d. Preparations and therapeutic uses (see Table 4-1). Lidocaine hydrochloride can be administered with or without epinephrine. The major clinical uses of lidocaine are as a local anesthetic and, intravenously, as an antiarrhythmic agent (see Chapter 5 II C).

5. Prilocaine
    a. Chemistry. Like lidocaine, prilocaine is an amide local anesthetic.
    b. Pharmacokinetics. The onset and duration of action of prilocaine are slightly longer than those of lidocaine.
    c. Preparations and therapeutic uses (see Table 4-1)
    d. Adverse effects. The major disadvantage of prilocaine is the production of methemoglobinemia and a shift to the left of the oxygen-dissociation curve for hemoglobin.

6. Etidocaine
    a. Pharmacokinetics. Etidocaine is similar to lidocaine except for its greater potency and longer duration of action.
    b. Preparations and therapeutic uses (see Table 4-1)
        (1) Etidocaine is used clinically in epidural, infiltrative, and regional anesthesia. The drug usually blocks motor fibers before sensory fibers.
        (2) Etidocaine hydrochloride is available both with and without epinephrine.

7. Mepivacaine
    a. Chemistry. Like lidocaine, mepivacaine is an amide-type local anesthetic.
    b. Pharmacokinetics
        (1) Mepivacaine is similar to lidocaine; however, it does not have antiarrhythmic activity.
        (2) In onset of action, mepivacaine is more rapid than lidocaine, and its duration of action is about 20% longer.
    c. Preparations and therapeutic uses (see Table 4-1). Epinephrine is rarely used with this drug.

8. Bupivacaine
    a. Chemistry. An amide local anesthetic, bupivacaine is structurally similar to mepivacaine.
    b. Pharmacokinetics. Bupivacaine is more potent and has a longer duration of action than mepivacaine, lasting for more than 24 hours in some situations, possibly as a result of increased tissue binding. The onset of action is slower than that of mepivacaine.
    c. Preparations and therapeutic uses (see Table 4-1).
    d. Adverse effects. Toxicity is similar to that of tetracaine; however, cardiac arrest has been reported in association with a 0.75% solution of bupivacaine used for obstetric epidural anesthesia.

9. **Dibucaine**
   a. **Chemistry.** Dibucaine is a substituted amide and a quinoline derivative.
   b. **Pharmacokinetics**
      (1) Dibucaine is a potent anesthetic with a long duration of action.
      (2) It has a high systemic toxicity and is used only as a topical anesthetic.
   c. **Preparations and therapeutic uses** (see Table 4-1)

D. **Adverse systemic effects of local anesthetics** result from absorption of toxic amounts of these agents into the bloodstream. Adding epinephrine to the optimal concentration of a local anesthetic reduces the rate of systemic absorption, thereby decreasing systemic toxicity.

1. **Seizures,** the result of absorption of the local anesthetic and stimulation of the CNS, are the most serious adverse effect. Convulsions, if they occur, are treated with basic supportive measures, including ventilation and oxygenation, and with intravenous diazepam.

2. **Respiratory failure** secondary to CNS depression is a late stage of intoxication.

3. A **quinidine-like effect on the myocardium** can be produced by local anesthetics.

4. **Hypotension** is a late effect that can occur as the result of myocardial depression and peripheral arterial vasodilation; affected patients are treated with appropriate parenteral vasopressor agents.

5. **Allergic reactions** to local anesthetic agents **rarely occur**.

III. GENERAL ANESTHETICS

A. **Inhalation anesthetics**

1. **General considerations** (Figure 4-2)
   a. The relationship between the administered dose of an inhalation anesthetic and the quantitative effect produced is described as the **minimum alveolar concentration (MAC)** of the anesthetic at 1 atm that will produce loss of movement in 50% of subjects exposed to a noxious stimulus. The MAC is used as the **measure of potency** for all inhalation anesthetics.
   b. The concentration of an inhalation anesthetic in blood or tissue is the product of its solubility and partial pressure. The **solubility** of an agent is expressed most commonly in terms of a blood:gas or a tissue:blood partition coefficient.
      (1) An agent with a **blood:gas partition coefficient** of 2 reaches twice the concentration in the blood phase as in the gas phase when the partial pressure is the same in both phases (i.e., at equilibrium). Very soluble agents (e.g., ether) have a blood:gas partition coefficient as high as 12; relatively insoluble agents (e.g., nitrous oxide) have a coefficient of less than 1. **The lower the blood:gas partition coefficient of an anesthetic, the more rapid the induction of anesthesia** with that agent, because high blood solubility constantly lowers the alveolar gas pressure.
      (2) Most inhalation agents are equally soluble in lean tissue and in blood, so that the **tissue:blood partition coefficient** often approximates 1. On the other hand, most anesthetics have a far greater concentration in fatty tissues than in blood at equilibrium.

2. **Halothane**
   a. **Pharmacokinetics**
      (1) Halothane, with a MAC of 0.75%, is a potent anesthetic agent.
      (2) **Excretion**
         (a) Approximately 70% of halothane is eliminated unchanged in exhaled gas in the first 24 hours after administration.

A. Blood:gas partition coefficient

0 — 0.42 Desflurane
— 0.47 Nitrous oxide
1 —
— 1.4 Isoflurane
2 — 1.9 Enflurane
— 2.3 Halothane
3 —
4 —
5 —

Solubility
Induction/recovery time
Least ··· Most

B. MAC

0 —
1 — 0.75 Halothane
— 1.15 Isoflurane
— 1.68 Enflurane
2 —
3 —
4 —
5 —
6 — 6 Desflurane
100 — 105.2 Nitrous oxide

Potency
Most ··· Least

FIGURE 4-2. (*A*) The solubility of an agent determines the concentration of the agent in the blood or tissue. The lower the blood:gas partition coefficient, the more rapid the induction of, and the recovery from, anesthesia. Desflurane has the lowest blood:gas partition coefficient of the agents shown; consequently, it achieves a maximum alveolar concentration very quickly. In contrast, halothane, with the highest blood:gas partition coefficient, never comes close to achieving an alveolar concentration of 100%, and induction and recovery are slow. (*B*) The minimum alveolar concentration (*MAC*) is a measure of potency. The higher the MAC, the lower the potency.

        (b) Approximately 5% is biotransformed by the cytochrome P-450 system in the endoplasmic reticulum of the liver.
    b. Pharmacologic effects. Halothane **lacks significant analgesic potency** and, thus, is most frequently used with another anesthetic.
      (1) Respiratory effects
        (a) Respirations become rapid and shallow, and there is a reduction in the minute volume.
        (b) Halothane produces bronchiolar dilation.
      (2) CNS effects. As halothane anesthesia deepens, fast, low-voltage electroencephalographic waves are replaced by slow, high-voltage waves.
      (3) Muscular effects
        (a) Halothane causes skeletal muscle relaxation by both central and peripheral mechanisms.
        (b) It appears to increase the sensitivity of end-plates to the action of competitive neuromuscular blocking agents.
        (c) It relaxes uterine smooth muscle.
    c. Preparations and therapeutic uses (Table 4-2)
      (1) Halothane is not irritating to the larynx; thus, induction of anesthesia with this agent is smooth and bronchospasm is uncommon.
      (2) Halothane administration is often supplemented with thiopental for induction of anesthesia. Nitrous oxide, oxygen, and muscle relaxants are normally used with halothane.

TABLE 4-2. Inhalation Anesthetics

Anesthetic	Advantages
Halothane	Nonflammable Potent Nonirritating
Enflurane	Little change in pulse or respiratory rate Smooth adjustments of depth of anesthesia are possible Adequate skeletal muscle relaxant
Isoflurane	Depth of anesthesia can be rapidly adjusted Cardiac output sustained; arrhythmias uncommon Potentiates action of skeletal muscle relaxants
Desflurane	Very rapid induction and recovery Organ toxicity is negligible
Nitrous oxide	Nonflammable Nonirritating Rapid onset and recovery Little toxicity
Diethyl ether	Good skeletal muscle relaxant

    (3) Halothane is a safe anesthetic for children and may be administered via a mask because it is the least pungent volatile agent.

d. Adverse effects

    (1) Halothane is a highly potent, nonflammable general anesthetic with a relatively high blood:gas partition coefficient; thus, induction of and recovery from anesthesia with this agent may be prolonged.

    (2) Respiratory effects. Halothane causes a reduction in the ventilatory response to carbon dioxide. This effect appears to result from depression of central chemoreceptors.

    (3) Cardiovascular effects

        (a) Halothane causes a dose-dependent decrease in arterial blood pressure.

        (b) Cutaneous blood flow may increase as blood vessels dilate.

        (c) Myocardial contractility is depressed with halothane administration.

        (d) Halothane interferes with the action of norepinephrine and, thus, antagonizes the sympathetic response to arterial hypertension.

        (e) Halothane anesthesia depresses cardiac sympathetic activity, which can result in a slow heart rate.

        (f) Although arrhythmias are uncommon, halothane can increase the automaticity of the heart. This condition is exacerbated by adrenergic agonists, cardiac disease, hypoxia, and electrolyte abnormalities.

    (4) CNS effects

        (a) Cerebral blood vessels dilate, increasing cerebral blood flow and cerebrospinal fluid pressure. A maldistribution of cerebral blood flow and altered metabolism can occur.

        (b) Shivering during recovery is common.

    (5) Renal effects

        (a) At a level of 1 MAC, halothane causes renal blood flow and glomerular filtration to drop to about 50% of normal.

        (b) These effects are mitigated by adequate hydration.

    (6) Hepatic effects

        (a) Halothane depresses liver function. This effect is rapidly reversed when administration of the anesthetic is stopped.

        (b) Hepatic necrosis that cannot be attributed to known causes can occur with halothane anesthesia. Two to five days postoperatively, an affected patient develops fever, anorexia, and vomiting. Eosinophilia and biochemical abnormalities characteristic of hepatitis occur. This syndrome is known as **halothane hepatitis**.

           (i) Halothane hepatitis has an incidence of 1 in 7000 individuals receiving halothane anesthesia, and it is associated with a 20%–50% mortality rate.

           (ii) It is likely that halothane-induced hepatic damage is metabolic in origin. The possibility of genetic susceptibility has been suggested and would provide evidence that the rate of halothane metabolism is genetically determined.

           (iii) Patient characteristics that increase the potential for liver damage include middle age, obesity, and female sex. Closely spaced, repeated administration of halothane increases the potential for liver damage. Preexisting liver disease is not exacerbated by halothane.

           (iv) Children do not appear to be susceptible to the liver damage associated with halothane.

    (7) Muscular effects. Halothane, like all potent inhalation agents, can trigger **malignant hyperthermia,** a potentially fatal condition believed to be autosomal dominant, in which, in response to anesthesia, a sudden, rapid rise in body temperature and signs of increased muscle metabolism occur.

3. Enflurane

  a. Pharmacokinetics

    (1) Enflurane has a MAC of 1.68%.

    (2) Excretion

      (a) Approximately 80% of enflurane is eliminated unchanged as expired gas.

      (b) Because enflurane's oil:gas partition is less than that of other halogenated anesthetics, enflurane leaves fatty tissues more rapidly.

      (c) Approximately 5% of enflurane is metabolized in the liver. Free fluoride ion is released, but poses little danger of renal toxicity.

  b. Pharmacologic effects

    (1) Respiratory effects. Enflurane causes bronchodilation and inhibits bronchoconstriction.

    (2) Muscular effects

      (a) Enflurane, which acts directly on the neuromuscular junction, provides adequate muscular relaxation for most surgical procedures.

      (b) Enflurane relaxes uterine smooth muscle.

  c. Therapeutic uses (see Table 4-2). Enflurane is a potent general anesthetic. It is a better skeletal relaxant than halothane, but, unlike halothane, enflurane can cause seizure activity.

  d. Adverse effects

    (1) Enflurane causes mild stimulation of salivation and tracheobronchial secretions. It suppresses laryngeal reflexes.

    (2) Respiratory effects

      (a) Enflurane produces dose-dependent respiratory depression.

      (b) With enflurane at a level of 1 MAC, respiratory responses to hypoxia and hypercapnia are less than those with halothane.

    (3) Cardiovascular effects

      (a) Dose-dependent depression of the arterial blood pressure and depressed baroreceptor responses are similar to those caused by halothane.

      (b) Dose-dependent myocardial depression also occurs and is similar to that caused by halothane.

      (c) Enflurane causes a lower incidence of arrhythmias and less sensitization of the myocardium to catecholamines than does halothane.

(4) CNS effects
- **(a)** Enflurane anesthesia can lead to an electroencephalographic pattern characteristic of seizure activity or to frank seizures.
  - **(i)** The seizures are self-limited and can be prevented by avoiding both high concentrations of enflurane and hyperventilation, which leads to hypocapnia.
  - **(ii)** Enflurane is contraindicated in patients who have known seizure disorders.
- **(b)** Enflurane causes cerebral vasodilation and increased intracranial pressure as long as the arterial blood pressure remains normal.

(5) Renal effects. At a level of 1 MAC, enflurane anesthesia causes a reduction in renal blood flow and glomerular filtration that is similar to that caused by halothane.

(6) Hepatic effects
- **(a)** Liver impairment has been reported but usually is reversible.
- **(b)** Hepatic necrosis also has been reported, especially after repeated administration of enflurane.

4. Isoflurane
- **a. Chemistry.** Isoflurane is a dialkyl-haloether. The general structure of these volatile anesthetics is shown in Figure 4-3.
- **b. Pharmacologic effects**
  - **(1)** Isoflurane is an isomer of enflurane and has similar physical properties. Isoflurane's MAC is 1.15%.
  - **(2)** Isoflurane is a better muscle relaxant than either halothane or enflurane.
- **c. Therapeutic use** (see Table 4-2). For adults, isoflurane has largely replaced halothane and enflurane as an anesthetic, because it offers rapid induction and emergence and has little postanesthetic organ toxicity. Unlike enflurane, isoflurane does not cause seizure activity; unlike halothane, isoflurane does not sensitize the myocardium to epinephrine or induce arrhythmias.
- **d. Adverse effects**
  - **(1)** Isoflurane produces significant respiratory depression.
  - **(2)** Because of hypercapnia resulting from respiratory depression, cardiac output may increase.
  - **(3)** Peripheral vascular resistance is decreased by isoflurane, resulting in a fall in arterial blood pressure.

5. Desflurane is a newly approved inhalation anesthetic that differs from isoflurane in that a fluorine atom is substituted for a chlorine atom.
- **a. Pharmacokinetics**
  - **(1)** Desflurane has the lowest blood:gas partition coefficient of any inhalation anesthetic, producing the most rapid induction.
  - **(2)** Recovery time is 5 minutes with desflurane, as opposed to 10 minutes with isoflurane.
- **b. Therapeutic use** (see Table 4-2). As a muscle relaxant, desflurane may offer some advantage over isoflurane in that induction and emergence are more rapid, permitting rapid anesthesia adjustment.
- **c. Adverse effects**
  - **(1)** Desflurane causes myocardial and respiratory depression.
  - **(2)** Desflurane dilates peripheral, coronary, and cerebral arteries.
  - **(3)** It is pungent, thus preventing mask induction in children.

FIGURE 4-3. Structure of the dialkyl-haloethers. The halide (X) can be either chlorine or fluorine.

6. Nitrous oxide
  a. Pharmacokinetics
   (1) Nitrous oxide is an inorganic inert gas that supports combustion.
   (2) The MAC for nitrous oxide is 105.2%, meaning that hyperbaric conditions would be required to reach a level of 1 MAC with this drug. For maintaining anesthesia, a concentration of 75%–80% nitrous oxide is required.
   (3) Nitrous oxide is not effective for anesthesia as a single agent, and attempting to use it in this manner is likely to induce hypoxia. To achieve "complete" anesthesia with this agent, administration of opioids to supplement analgesia, the use of thiopental for narcosis, and a neuromuscular blocking agent for muscular relaxation are all required.
   (4) Excretion
      (a) Nitrous oxide is eliminated primarily as an expired gas.
      (b) The amount of nitrous oxide subject to biotransformation is not known.
  b. Therapeutic uses (see Table 4-2)
   (1) Nitrous oxide is an important and **powerful analgesic** that is well tolerated. Its onset of action is rapid, as is recovery from its effects. Because of this, it is frequently used for **outpatient dental procedures**.
   (2) Nitrous oxide is used as a **supplement to more potent anesthetic agents** and, in this capacity, is probably the most widely used general anesthetic agent. The effects of nitrous oxide on respiration are minimal when a concentration of 50% is used. However, when nitrous oxide is combined with thiopental or another anesthetic agent for induction of anesthesia, the respiratory stimulant response to carbon dioxide is depressed more than when thiopental or the other anesthetic agent is used alone.
  c. Adverse effects
   (1) Cardiovascular effects. When nitrous oxide is combined with a potent inhalation anesthetic, activation of the sympathetic nervous system results; blood pressure and total peripheral vascular resistance rise, and cardiac output is reduced.
   (2) Because of its high partial pressure in blood and its low blood:gas partition coefficient, nitrous oxide diffuses into air-containing body cavities and **can increase the pressure or expand the volume of gas in air pockets**. This action can result in:
      (a) Distention of the bowel
      (b) Expansion or rupture of a pulmonary cyst
      (c) Rupture of the tympanic membrane in an occluded middle ear
      (d) Pneumocephalus
   (3) When nitrous oxide is dissolved in blood, it **can enlarge the volume of air emobli**.
   (4) Diffusion hypoxia can occur at the termination of nitrous oxide anesthesia if a patient abruptly begins to breathe room air. This hypoxia is caused by a rapid outward diffusion of nitrous oxide from tissues into the bloodstream and then into the alveoli, where it decreases alveolar tension and consequently lowers arterial oxygen levels. This problem can be avoided by administration of 100% oxygen for a short period following nitrous oxide anesthesia.
   (5) Nitrous oxide is associated with a high incidence of postoperative **nausea and vomiting**.
   (6) Inactivation of vitamin B$_{12}$ can occur.
   (7) Leukopenia has been reported with chronic nitrous oxide abuse.
   (8) Nitrous oxide is **contraindicated in pregnant women, immunosuppressed patients,** and **patients with pernicious anemia**.

7. Diethyl ether
  a. Chemistry. Diethyl ether is a highly flammable and explosive anesthetic agent that essentially has been replaced by halogenated anesthetics.
  b. Pharmacologic effects
   (1) Respiratory effects
      (a) Increased sympathetic activity produced by diethyl ether results in bronchodilation.

(b) The respiratory response to carbon dioxide, although reduced, is maintained spontaneously by reflex excitation at peripheral sites.

(2) Cardiovascular effects. Although diethyl ether is a myocardial depressant, cardiac output and arterial blood pressure are maintained because of sympathetic activation.

(3) Muscular effects

  (a) Diethyl ether is a good skeletal muscle relaxant because it causes CNS depression at synaptic pathways in the spinal cord.

  (b) In addition, diethyl ether has a curare-like action, allowing a lower dose of neuromuscular blockers; several aminoglycoside antibiotics augment this effect.

c. Adverse effects

  (1) When used as a sole agent to induce anesthesia, diethyl ether increases salivary secretions, vomiting, and laryngospasm.

  (2) Vagal blockade occurs with diethyl ether administration, resulting in tachycardia.

  (3) Diethyl ether is a strong stimulant of antidiuretic hormone.

  (4) Sympathetic activation results in increased hepatic glycogenolysis.

B. Intravenous anesthetics

1. Neuroleptanesthesia

  a. General considerations

   (1) When a neuroleptic agent is combined with a powerful narcotic, **neuroleptanalgesia** is produced. Diagnostic and minor surgical procedures can be accomplished under neuroleptanalgesia. When these procedures require anesthesia, neuroleptanalgesia can be converted to **neuroleptanesthesia** by the concurrent administration of 65% nitrous oxide in oxygen.

   (2) The agents most frequently used to achieve neuroleptanalgesia are **droperidol** (a butyrophenone derivative—see Chapter 3 V D) and **fentanyl** (an opioid—see Chapter 3 IX C 3). A premixed combination of the two drugs is available as a product called **Innovar**.

  b. Pharmacologic effects

   (1) Respiratory effects

    (a) Droperidol slightly decreases the respiratory rate but increases tidal volume.

    (b) Fentanyl reduces both respiratory rate and tidal volume.

    (c) The marked respiratory depressant effect of the two drugs outlasts the analgesic effect.

   (2) Cardiovascular effects

    (a) Droperidol can produce mild α-adrenergic blockade, causing some hypotension.

    (b) Fentanyl has a parasympathomimetic effect that can cause bradycardia and hypotension.

    (c) Innovar can cause bradycardia. However, it rarely causes other cardiac arrhythmias, and, in general, it has little effect on the cardiovascular system.

  c. Preparations and therapeutic uses

   (1) Fentanyl should be administered as a slow intravenous infusion (given over 5–10 minutes), because rapid injection may cause respiratory muscle spasm.

   (2) After induction of neuroleptanalgesia, nitrous oxide administration is begun. Supplementary fentanyl may be required for prolonged analgesia because fentanyl has a short duration of action.

  d. Adverse effects

   (1) Confusion and mental depression are the most common complaints after neuroleptanesthesia.

   (2) Respiratory depression is a frequent occurrence, and adequate ventilation and oxygenation may require use of mechanical measures.

   (3) Extrapyramidal symptoms occur rarely.

2. **Dissociative anesthesia**
    a. **General considerations.** Dissociative anesthesia is a state similar to neuroleptanalgesia in which anesthetized patients feel totally dissociated from their surroundings. **Phencyclidine** was the original dissociative anesthetic; however, the structurally similar **ketamine** is the only drug presently used to produce this state.
    b. **Pharmacologic effects**
        (1) Ketamine produces profound analgesia and amnesia.
        (2) It has no effect on laryngeal reflexes.
        (3) Skeletal muscle tone, heart rate, arterial blood pressure, and cerebrospinal fluid pressure can be increased by ketamine.
        (4) The respiratory cycle is maintained near normal.
    c. **Preparations and therapeutic uses**
        (1) Ketamine is used mainly in children and young adults for diagnostic procedures of short duration.
        (2) Premedication with atropine reduces salivary secretions; premedication with a narcotic analgesic decreases the dose of ketamine needed for anesthesia.
    d. **Adverse effects**
        (1) Because of its hallucinogen-like structure, ketamine frequently produces unpleasant dreams, especially in adults. Recovery from ketamine anesthesia often is accompanied by emergence delirium and psychomotor activity.
        (2) Contraindications to the use of ketamine include psychiatric disorders, a history of cerebrovascular disease (to avoid the risk of hypertension-induced stroke), and respiratory infection.

3. **Barbiturates**
    a. **General considerations**
        (1) **Thiopental** is the barbiturate most frequently used for general anesthesia. It provides rapid and pleasant induction and, thus, often is used before administration of stronger agents. It can be used alone to provide anesthesia for short procedures, but thiopental and other barbiturates are poor analgesics.
        (2) Once a barbiturate is injected, little can be done to facilitate its removal. Termination of its effects depends on redistribution of the drug from the brain to other tissues and, to a lesser extent, on biotransformation.
    b. The **pharmacology** and **therapeutic uses** of barbiturates are presented in Chapter 3 II A.

4. **Propofol**
    a. **Pharmacokinetics.** Onset of unconsciousness occurs within 1 minute, and duration of action is only 3–5 minutes because of rapid redistribution.
    b. **Pharmacologic effects.** The hemodynamic and respiratory effects are similar to those occurring with barbiturate induction.
    c. **Therapeutic uses**
        (1) Propofol is a short-acting intravenous anesthetic that can be used for induction of anesthesia or maintenance as part of a balanced anesthesia regimen.
        (2) The clarity of mental status upon recovery makes propofol particularly useful for ambulatory surgical patients.
    d. **Adverse effects**
        (1) Hypotension can be particularly severe in older patients.
        (2) Intravenous administration of propofol can be irritating.

5. **Medazolam**
    a. **General considerations.** Medazolam is a parenteral benzodiazepine that is three to four times as potent as diazepam, but unlike diazepam, it does not cause local irritation after intramuscular or intravenous injection.
    b. **Pharmacokinetics**
        (1) Medazolam is highly lipid-soluble and rapidly crosses the blood–brain barrier.
        (2) It is metabolized in the liver and has a half-life of 1–4 hours.
    c. **Therapeutic uses.** Medazolam is used for sedation during short procedures, sedation before general anesthesia, induction of general anesthesia, and as a hypnotic drug in balanced anesthesia regimens.

    d. Adverse effects. Medazolam can cause respiratory depression, and anterograde amnesia lasts for at least 2 hours.

  6. Etomidate
    a. General considerations
      (1) Etomidate is an ultra–short-acting hypnotic used for induction of anesthesia.
      (2) Cardiovascular effects are virtually absent.
    b. Adverse effects
      (1) Etomidate can cause pain on injection, myoclonic movements, and postoperative nausea and vomiting, especially with opioid use.
      (2) Etomidate has embryocidal activity.

C. **Preanesthetic medications** can foster an uncomplicated anesthetic and operative course by improving the rapidity and smoothness of induction, reducing anxiety, providing analgesia and amnesia, and compensating for the salivation, bradycardia, and other side effects of anesthesia. Agents used as preanesthetic medications include sedatives, opioids, tranquilizers, and anticholinergic agents. The pharmacology, therapeutic uses, and undesirable effects of barbiturates, opioids, and tranquilizers are discussed in Chapter 3; anticholinergic agents are discussed in Chapter 2.

  1. Barbiturates, such as **secobarbital** and **pentobarbital,** are the preoperative sedatives most frequently employed. These agents produce less postoperative nausea and vomiting than opioids.

  2. Opioids, such as **morphine, fentanyl,** and **alfentanil,** often are given to patients who are to be anesthetized with general anesthetics of fairly low potency, such as the combination of nitrous oxide and thiopental. In addition, they can be administered with a barbiturate or diazepam for regional anesthesia. In both instances, they provide analgesia. Alfentanil may offer advantages over fentanyl for longer procedures. Response and recovery appear to be more rapid.

  3. Phenothiazine derivatives, such as **promethazine** and the antihistamine **hydroxyzine,** often are administered concomitantly with opioids because they potentiate the analgesic effect without increasing side effects.

  4. Tranquilizers, such as **diazepam,** are useful in a wide variety of anesthetic situations. They can provide preoperative sedation, help to prevent and treat the CNS stimulation caused by local anesthetics, and provide amnesia.

  5. Anticholinergic agents. Atropine and **scopolamine,** as well as the quaternary ammonium compound **glycopyrrolate,** are used routinely to decrease the flow of saliva. Because of a lower incidence of undesirable side effects, glycopyrrolate is recommended as the anticholinergic agent of choice for bronchoscopy.

DIRECTIONS: Each of the numbered items or incomplete statements in this section is negatively phrased, as indicated by a capitalized word such as NOT, LEAST, or EXCEPT. Select the ONE lettered answer or completion that is BEST in each case.

1. A patient who has an untreatable hepatic carcinoma must undergo foot surgery. All of the following local anesthetic agents may be deleterious to this patient based on his history EXCEPT

(A) lidocaine
(B) prilocaine
(C) mepivacaine
(D) procaine
(E) etidocaine

2. Lidocaine has all of the following properties EXCEPT

(A) it is a therapeutically useful local anesthetic
(B) it has a rapid onset of activity
(C) it has an esteratic linkage
(D) it is metabolized in the liver
(E) epinephrine is not required when lidocaine is administered

3. Correct statements concerning procaine include all of the following EXCEPT

(A) it has an ester linkage
(B) it interferes with sodium influx during depolarization
(C) it is relatively short-acting
(D) it can produce a lupus-like syndrome
(E) its metabolic product can inhibit the action of sulfonamides

4. A 72-year-old man is scheduled to undergo a transurethral prostatic resection. He refuses general anesthesia, so spinal anesthesia is selected. All of the following statements are correct EXCEPT

(A) procaine and epinephrine should not be used topically to numb the skin surface for spinal anesthetic administration
(B) tetracaine combined with 10% dextrose to increase the specific gravity would be a very effective spinal anesthetic in this patient
(C) dibucaine should not be given as a spinal anesthetic because it has a high systemic toxicity
(D) If the spinal anesthetic produces a C-4 block causing the patient to experience respiratory difficulty, the spinal should be converted to a general anesthetic
(E) dissociative anesthesia is the anesthesia of choice for this procedure

5. A patient with a pseudocholinesterase deficiency requires minor surgery. A local anesthetic will be used. All of the following statements regarding the choice of an anesthetic agent for this patient are true EXCEPT

(A) procaine should not be used in this patient because a pseudocholinesterase deficiency would lengthen its duration of action
(B) tetracaine should not be used because it is most commonly used for spinal anesthesia
(C) the chemical structure of lidocaine would most likely explain its therapeutic usefulness in this case
(D) dibucaine would not be contraindicated because it is a surface anesthetic
(E) although cocaine has abuse potential, because it is metabolized in the liver, it would be of therapeutic value in this case

6. Isoflurane has largely replaced halothane and enflurane as the most frequently used inhalation anesthetic in adults for all of the following reasons EXCEPT

(A) it offers rapid induction
(B) it offers rapid emergence
(C) it is a better muscle relaxant
(D) it maintains arterial blood pressure by increasing peripheral vascular resistance
(E) it has little post-anesthetic organ toxicity

7. A toxic dose of lidocaine is inadvertently administered locally into the dorsalis pedis artery of a patient. All of the following effects may occur EXCEPT

(A) convulsions
(B) respiratory depression
(C) hypotension
(D) increased inotropic effect
(E) reduced oxygen tension

8. A patient is given an inhalation anesthetic, an inert gas that supports combustion. Although it is not effective as a single agent, when combined with more potent inhalation agents, it provides significant analgesia. Because of its high partial pressure in blood, this agent could result in all of the following EXCEPT

(A) distention of the bowel
(B) leukocytosis
(C) pneumocephalus
(D) rupture of a pulmonary cyst
(E) rupture of a tympanic membrane in an occluded middle ear

9. Neuroleptanalgesia has all of the following properties EXCEPT

(A) it is used chiefly for diagnostic and minor surgical procedures
(B) droperidol and fentanyl are commonly used agents
(C) hypertension is a common consequence
(D) it can be used with nitrous oxide
(E) confusion can occur as an adverse effect

DIRECTIONS: Each set of matching questions in this section consists of a list of four to twenty-six lettered options (some of which may be in figures) followed by several numbered items. For each numbered item, select the ONE lettered option that is most closely associated with it. To avoid spending too much time on matching sets with large numbers of options, it is generally advisable to begin each set by reading the list of options. Then, for each item in the set, try to generate the correct answer and locate it in the option list, rather than evaluating each option individually. Each lettered option may be selected once, more than once, or not at all.

Questions 10–13

Match each type of anesthesia with the correct anesthetic agent.

(A) Ketamine
(B) Halothane
(C) Droperidol, fentanyl, nitrous oxide, and oxygen
(D) Thiopental

10. Dissociative anesthesia

11. Neuroleptanesthesia

12. Inhalation anesthesia

13. Intravenous induction anesthesia

Questions 14–17

Match each description with the local anesthetic it describes.

(A) Cocaine
(B) Lidocaine
(C) Procaine
(D) Dibucaine
(E) Tetracaine

14. Commonly used spinal anesthetic that is ten times more potent than procaine

15. Provides good topical anesthesia of nose, pharynx, and tracheobronchial tube

16. Its metabolic product inhibits the action of sulfonamides

17. Widely used as an antiarrhythmic agent as well

Questions 18–20

Match the stated advantage with the correct inhalation anesthetic.

(A) Nitrous oxide
(B) Isoflurane
(C) Halothane
(D) Desflurane
(E) Enflurane

18. Produces the most rapid induction and has the lowest blood:gas partition coefficient

19. Nonirritating to the larynx and produces bronchiolar dilation

20. Powerful analgesic used to supplement more potent anesthetic agents

1. The answer is D *[II A 1, C 2 b, 4 b, 6 b, 7 a]*. Procaine is metabolized systemically by pseudocholinesterase, whereas lidocaine, prilocaine, mepivacaine, and etidocaine are metabolized in the liver by microsomal mixed-function oxidases. Thus, for a patient with liver disease, procaine would be the anesthetic agent of choice among this group.

2. The answer is C *[II C 4]*. Lidocaine has an amide, not an esteratic, linkage. Possessing an amide linkage gives it a greater duration of action than procaine, which is metabolized by ester hydrolysis. Lidocaine is a therapeutically useful local anesthetic with a rapid onset of activity. Metabolism of the drug takes place in the liver. It can be administered with or without epinephrine.

3. The answer is D *[II B 1 b, C 2]*. Unlike procainamide, procaine does not cause a lupus-like syndrome. Procaine is an ester of diethyl-aminoethanol and para-aminobenzoic acid (PABA), which can inhibit the action of sulfon-amides. It does interfere with sodium influx during depolarization. It has a short duration of action and is metabolized by pseudo-cholinesterase.

4. The answer is E *[II C 2–3, 9; III B 2]*. Disso-ciative anesthesia is used mainly for short diagnostic procedures, not longer operative procedures. Procaine does not possess topical activity and would not numb the skin surface. Tetracaine is usually combined with 10% dex-trose and is an excellent agent for spinal anes-thesia. Dibucaine, because of its high systemic toxicity, is not used for spinal anesthesia. It is used topically. If spinal anesthesia results in respiratory difficulty because of a "high block," conversion to a general anesthesia and excellent oxygenation are required. Little anes-thesia is required to produce analgesia in the presence of this "high spinal." Oxygenation should continue until motor and sensory func-tion return.

5. The answer is E *[II C 1 b (2), 2, 3 c, 4 a, b; Table 4-1]*. Patients with cholinesterase defi-ciency would have difficulty metabolizing local anesthetics possessing ester linkages. Thus, cocaine, which is an ester of benzoic acid, is metabolized via ester hydrolysis in the blood by pseudocholinesterase; it is not

metabolized in the liver. Procaine is also metab-olized by pseudocholinesterase; therefore, a pseudocholinesterase deficiency would lengthen its duration of action. Tetracaine is commonly used for spinal anesthesia and, therefore, is inappropriate for this patient. Lido-caine, which has an amide bond, is metabo-lized in the liver and therefore would be of ther-apeutic use in this case. Dibucaine, a surface anesthetic, would not be contraindicated.

6. The answer is D *[III A 4 c]*. For adults, isoflurane has largely replaced halothane and enflurane as the inhalation anesthetic of choice because it offers rapid induction and emergence and has little post-anesthetic organ toxicity. Isoflurane is a better muscle relaxant than either halothane or enflurane. Isoflurane decreases, rather than increases, peripheral vascular resistance, resulting in a fall in arterial blood pressure.

7. The answer is D *[II C 4, D]*. Local anes-thetic toxicity (e.g., lidocaine toxicity) can pro-duce myocardial depression (a negative inotropic effect). In addition, lidocaine toxicity can cause convulsions, followed by a central nervous system (CNS) depression that results in respiratory depression, reduced oxygen lev-els, and hypotension.

8. The answer is B *[III A 6 c (2), (7)]*. The inhalation anesthetic described in the question is nitrous oxide. Leukopenia, not leukocytosis, has been reported with chronic nitrous oxide abuse. Because of its high partial pressure in blood and its low blood:gas partition coeffi-cient, nitrous oxide diffuses into air-containing body cavities and can increase the pressure or expand the volume of gas in air pockets, resulting in distention of the bowel, rupture of a tympanic membrane in an occluded middle ear, rupture of a pulmonary cyst, and pneumo-cephalus.

9. The answer is C *[III B 1]*. Neuroleptanalge-sia is produced when a neuroleptic agent is combined with a powerful narcotic. The agents most commonly used are droperidol (a butyrophenone) and fentanyl (an opioid). When nitrous oxide and oxygen are added after neuroleptanalgesia is achieved, neuro-leptanesthesia results. Droperidol and fentanyl can both cause hypotension, not hypertension;

however, use of these agents for neurolept-analgesia generally has little effect on the cardiovascular system. Confusion and mental depression are the most common complaints. Neuroleptanalgesia is used chiefly for diagnostic procedures (e.g., endoscopy) and minor surgical procedures.

10–13. The answers are: 10-A *[III B 2]*, **11-C** *[III B 1]*, **12-B** *[III A 2]*, **13-D** *[III B 3]*. Dissociative anesthesia, such as that caused by ketamine, produces rapid analgesia and amnesia while maintaining laryngeal reflexes.

Neuroleptanesthesia is induced by combining a powerful narcotic analgesic (fentanyl) with a neuroleptic agent (droperidol) together with the inhalation of nitrous oxide and oxygen.

Inhalation anesthesia, such as that induced by halothane, diffuses across the alveolus and depresses the central nervous system (CNS). Intravenous anesthetics (e.g., thiopental) are mostly used for induction of anesthesia before the administration of more potent anesthetic agents.

14–17. The answers are: 14-E *[II C 3 c (1)]*, **15-A** *[II C 1; Table 4-1]*, **16-C** *[II C 2 b (2)]*, **17-B** *[II C 4 d]*. Tetracaine, a commonly used

spinal anesthetic, is ten times more potent and toxic than procaine.

Cocaine has excellent topical local anesthetic properties and has been used extensively for nasotracheal intubations; however, its significant abuse potential limits its use.

The metabolic product of procaine hydrolysis is para-aminobenzoic acid (PABA), which inhibits the action of sulfonamides.

The major clinical uses of lidocaine are as a local anesthetic and intravenously as an antiarrhythmic agent.

18–20. The answers are 18-D *[III A 5 a (1)]*, **19-C** *[III A 2 c (1)]*, **20-A** *[III A 6 b (1)–(2)]*. Desflurane is a recently approved inhalation anesthetic that has the lowest blood:gas partition coefficient of all the inhalation anesthetics, resulting in rapid induction.

Halothane is not irritating to the larynx and thus induction is smooth and bronchospasm uncommon. It produces bronchiolar dilation.

Nitrous oxide is an important and powerful analgesic that is used as a supplement to more potent anesthetic agents.

Chapter 5

Cardiovascular Agents

I. DRUGS USED IN THE TREATMENT OF CONGESTIVE HEART FAILURE (CHF)

A. Introduction

1. **Definition.** CHF is defined as the inability of the heart to meet the metabolic requirements of the peripheral systems.

2. **Pathophysiology**
   a. **Myocardial cell loss** resulting from regional ischemia or myopathy leads to deterioration of systolic and diastolic performance.
   b. When confronted by an increased load, the remaining normal heart hypertrophies to maintain adequate cardiac performance.
      (1) **Hypertrophy** results in a fall in stroke volume index and a rise in left ventricular filling pressure.
      (2) Peripheral vascular resistance increases and **pulmonary congestion** develops.
   c. Vasoconstrictor compensatory mechanisms develop to maintain cerebral and coronary perfusion. These include:
      (1) Stimulation of the sympathetic nervous system
      (2) Stimulation of the renin–angiotensin system

3. **Symptoms.** Major symptoms include weakness, fatigue, and dyspnea.

B. Cardiac glycosides

1. **Chemistry**
   a. Cardiac glycosides are the combination of an aglycone, or genin, and one to four sugars.
      (1) The **aglycone** is chemically similar to bile acids and to steroids, such as adrenocortical and sex hormones. It is the pharmacologically active portion of the glycosides.
      (2) The **sugars** modify the water- and lipid-solubility of the glycoside molecule and, thus, affect its potency and duration of action.
   b. Glycosides are obtained from dried leaves of the foxglove, *Digitalis purpurea* (digitoxin) or *Digitalis lanata* (digitoxin, digoxin), and from the seeds of *Strophanthus gratus* (ouabain). The term **digitalis** is frequently used to refer to the entire group of cardiac glycosides.

2. **Pharmacokinetics** (Table 5-1)
   a. **Digoxin** is the most commonly used digitalis glycoside.
      (1) The bioavailability varies widely for different proprietary preparations of digoxin; intestinal absorption of the drug may be as low as 40%.
      (2) The serum half-life is normally about 36 hours but is significantly prolonged by impaired renal function.
      (3) Digoxin is not metabolized and is eliminated principally by the kidneys in almost unchanged form.
   b. **Digitoxin**
      (1) Digitoxin is well absorbed (90%–100%) from the gastrointestinal tract and does not have the variable bioavailability seen with digoxin.

TABLE 5-1. Pharmacokinetics of Commonly Used Cardiac Glycoside Preparations

Drug	Gastrointestinal Absorption	Protein Binding	Serum Half-life ($t_{1/2}$)	Principal Metabolic Route	Serum Concentration (ng/ml)
Digoxin	Approx. 75%	< 30%	36 hours	Kidney	Therapeutic: 0.5–2.5 Toxic: > 2
Digitoxin	90%–100%	97%	5–7 days	Liver	Therapeutic: 10–35 Toxic: > 35

    (2) The serum half-life of digitoxin is 5–7 days.
    (3) Digitoxin is metabolized by the liver, and drugs that increase the activity of hepatic microsomal enzymes, such as phenobarbital and phenytoin, accelerate its metabolism.
    (4) In contrast to digoxin, digitoxin is approximately 97% bound to plasma albumin.

  3. Pharmacologic effects
    a. General considerations
      (1) The most important property of cardiac glycosides is their **positive inotropic effect,** that is, their ability to increase the force of myocardial contraction. The result is increased cardiac work at reduced metabolic cost.
      (2) Glycosides also have effects on the **electrophysiologic properties** of the heart (conductivity, refractory period, automaticity).
      (3) In addition, glycosides have **extracardiac effects** on vascular smooth muscle, neural tissue, and other tissues.
      (4) Factors that influence the effects of cardiac glycosides on the heart include:
        (a) The dose of the agent (see I B 5)
        (b) The interaction of direct cardiac effects with reflex changes in the autonomic and hormonal regulation of cardiovascular function
        (c) The underlying cardiovascular pathophysiology
    b. Effects of cardiac glycosides on the heart (Table 5-2)
      (1) Myocardial contractility
        (a) Cardiac glycosides **increase the contractility of cardiac muscle** by increasing both the velocity of muscle contraction and the maximum force that is developed. Cardiac glycosides do not prolong the duration of the contraction and they do not directly affect myocardial contractile proteins or alter cellular mechanisms that provide energy for contraction. However, digitalis may interfere with Ca^{2+} binding to the sarcoplasmic reticulum, making more Ca^{2+} available for interaction with contractile proteins. Cardiac glycosides appear to exert their positive inotropic effect by **two mechanisms:**
          (i) Digitalis inhibits membrane-bound Na^+,K^+-activated adenosine triphosphatase (Na^+,K^+-ATPase) thus increasing intracellular Ca^{2+} levels.
          (ii) The movement of Ca^{2+} into the cell causes an increase in the slow inward Ca^{2+} current during the action potential.
        (b) In CHF patients, glycosides increase cardiac output, decrease cardiac filling pressures, decrease heart size, and decrease venous and capillary pressures, which is reflected by a downward shift in the ventricular curve.
      (2) Myocardial oxygen consumption
        (a) The digitalis-induced increase in myocardial contractility causes an increase in myocardial oxygen consumption.
        (b) Decreased ventricular volume, resulting from the digitalis-induced increase in muscle tone and cardiac output, decreases the myocardial oxygen consumption.

TABLE 5-2. Effects of Cardiac Glycosides on the Heart

Effects	Atria	A-V Node	Ventricles
Direct			
Contractility	↑	→	↑
ERP*	↑	↑	↓
Conduction velocity†	↓	↓	→
Automaticity‡	→	→	↑
Indirect§			
ERP	↓	↑	→
Conduction velocity	↑	↓	→
Effects on electrocardiogram	P changes	PR ↑	QT ↓ T and ST depressed
Adverse effects	Extrasystole Tachycardia	A-V depression or block	Fibrillation Extrasystole Tachycardia

A-V = atrioventricular; ERP = effective refractory period; ↑ = increased; ↓ = decreased; → = no change.
*Defined as the period during which no normal action potential can be elicited.
†Defined as the speed at which an impulse is propagated.
‡Defined as the ability of a cardiac cell to reach threshold potential and generate impulses spontaneously.
§Mediated primarily through the vagus.

- **(3) Electrophysiologic activity**
    - **(a)** The electrophysiologic effects of cardiac glycosides vary in different parts of the heart (see Table 5-2).
    - **(b)** Cardiac glycosides indirectly increase the vagal tone of the heart. They prolong the refractory period of the atrioventricular (A-V) node and decrease conduction velocity (both directly and indirectly) through the A-V node.
- **(4) Heart rate.** In normal individuals, digitalis has little effect on the heart rate.
    - **(a)** In **CHF patients,** digitalis slows the heart rate (a **negative chronotropic effect**). This results from vagal nerve stimulation, which slows pacemaker activity at the sinoatrial (S-A) node.
    - **(b) Excessive doses** of digitalis can produce **tachycardia**.
- **c. Extracardiac effects**
    - **(1)** When cardiac glycosides increase the cardiac output **in CHF patients, there is a drop in peripheral vascular resistance and venomotor tone as well as an increase in blood flow**. In normal individuals, digitalis produces venous and arterial constriction.
    - **(2)** Because digitalis increases the stroke volume **in CHF patients, systolic blood pressure may rise**.
    - **(3) Diastolic pressure may fall** because of improved circulation, increased tissue oxygenation, and diminished reflex vasoconstriction.
    - **(4)** A **diuretic effect** occurs because the increased cardiac output and renal blood flow combine to reduce the neurohumoral factors that inhibit the excretion of salt and water.
- **4. Therapeutic uses and contraindications**
    - **a.** Cardiac glycosides are of greatest value for treating **low-output cardiac failure**.
    - **b.** They are also of great value in the **control of atrial fibrillation and flutter** because of the ability to reduce the ventricular rate by prolonging the refractory period of conduction tissue. Digitalis may convert atrial flutter to atrial fibrillation.
    - **c. Paroxysmal atrial tachycardia** frequently responds to digitalis therapy, presumably as a result of reflex vagal stimulation.

d. The use of cardiac glycosides is **contraindicated** in **cardiac tamponade, high-output CHF, constrictive pericarditis,** and **idiopathic hypertrophic subaortic stenosis** with outlet obstruction.

5. Digitalization and maintenance dosage
  a. General considerations
    (1) Because digitalis glycosides are used almost exclusively either to restore adequate circulation in patients with CHF or to slow ventricular rate in patients with atrial fibrillation or flutter, **long-term therapy is frequently necessary** to maintain therapeutic myocardial concentrations.
    (2) The **low margin of safety** (see I B 6) increases the critical nature of dosage and administration.
  b. Digoxin
    (1) When there is no urgency, an **oral digitalizing dose** is first administered, and then the maintenance dose is adjusted on the basis of clinical and laboratory assessment. Usually, a steady-state level is achieved in 5 half-lives (about 8 days).
    (2) When digitalization must be achieved rapidly, digoxin can be administered intravenously over a period of several minutes. The onset of action is within 5–30 minutes; the maximal effect is reached within 1–5 hours.
  c. Digitoxin
    (1) The total **oral loading (digitalizing) dose** of digitoxin is divided into doses given every 6 hours and administered over the course of 36–48 hours.
    (2) The maximal effect of a dose of digitoxin is reached approximately 9 hours after oral administration.
    (3) Once optimal benefit has been achieved, the maintenance dose usually is adjusted to 10% of the digitalizing dose.
    (4) Although digitoxin is available for intravenous administration, its long latency period precludes its use in emergency situations.

6. Adverse effects. Digitalis glycosides have a **low margin of safety,** and intoxication from an excess of the drug is a common and potentially fatal problem.
  a. In most CHF patients, the lethal dose of a digitalis glycoside is likely to be only 5–10 times the minimal effective dose.
  b. The **therapeutic:toxic ratio** does not vary from one glycoside to another, and the only difference among the drugs lies in the **duration of toxicity**.
  c. Intoxication is most frequently **precipitated by the depletion of serum K^+** caused by diuretic therapy, but it can also occur from **accumulation of maintenance glycoside doses** taken over a long period of time. Intoxication from hypokalemia may also occur as a result of prolonged administration of corticosteroids, protracted vomiting, and protracted diarrhea.
  d. Decreased renal function and hypothyroidism predispose patients to digitalis glycoside toxicity because they reduce the excretion or the metabolism of the glycoside. Hence, excessive glycoside accumulates.
  e. When the concentrations of digoxin and digitoxin rise above 2 ng/ml and 35 ng/ml of blood, respectively, **signs of systemic toxicity** often appear, and therapy must be discontinued. Signs of toxicity include:
    (1) Anorexia (often the earliest sign)
    (2) Nausea, vomiting, and diarrhea
    (3) Headache, fatigue, malaise, neuralgias, and delirium
    (4) Vision changes, including abnormal color perception
    (5) Gynecomastia (rare)
    (6) Cardiac effects
      (a) Premature ventricular contractions (PVCs) and ventricular tachycardia and fibrillation
      (b) A-V dissociation and block
      (c) Sinus arrhythmia and S-A block
      (d) Paroxysmal and nonparoxysmal atrial tachycardia, often with A-V block

7. Treatment of digitalis toxicity
 a. Cardiac glycosides and K+-depleting diuretics are discontinued.
 b. KCl is administered orally or by slow, careful intravenous infusion if hypokalemia is present; K+ is **not** given, however, if there is severe A-V block or if serum K+ levels are high.
 c. Because hypomagnesemia may accompany hypokalemia, magnesium replacement may also be necessary.
 d. Phenytoin can be given for ventricular and atrial arrhythmias.
 e. Lidocaine and procainamide can be used to treat ventricular tachyarrhythmias.
 f. Propranolol can be used for ventricular and supraventricular tachycardia but **not** in the presence of A-V block.
 g. Atropine can be used to control sinus bradycardia and various degrees of A-V block.
 h. Cholestyramine binds to cardiac glycosides and has been used to hasten their elimination.
 i. A digoxin-specific antibody fragment from immunized sheep is available for the treatment of life-threatening digoxin or digitoxin overdosage. Its use is reserved for patients exhibiting shock or cardiac arrest, ventricular arrhythmias, progressive bradyarrhythmias, or severe hyperkalemia.
 j. Electrical conversion is often hazardous in the treatment of digitalis-induced arrhythmias because it can precipitate ventricular fibrillation.

C. Angiotensin-converting enzyme (ACE) inhibitors (see IV I 1; Chapter 8 V C 2)

1. Chemistry, mechanism of action, and pharmacokinetics (see IV I)

2. Pharmacologic effects
 a. ACE inhibitors (e.g., captopril, enalapril, lisinopril) produce beneficial hemodynamic effects by decreasing the conversion of angiotensin I to angiotensin II. They also inhibit the degradation of bradykinin.
 b. Hemodynamically, these agents increase cardiac output by reducing afterload and by decreasing total peripheral resistance, pulmonary resistance, and preload.

3. Therapeutic uses
 a. Initially, ACE inhibitors were used in patients not responding adequately to digitalis and diuretics. Today, ACE inhibitors are used as first-line agents for CHF therapy.
 b. Adding an ACE inhibitor to therapy with diuretics and digitalis has increased the survival rate among patients with mild to severe CHF.
 c. After myocardial infarction, ACE inhibitors may lessen the progressive enlargement of the left ventricle.

4. Adverse effects
 a. Severe persistent cough occasionally occurs.
 b. Hypotension and deterioration of renal function can occur with an ACE inhibitor–diuretic combination.
 c. Hypokalemia and ventricular arrhythmias occur in CHF patients given an ACE inhibitor combined with a diuretic, although less frequently than in those treated with digoxin.
 d. Adverse effects associated with captopril, such as rash, taste disturbances, proteinuria, and leukopenia, may be related to the sulfhydryl moiety of captopril.

D. Other drugs

1. Diuretic therapy (see Chapter 6) **and Na+ restriction** play an important role in reducing extracellular fluid volume. Diuretics relieve symptoms of heart failure more rapidly than any other oral agent and, along with digoxin, are first-line drugs in the treatment of CHF.

2. α-Adrenergic blocking agents (see Chapter 2 III A) may be used in CHF to improve cardiac function by inducing vasodilation through both direct and reflex actions.

3. **Other vasodilators** (see III) may be used for patients not responding to digitalis glyco-sides and diuretics.
   a. **Arteriolar dilators** decrease afterload, whereas **venous vasodilators** reduce preload. The decrease in preload and afterload increases cardiac output while reducing pulmonary congestion.
   b. **Isosorbide dinitrate, hydralazine,** and **prazosin** (see III A; IV E 2, F 2) have all been used in the treatment of CHF. Isosorbide improves cardiac function, but it has not been shown to improve survival rates when used alone. Increased survival rates have been demonstrated with isosorbide and hydralazine used together.

4. **Amrinone** is a bipyridine derivative that inhibits phosphodiesterase type III. It is reserved for the short-term therapy of CHF that is refractory to other agents.
   a. **Pharmacologic effects.** Amrinone exerts a positive inotropic effect and increases systemic vasodilation.
   b. **Route of administration.** This agent is administered intravenously.
   c. **Adverse effects**
      (1) A dose-related thrombocytopenia may occur.
      (2) Amrinone may increase the ventricular rate in patients with atrial flutter or fibrillation.

II. DRUGS USED IN THE TREATMENT OF ARRHYTHMIA

A. General considerations

1. **Cardiac arrhythmias** are abnormalities in the rate, regularity, or site of origin of the cardiac impulse, or a disturbance in conduction of the impulse such that the normal sequence of activation of atria and ventricles is altered.
   a. Arrhythmias may result from:
      (1) Faulty impulse initiation
      (2) Faulty impulse conduction
      (3) Combinations of the above
   b. The change in the impulse upsets the normal relationship between the duration of the refractory period and the conduction velocity in myocardial tissue. Changes in the normal relationship between refractoriness and conduction velocity may be critical, because of the heterogeneity of electrophysiologic and mechanical properties of the heart.

2. **Cardiac electrophysiology**
   a. **Action potential phases** (Table 5-3)
   b. **Automaticity.** In cardiac cells, the resting potential depolarizes during phase 4 until a threshold potential is reached and an action potential is initiated. **Abnormalities in cardiac rhythms** arise from **alterations in the site of normal automaticity** and **abnormal generation of impulses**. Inhibition of automaticity may also result from a **decreased threshold potential** or **decreased excitability of pacemaker cells**.
      (1) In humans, the **S-A node** is the **normal pacemaker** because it has the steepest slope of phase 4 and the most rapid firing rate. However, **specialized atrial conduction fibers, distal cells of the A-V node,** and **His–Purkinje fibers** are **latent pacemakers**.
      (2) Most antiarrhythmic agents have more effect on latent pacemakers than on the S-A node pacemaker.
   c. **Conduction velocity and effective refractory period (ERP).** Depolarization of the membrane is associated with a decrease in conduction velocity.
      (1) Conduction velocity is a function of:
         (a) The maximum rate ($\dot{V}_{max}$) of depolarization of phase 0

TABLE 5-3. Cardiac Action Potential

Phase		Event	Ionic Current
	0	Rapid depolarization	Na^+ enters cell
	1	Rapid repolarization	K^+ briefly leaves cell
	2	Sustained depolariza-tion (plateau)	Ca^+ enters cell
	3	Rapid repolarization	K^+ leaves cell
	4	Slow depolarization (diastole)	Gradual increase in Na^+ permeability

        (b) The threshold potential
        (c) The resting membrane potential
    (2) In areas of injured myocardium, conduction may be slow, or refractoriness short-ened, or both, resulting in the **reentry of aberrant impulses** and, hence, a car-diac arrhythmia.

3. Classes of antiarrhythmic drugs (Table 5-4)

B. | **Class IA antiarrhythmic agents**

1. Quinidine
  a. Chemistry. Quinidine, an alkaloid isolated from cinchona bark, is the d-isomer of quinine.
  b. Pharmacokinetics
    (1) Quinidine, as the sulfate or gluconate, is well absorbed after oral administration. It exerts a maximum effect within 1–2 hours after administration by this route.
    (2) Quinidine is given intramuscularly as the gluconate.
    (3) Approximately 80% of the drug is bound to plasma albumin.
    (4) Quinidine is metabolized in the liver and excreted by the kidneys.
  c. Pharmacologic effects
    (1) Effects on the heart (Table 5-5). At high concentrations, quinidine has direct effects on most cells of the heart. At lower concentrations, indirect (anticholin-ergic) effects may significantly contribute to the overall action of quinidine on the heart.
      (a) Responsiveness, conduction, and refractoriness. Quinidine is believed to block Na^+ channels. The major effect of quinidine is to reduce the V_{max} of depolarization during phase 0 at all transmembrane voltages in atrial, ventric-ular, and Purkinje fibers. Thus, conduction velocity decreases and ERP increases in all of these tissues.
      (b) Automaticity is decreased in ventricular tissue by depression of the slope of phase 4. Quinidine has little effect on automaticity of the sinus node.
      (c) Electrocardiographic effects (Table 5-6)
        (i) Because quinidine depresses conduction in the bundle of His and Purkinje fibers, it produces progressive prolongation of the QRS complex.
        (ii) Prolongation of the QT interval and alterations in T waves are related to delayed repolarization.
        (iii) Prolongation of the PR interval is caused by the direct effect of the drug on A-V conduction and the refractoriness of the A-V system.
    (2) Extracardiac effects. Quinidine can depress vascular smooth muscle tone, in part by α-receptor blockade. This may contribute to a reduction in peripheral vascular resistance.
  d. Therapeutic uses (Table 5-7)
    (1) Supraventricular arrhythmias

TABLE 5-4. Antiarrhythmic Agents

Class		Major Electrophysiologic Properties	Specific Agents	Major Side Effects
Sodium channel blockers	IA	Inhibit rapid inward current Prolong repolarization	Quinidine	Proarrhythmia Diarrhea
			Procainamide	Proarrhythmia Lupus-like syndrome
			Disopyramide	Proarrhythmia CHF Anticholinergic effects
	IB	Inhibit rapid inward current Accelerate repolarization	Lidocaine	CNS effects
			Tocainide	Proarrhythmia CNS effects Neutropenia
			Mexiletine	CNS effects
			Phenytoin	CNS effects
	IC	Inhibit rapid inward current Little effect on repolarization	Flecainide	CHF Proarrhythmia
			Moricizine	Proarrhythmia
Beta blockers	II	Accelerate repolarization	Propranolol	Bradycardia
	II	Reduce ischemia Reduce sympathetic arrhythmogenicity		Bronchospasm CHF
			Acebutolol	CHF
			Esmolol	Hypotension, brady-arrhythmias
			Sotalol	Proarrhythmic effects, CHF, hypotension
	III	Delay repolarization Lengthen phase 2	Amiodarone	Pulmonary fibrosis Hypo- and hyper-thyroidism
			Bretylium	Orthostatic hypotension
			Sotalol	Proarrhythmic effects, CHF, hypotension
Calcium channel blockers	IV	Depress slow inward current	Verapamil (atrial arrhyth-mias)	Bradycardia CHF

Adapted with permission from *NMS Medicine,* 2e. Baltimore, Williams & Wilkins, 1994, p 12.
CHF = congestive heart failure; CNS = central nervous system.

    (a) Quinidine is primarily used chronically and prophylactically to prevent recurrences of paroxysmal supraventricular tachycardia due to A-V nodal reciprocating tachycardia or to Wolff-Parkinson-White syndrome.

    (b) Quinidine can also be used to convert atrial flutter or fibrillation to normal sinus rhythm, but direct-current cardioversion is the procedure of choice for this problem. Quinidine is more frequently used to prevent recurrence of atrial flutter or fibrillation.

    (c) Quinidine should not be used without prior digitalization because its vagolytic action may increase the frequency of impulse transmission across the A-V node.

  (2) Ventricular arrhythmias. Quinidine is very useful for long-term treatment of ventricular premature depolarization or to prevent recurrences of ventricular tachycardia after cardioversion of this arrhythmia.

e. Route of administration

  (1) Quinidine is usually given orally three or four times a day.

TABLE 5-5. Effects of Antiarrhythmic Drugs on Electrophysiologic Properties of the Heart

	Automaticity		Effective Refractory Period		Membrane Responsiveness (Purkinje Fibers)
Drug	Sinus Node	Purkinje Fibers	A-V Node	Purkinje Fibers	
Quinidine Procainamide Amiodarone Disopyramide	→	↓	↑→↓	↓	↓
Lidocaine Phenytoin Tocainide Mexiletine	→	↓	↑→↓	↓	↓
Propranolol	↓	↓	↑	↑	↓
Esmolol	↓	↓	↑	↑	↓
Acebutolol	↓	↓	↑	↑	↓
Bretylium	↑↓	↑↓	↓→↑	↑	→
Verapamil	↓	→↓	↑	→	→

Arrows indicate changes: ↑ = increased; ↓ = decreased; → = no change.

(2) For intravenous use, the dose must be diluted in glucose solution and injected slowly, and the patient's electrocardiogram must be carefully monitored.

f. Adverse effects

(1) Cardiotoxicity includes A-V block, ventricular tachyarrhythmias, and depression of myocardial contractility.

    (a) A 50% increase in the QRS complex indicates the need for a prompt reduction in dosage.

    (b) Ventricular arrhythmias are life-threatening, and if the therapist can distinguish this adverse effect of quinidine from the underlying disease,

TABLE 5-6. Major Effects of Antiarrhythmic Drugs on Electrocardiogram

Drug	QRS	QT	PR*
Quinidine Procainamide Amiodarone	↑	↑	→↑
Disopyramide	↑	↑	→
Lidocaine Phenytoin Tocainide Mexiletine	→	↓	→↑↓
Flecainide	↑	↑	↑
Verapamil	→	→	↑
Adenosine	→	→	↑
Digoxin	Depresses ST	Flattens T	↑
Propranolol	→	↓	→↑
Sotalol	→	↑	↑

Arrows indicate changes: ↑ = increased; ↓ = decreased; → = no change.
*PR intervals: All antiarrhythmic drugs have a variable response, usually with little observable effect. However, lidocaine hardly ever affects the PR interval, while phenytoin and propranolol usually increase the PR interval.

TABLE 5-7. Uses of Antiarrhythmic Drugs in Common Cardiac Arrhythmias

Arrhythmia	Treatment of Choice	Alternatives
I. Supraventricular		
Atrial fibrillation or flutter	Digitalis to control ventricular rate; direct-current shock for conversion	Verapamil or β blocker to slow ventricular response; quinidine to suppress recurrences after direct-current shock
Paroxysmal atrial or nodal tachycardia	Vagotonic maneuver; intravenous adenosine or verapamil for termination	Digoxin and β blockers may be useful, especially prophylactically
II. Ventricular		
Ventricular premature complexes	β Blockers for symptomatic patients	No evidence that prolonged suppression with procainamide, quinidine, or disopyramide prevents sudden cardiac death; after myocardial infarction, β blockers decrease mortality
Ventricular tachycardia	Direct-current shock, lidocaine	Procainamide, mexiletine, β blockers
III. Digitalis-induced	Lidocaine	Phenytoin, procainamide, β blockers
IV. Torsades de pointes	Magnesium	Cardiac pacing, isoproterenol

treatment (in addition to cessation of quinidine) may be either of the following:
  (i) Na+ lactate or NaHCO$_3$, catecholamines (see Chapter 2 II A) or glucagon
  (ii) Removal of quinidine by dialysis
  (c) "Quinidine syncope" caused by ventricular tachyarrhythmias of polymorphic form (**torsades de pointes**) can occur, especially in patients whose QT interval is prolonged by the drug.
  (d) Quinidine increases serum levels of digitalis and can lead to digitalis toxicity.
  (2) Diarrhea, vomiting, nausea, and anorexia are the most common side effects and, when severe, may force discontinuation of quinidine.
  (3) Quinidine can cause cinchonism. Mild symptoms of this condition include tinnitus, hearing loss, vomiting, and diarrhea; severe symptoms include headache, diplopia, photophobia, altered perception of color, confusion, and psychosis.

2. **Procainamide**
  a. **Chemistry.** Procainamide differs from procaine only in that it contains an amide structure rather than an ester linkage; this difference protects it from enzymatic hydrolysis and frees it from most of the central nervous system (CNS) effects of procaine.
  b. **Pharmacokinetics**
    (1) Procainamide may be administered orally, intravenously, or intramuscularly.
    (2) It is rapidly absorbed after oral administration and, when capsules are used, normally has a peak effect in about 1 hour. However, absorption of the drug from the gastrointestinal tract may be impaired immediately after an acute myocardial infarction.
    (3) The half-life of procainamide is approximately 3 hours.
    (4) Procainamide is eliminated by both hepatic metabolism and renal excretion, and renal failure can produce toxicity.
      (a) There is a marked variation among individuals in the rate of acetylation and excretion.
      (b) From 50%–60% of an administered dose is excreted unchanged in the urine.
  c. **Pharmacologic effects**
    (1) Effects on the heart (see Table 5-5)
      (a) The direct cardiac effects of procainamide are similar to those of quinidine.
      (b) Electrocardiographic effects are also similar to those of quinidine (see Table 5-6).

(2) Extracardiac effects
  (a) Procainamide, especially when given intravenously, can cause a drop in blood pressure, probably from peripheral vasodilation.
  (b) Unlike quinidine, procainamide does not have α-adrenergic blocking properties.
d. Therapeutic uses (see Table 5-7)
  (1) The clinical uses of procainamide are similar to those of quinidine. Patients may respond to one drug after failing to respond to the other.
  (2) Ventricular arrhythmias. Procainamide is particularly effective in promptly abolishing ventricular premature depolarizations and paroxysmal ventricular tachycardia.
  (3) Supraventricular arrhythmias. Procainamide is believed to be as effective as quinidine for the management of atrial arrhythmias; however, higher doses of procainamide than of quinidine may be necessary.
e. Route of administration
  (1) Procainamide may be given orally, both initially and for maintenance.
  (2) The intravenous dose, which is reserved for life-threatening situations, must be administered slowly. When the arrhythmia has been interrupted, infusion is stopped.
f. Adverse effects
  (1) Acute procainamide toxicity can cause ventricular arrhythmia, ventricular fibrillation, and cardiac depression (see II B 1 f).
  (2) Nausea, vomiting, diarrhea, and anorexia occur fairly frequently with oral administration of procainamide, but they occur much less commonly than with quinidine therapy.
  (3) Mental confusion and psychosis have been reported but occur less commonly than with the chemically similar compounds procaine and lidocaine.
  (4) Hypersensitivity reactions are much more common than with quinidine.
    (a) Fever, joint and muscle pain, and skin rashes can occur.
    (b) Fatal agranulocytosis has occurred.
    (c) A syndrome resembling systemic lupus erythematosus, which is reversible on discontinuation of procainamide, develops in as many as 30% of patients taking procainamide for long periods of time. As many as 70% of patients taking procainamide develop positive antinuclear antibody tests. The latter occurs more rapidly in slow acetylators.
  (5) Hypotension can result, especially after intravenous administration.
  (6) Procainamide can precipitate acute glaucoma and urinary retention.

3. Disopyramide
  a. Pharmacokinetics
    (1) Disopyramide is well absorbed (83%) after oral administration.
    (2) Approximately 50% of a dose of disopyramide is excreted in the urine in unchanged form. Disappearance from the plasma is a function of both renal and hepatic clearance.
    (3) The half-life of disopyramide in plasma is 5–7 hours but may be prolonged in patients with renal disease.
  b. Pharmacologic effects
    (1) Effects on the heart (see Table 5-5). Disopyramide has both direct and indirect actions on the heart, which resemble those of quinidine.
      (a) Responsiveness, conduction, and refractoriness
        (i) Disopyramide reduces membrane responsiveness, amplitude of the action potential, and excitability of atrial and ventricular muscle.
        (ii) Accordingly, conduction velocity is decreased and ERP is increased in these tissues.
        (iii) Unlike either quinidine or procainamide, disopyramide produces a greater reduction in the V_{max} of phase 0 depolarization at depressed membrane potentials than at normal resting membrane potentials.
      (b) Automaticity. Concentrations of disopyramide that do not affect conduction velocity or ERP can reduce automaticity in atrial and ventricular tissue.

   (c) Electrocardiographic changes are similar to but milder than those of quinidine and procainamide (see Table 5-6).

   (2) Extracardiac effects. Disopyramide has a mild atropine-like action. It is neither
   an α-receptor antagonist nor a β-receptor antagonist.

c. Therapeutic uses (see Table 5-7)

   (1) Disopyramide is approved in the United States for oral administration in the
   treatment of ventricular arrhythmias as an alternative to quinidine and
   procainamide.

   (2) It may be as effective as quinidine and procainamide against atrial arrhythmias,
   but it has not been approved for this use.

d. Adverse effects

   (1) Major untoward effects are related to the action of disopyramide on the heart
   and may include conduction disturbances, CHF, or hypotension. Disopyramide
   has a negative inotropic action that can be especially troublesome in patients
   with preexisting ventricular failure.

   (2) Other adverse effects relate to its anticholinergic action. These effects include
   dry mouth, constipation, blurred vision, and urinary retention. Consequently,
   patients with glaucoma or with conditions causing urinary retention should not
   take the drug.

C. | **Class IB antiarrhythmic agents**

1. Lidocaine

a. Chemistry. Lidocaine is an amide local anesthetic (see Chapter 4 II C 4).

b. Pharmacokinetics

   (1) Lidocaine is rapidly metabolized by the hepatic microsomal enzyme system
   with 70% of the amount that enters the liver being metabolized in a single pass
   (**first-pass metabolism**). Reductions in hepatic blood flow or function reduce
   lidocaine plasma clearance.

   (2) Oral administration of lidocaine results in a very low plasma concentration
   because of the high percentage of the drug that is removed by hepatic metabolism before reaching the general circulation.

   (3) Lidocaine has an elimination half-life of approximately 1½ hours.

c. Pharmacologic effects

   (1) Effects on the heart (see Table 5-5)

      (a) Automaticity. Lidocaine does not affect sinus nodal pacemaker discharge. It
      depresses the rate of phase 4 depolarization of Purkinje and atrial muscle
      fibers, depressing automaticity at these sites.

      (b) Responsiveness, conduction, and refractoriness

         (i) Lidocaine has little effect on these electrophysiologic properties of the
         atria.

         (ii) In the His–Purkinje system, lidocaine reduces action potential ampli-
         tude and membrane responsiveness.

         (iii) The V_{max} of phase 0 depolarization in normal Purkinje fibers is not as
         greatly depressed with lidocaine as it is with procainamide or quini-
         dine. However, the V_{max} of phase 0 is severely depressed in fibers with
         reduced resting membrane potentials and elevated extracellular K^+.

         (iv) Lidocaine decreases the action potential duration by blocking the Na^+
         channel in depolarized cells; it also shortens the ERP of Purkinje fibers.

      (c) Electrocardiographic effects. Unlike quinidine and procainamide, lidocaine
      produces few changes in the electrocardiogram (see Table 5-6).

   (2) Extracardiac effects. Lidocaine has little effect on autonomic tone.

d. Therapeutic uses (see Table 5-7). The use of lidocaine as an antiarrhythmic agent is
limited, even though lidocaine is effective in treating ventricular arrhythmias.
Because of its rapid onset and short duration of action, lidocaine is particularly useful in treating these arrhythmias when they arise in emergency situations, such as:

   (1) Open-heart surgery

(2) Digitalis intoxication

(3) Myocardial infarction

e. Route of administration. Lidocaine can be administered intravenously or intramuscularly.

(1) The usual intravenous dose is given until the arrhythmia is abolished.

(2) Lidocaine can also be given by continuous intravenous infusion. Because its half-life is short, a steady-state plasma concentration can be reached quickly by this method.

(3) Lidocaine may be given intramuscularly to achieve rapid plasma levels during emergencies.

f. Adverse effects

(1) CNS side effects of lidocaine can include drowsiness, paresthesias, decreased auditory function, convulsions, and respiratory arrest.

(2) Circulatory collapse can occur in patients with an acute myocardial infarction after a rapid, large intravenous injection.

(3) Propranolol or cimetidine can decrease the plasma clearance of lidocaine.

(4) The concurrent use of tocainide and lidocaine can cause seizures.

2. Mexiletine

a. Chemistry. Mexiletine is an orally active congener of lidocaine.

b. Pharmacokinetics

(1) Mexiletine is well absorbed when given orally.

(2) Unlike lidocaine, its first-pass metabolism is low.

(3) Its plasma elimination half-life is 10–12 hours.

(4) Mexiletine is metabolized in the liver. Only 10% is excreted unchanged in the urine.

c. Pharmacologic effects (see Table 5-5). The prominent effects of mexiletine on the heart are similar to the effects of lidocaine; and, like lidocaine, the electrocardiographic effects of mexiletine are minimal (see Table 5-6).

d. Therapeutic uses (see Table 5-7). Mexiletine is most useful in suppressing symptomatic ventricular arrhythmias.

e. Route of administration

(1) Mexiletine is given orally; administration with food and antacid is recommended.

(2) A minimum of 2–3 days between dose adjustments is recommended.

(3) Patients with liver disease may require lower doses.

f. Adverse effects

(1) In controlled trials, up to 40% of patients discontinued treatment because of gastrointestinal or neurologic adverse effects.

(2) Mexiletine may aggravate preexisting sinus node or intraventricular conduction defects.

(3) Hepatic enzyme inducers (e.g., phenobarbital) can lower mexiletine plasma levels.

3. Tocainide, a lidocaine analog, is also an amide local anesthetic. Unlike lidocaine, tocainide can be given orally.

a. Tocainide, like lidocaine, can suppress ventricular arrhythmias.

b. Tocainide shortens the action potential duration and the ERP.

c. Uncommonly, tocainide may aggravate ventricular arrhythmias.

d. Other side effects include gastrointestinal distress, CNS disturbances, and allergic reactions, most frequently a maculopapular rash.

4. Phenytoin (diphenylhydantoin) is closely related in structure to phenobarbital and is effective in treating epileptic seizures (see Chapter 3 III C 1). As an antiarrhythmic agent, phenytoin resembles lidocaine.

a. Pharmacokinetics

(1) Phenytoin is slowly and somewhat variably absorbed after oral administration.

(2) It is inactivated by microsomal enzymes in the liver, with considerable variability in this process among individuals.

(3) The plasma elimination half-life is prolonged with increasing doses and is about 17 hours for a single 300-mg dose.

b. Pharmacologic effects

(1) **Effects on the heart** (see Table 5-5)

(a) The prominent effects of phenytoin on the heart are similar to the effects of lidocaine.

(b) **Electrocardiographic effects** of phenytoin, like those of lidocaine, are minimal (see Table 5-6).

(2) **Extracardiac effects.** Phenytoin exerts a depressant action on the sympathetic centers in the CNS, which may contribute to its antiarrhythmic effects.

c. Therapeutic uses (see Table 5-7). Phenytoin is most useful in treating ventricular arrhythmias. It is particularly useful for ventricular arrhythmias associated with digitalis toxicity or acute myocardial infarction.

d. Route of administration

(1) Phenytoin is most often administered by intermittent intravenous injection, until either a therapeutic effect is achieved or a toxic effect results. (Intravenous administration is dangerous and should be undertaken only in severe acute arrhythmia and with continuous monitoring of the patient.)

(2) Orally, therapy is initiated with a loading dose, followed by maintenance oral therapy.

e. Adverse effects (see Chapter 3 III C 1 c)

(1) CNS side effects are the most common problems encountered with phenytoin and include nystagmus, vertigo, and loss of mental acuity.

(2) Large intravenous doses can alter hemodynamic function and produce both a fall in cardiac output and hypotension, resulting in death.

D. | **Class IC antiarrhythmic agents**

1. **Flecainide** and **moricizine** are indicated for use in patients with life-threatening arrhythmias, such as sustained ventricular tachycardia.

2. These agents are no longer indicated for less severe ventricular arrhythmias because they can precipitate cardiac arrest.

3. Both agents are administered orally.

E. | **Class II antiarrhythmic agents: β-adrenergic antagonists (β blockers)**

1. **Propranolol** is a β-adrenergic receptor blocking agent (see Chapter 2 III B 1). Its antiarrhythmic action and its uses in treating angina and hypertension are discussed in this chapter.

a. Pharmacokinetics. Propranolol is a nonselective β-adrenergic antagonist, blocking both β_1 and β_2 receptors (see Chapter 2 III B 1 b).

b. Pharmacologic effects

(1) **Effects on the heart** (see Table 5-5). The antiarrhythmic effects of propranolol result primarily from β-receptor blockade but also result from a direct membrane effect.

(a) **Automaticity.** Propranolol, by blocking β receptors in the S-A node and blocking sympathetic and hormonal influences on this structure, depresses S-A node firing and causes bradycardia. Automaticity is also depressed in Purkinje fibers.

(b) **Responsiveness and conduction velocity** are not greatly affected by propranolol.

(c) **Action potential duration and refractoriness.** The major effect of propranolol, which underlies its use as an antiarrhythmic agent, is that it causes a substantial increase in the ERP of the A-V node because of the β blockade. The refractoriness of the S-A node and of atrial and ventricular muscle is not greatly affected, whereas the ERP of Purkinje fibers is shortened substantially.

   (2) Electrocardiographic effects. Propranolol prolongs the PR interval by its action on the A-V node (see Table 5-6).

   (3) Hemodynamic effects are discussed in Chapter 2 III B 1.

  c. Route of administration

   (1) For intravenous administration, propranolol is given slowly, with additional doses usually given every 3–5 minutes.

   (2) Oral medication usually is begun with relatively small divided doses. The total amount may need to be increased significantly to produce a therapeutic effect.

  d. Therapeutic uses (see Table 5-7)

   (1) Propranolol is used to control supraventricular tachyarrhythmias, including atrial fibrillation, atrial flutter, and paroxysmal supraventricular tachycardia. By decreasing conduction through the A-V node, propranolol decreases the response of the ventricles to atrial flutter and fibrillation but does not usually convert these arrhythmias to sinus rhythm.

   (2) Propranolol is useful in ventricular arrhythmias that are caused by enhanced adrenergic stimulation (from emotional stress, exercise).

   (3) Propranolol is sometimes used to abolish ventricular arrhythmias caused by digitalis excess, but it can cause conduction problems in this context, resulting in A-V dissociation. Furthermore, propranolol, by itself, can depress myocardial contractility.

  e. Adverse effects

   (1) Because propranolol decreases sympathetic activity, it can produce severe hypotension, significantly worsen CHF, and cause cardiac arrest.

   (2) Because it impairs A-V conduction and depresses ventricular pacemaker activity, propranolol can produce asystole.

   (3) Propranolol can induce significant bronchospasm in asthmatic patients and can mask signs and symptoms of acute hypoglycemia.

   (4) Sudden withdrawal of the drug can produce angina, arrhythmias, and infarction.

 2. β_1-selective (cardioselective) adrenergic antagonists

  a. Acebutolol is a β_1-selective adrenergic receptor blocker with some sympathomimetic (adrenergic) activity.

   (1) Therapeutic uses. Acebutolol is used chiefly for controlling ventricular premature beats.

   (2) Adverse effects (see Chapter 2 III B 6)

  b. Esmolol is a cardioselective β-adrenergic blocking agent with a short duration of action.

   (1) Therapeutic uses. Esmolol is given by intravenous infusion to provide rapid control of supraventricular arrhythmias.

   (2) Adverse effects. Dose-related hypotension and bradyarrhythmias can occur.

F. | **Class II/III antiarrhythmic agent: sotalol**

 1. Pharmacokinetics. Sotalol is rapidly and completely absorbed from the gastrointestinal tract after oral administration and is eliminated in the urine. Its elimination half-life is 12 hours.

 2. Pharmacologic effects

  a. Sotalol **prolongs repolarization (a Class III effect)** and also has nonselective β-adrenergic-blocking activity (**a Class II effect**).

  b. Sotalol slows the heart rate and prolongs the QT interval.

 3. Therapeutic uses

  a. Sotalol is effective in preventing life-threatening ventricular arrhythmias.

  b. Sotalol may be useful for the treatment of supraventricular arrhythmias.

 4. Adverse effects. Sotalol is better tolerated than sodium-channel blocking drugs.

  a. Adverse effects of sotalol are similar to those of β blockers.

  b. Sotalol has a proarrhythmic effect, which can include torsades de pointes.

G. | **Class III antiarrhythmic agents**

1. **Bretylium**
   a. **Mechanism of action**
      (1) Bretylium, a quaternary ammonium salt, is an adrenergic neuronal blocking agent (see Chapter 2 III C 4). It accumulates in postganglionic adrenergic nerve terminals, where it initially stimulates norepinephrine release but then inhibits the release of norepinephrine in response to neuronal stimulation. Bretylium does not impair the postsynaptic response to exogenous catecholamines.
      (2) The drug also has direct electrophysiologic effects on the heart.
   b. **Pharmacokinetics**
      (1) Oral absorption of bretylium is poor; however, it is well absorbed after intramuscular administration.
      (2) Bretylium is excreted unchanged in the urine.
      (3) Its elimination half-life is approximately 6–10 hours.
   c. **Pharmacologic effects**
      (1) **Effects on the heart** (see Table 5-5)
         (a) **Automaticity.** Bretylium does not directly affect automaticity. It is one of the few antiarrhythmic agents that does not affect automaticity in His–Purkinje systems.
         (b) **Excitability and threshold.** Resting membrane potentials are not greatly affected in any cardiac cell. However, bretylium increases the ventricular fibrillation threshold.
         (c) **Responsiveness, conduction, and refractoriness.** In therapeutic doses, bretylium does not affect either responsiveness or conduction in cardiac tissue. Bretylium prolongs the duration of action potentials and the ERP of atrial and ventricular muscle and the A-V node.
      (2) **Electrocardiographic effects.** Bretylium decreases the sinus rate and increases the PR and QT intervals.
   d. **Route of administration.** Bretylium tosylate is for **short-term use only** and is administered with patients in the supine position.
      (1) For **intravenous use,** the drug usually is diluted and infused over 10–20 minutes. For immediately life-threatening arrhythmias, undiluted bretylium can be injected intravenously every 15–30 minutes.
      (2) For **intramuscular use,** undiluted bretylium is used.
   e. **Therapeutic uses.** Bretylium is reserved for life-threatening ventricular arrhythmias that are refractory to other therapy. Its use is confined to intensive care units.
   f. **Adverse effects**
      (1) Intravenous bretylium causes orthostatic hypotension and some degree of supine hypotension.
      (2) Nausea and vomiting can occur with rapid intravenous administration.

2. **Amiodarone** is an iodinated benzofuran derivative.
   a. **Pharmacokinetics.** Amiodarone is highly lipid-soluble; its half-life is 20–100 days.
   b. **Pharmacologic effects on the heart**
      (1) Amiodarone increases both the action potential duration and the ERP in ventricular and atrial muscle.
      (2) It increases the PR, QRS, and QT intervals.
      (3) It decreases S-A node automaticity.
      (4) It induces α- and β-adrenergic blockade by noncompetitive antagonism; therefore, it causes both systemic and coronary vasodilation.
   c. **Therapeutic use.** Amiodarone suppresses premature ventricular contractions and ventricular tachycardia. Its use is reserved for the treatment of life-threatening ventricular arrhythmias refractory to other treatment.
   d. **Adverse effects**
      (1) Pulmonary fibrosis, which is usually reversible, is caused by amiodarone therapy.
      (2) Cardiac effects, including sinus bradycardia, A-V block, and paradoxical ventricular arrhythmias (torsades de pointes), are results of amiodarone therapy.

(3) Photosensitivity can occur.

(4) Amiodarone causes corneal microdeposits and blurred vision.

(5) Amiodarone interferes with conversion of thyroxine (T_4) to triiodothyronine (T_3), causing hyperthyroidism or hypothyroidism.

(6) Amiodarone causes neurologic effects, such as ataxia, dizziness, tremor, peripheral neuropathy, and proximal myopathy.

(7) Anorexia, nausea, and vomiting occur.

(8) Serum levels of digitalis, diltiazem, quinidine, and procainamide are increased with amiodarone use.

H. | **Class IV antiarrhythmic agents: calcium (Ca^{2+})-channel blockers**

1. **Verapamil,** a Ca^{2+}-channel blocker (see III C), is the drug of choice for supraventricular tachycardia treated intravenously.

   a. Pharmacologic effects on the heart and therapeutic uses

   (1) Verapamil significantly depresses A-V nodal conduction.

       (a) It is, therefore, very effective in paroxysmal supraventricular tachycardia.

       (b) It is also used to reduce the ventricular response in atrial fibrillation or flutter.

   (2) It is less useful than other agents for ventricular arrhythmias.

   b. Adverse effects

   (1) Because of its effects on the A-V node, verapamil should not be used in patients with A-V nodal dysfunction.

   (2) Verapamil can depress myocardial contractility; therefore, care should be exercised when administering it to patients with CHF.

   (3) Verapamil is contraindicated in patients with atrial fibrillation who have Wolff-Parkinson-White syndrome.

2. Other Ca^{2+}-channel blockers (e.g., diltiazem) are not yet approved for use as antiarrhythmic agents.

III. | **DRUGS USED IN THE TREATMENT OF ANGINA AND OTHER VASODILATORS.** The nitrates, the β-adrenergic antagonists, and the Ca^{2+}-channel blockers are useful in treating the pain resulting from ischemic heart disease. They provide symptomatic treatment of angina pectoris but do not affect the course of the disorder. Several vasodilators that are not used in the treatment of angina are also discussed here.

A. | **Nitrates**

1. **Chemistry**

   a. The term **nitrates** is used in this chapter to encompass both **nitrites** (esters of nitrous acid) and **nitrates** (polyol esters of nitric acid).

   b. Glyceryl trinitrate (**nitroglycerin**) is the prototype of this group.

   c. **Nitroglycerin** and **amyl nitrite** are volatile liquids at room temperature. Other nitrates [**isosorbide dinitrate, isosorbide mononitrate** (the active metabolite of dinitrate) **pentaerythritol tetranitrate, erythrityl tetranitrate**] are solids.

2. **Mechanism of action**

   a. The nitrates relax all smooth muscle, including vascular smooth muscle. The proposed biochemical action involves the formation of free radical nitric oxide (NO), which stimulates guanylate cyclase. The resultant guanosine 3′,5′-monophosphate (cyclic GMP) activates a protein kinase, which mediates dephosphorylation of myosin. The formation of endothelial-derived relaxation factor (EDRF) is also a contributory action.

   b. Nitrates reduce venous tone, thereby increasing venous capacitance and decreasing venous return to the heart.

   c. Nitrates decrease peripheral arteriolar resistance.

3. **Pharmacokinetics**
   a. The nitrates are readily absorbed through the buccal mucous membranes, the skin, the gastrointestinal tract, and the lungs.
      (1) Sublingual administration produces rapid onset (2–5 minutes) and short duration of action (less than 30 minutes) and, thus, provides the best treatment for acute attacks of angina.
      (2) Oral preparations, which often come in a sustained-release form, can provide more prolonged prophylaxis against angina than sublingual forms.
   b. The nitrates are broken down in the liver by a glutathione-dependent organic nitrate reductase and are excreted as various nitrites and nitrates.

4. **Pharmacologic effects**
   a. **Effects on the heart**
      (1) The major effect of the nitrates on the heart is to reduce myocardial oxygen requirements relative to myocardial oxygen delivery.
         (a) The arterial dilation produced by nitrates causes a reduction in the mean systemic arterial pressure, which reduces the afterload of the heart and, thus, diminishes the oxygen requirements of the heart.
         (b) The venous dilation produced by nitrates results in increased peripheral pooling of blood, which decreases ventricular end-diastolic pressure and volume (decreased preload). This reduction in ventricular pressure and size results in a decreased myocardial wall tension and, therefore, in decreased oxygen requirements.
         (c) In addition, the decrease in left ventricular end-diastolic pressure reduces tissue pressure around subendocardial vessels, favoring the redistribution of coronary blood flow to this area.
      (2) Nitrates are believed to dilate the large epicardial and collateral coronary arteries selectively, an action that favors the distribution of blood to ischemic areas. (They do **not** increase the total coronary blood flow in patients with atherosclerosis.)
   b. **Extracardiac effects**
      (1) Vasodilation of cerebral vessels produced by nitrates results in increased intracerebral pressure and sometimes in headache.
      (2) The nitrates dilate vessels in the skin, resulting in flushing.
      (3) They relax bronchial and biliary tract smooth muscle with the latter action resulting in a reduction of biliary pressure.

5. **Route of administration**
   a. Nitroglycerin is usually given **sublingually**. However, for long-lasting effects, nitroglycerin may be administered either orally or topically (**transdermally**) via ointment or patch.
      (1) Transdermal nitroglycerin patches become ineffective if they are left in place for 24 hours and reapplied daily, even if the dosage is increased.
      (2) Nitroglycerin patches delivering 10 mg or more remain effective if removed for 12 hours daily.
   b. Nitroglycerin may also be given intravenously in medical emergencies.
   c. Nitroglycerin tablets quickly lose potency when stored in contact with cotton, paper, or plastic and should be kept in a dark glass container.

6. **Therapeutic uses**
   a. The primary use of nitrates is to treat acute attacks of angina pectoris and, in anticipation of attacks, to prevent their occurrence. Patients with frequent angina require a second drug, such as a β blocker or Ca^{2+}-channel blocker.
   b. Paroxysmal nocturnal dyspnea can be relieved with nitroglycerin by improving left ventricular pressure and reducing pulmonary pressure.

7. **Adverse effects**
   a. Headache is a common early side effect of nitrates that usually decreases after the first few days of treatment (i.e., patients usually develop a tolerance to headache).

(1) Temporarily discontinuing the drugs for a few days causes a recurrence of susceptibility to headache (as well as to the direct vascular effect of the drugs) when the nitrates are readministered.

(2) Decreasing the dose of nitrates is sometimes beneficial for headache.

b. Dizziness, weakness, and cerebral ischemia associated with postural hypotension occasionally occur.

c. Nitrite ions, when present in large amounts, can oxidize enough hemoglobin to methemoglobin to result in hypoxia.

d. Death can occur with acute nitrate poisoning from circulatory collapse or respiratory failure.

8. **Tolerance.** When nitrates are appropriately administered intermittently, tolerance does not occur (see III A 5 a).

B. Propranolol

1. **Mechanism of action**
   a. The β-adrenergic blocking action of propranolol (see Chapter 2 III B 1) decreases sympathetic stimulation of the heart and, thus, reduces the heart rate, especially during exercise, and decreases myocardial contractility. These effects, in turn, decrease the oxygen requirements of the myocardium, both during exercise and at rest.
   b. Propranolol may also decrease arterial pressure.

2. **Route of administration.** Propranolol is usually administered orally for the treatment of angina.

3. **Therapeutic uses**
   a. Propranolol is used prophylactically to decrease the severity and frequency of anginal attacks.
   b. Propranolol can be administered concomitantly with nitroglycerin, in which case it reduces the amount of nitroglycerin needed to control angina. Although no data conclusively show a synergistic effect of these drugs, the two drugs tend to counteract each other's nontherapeutic effects; for example, the ability of nitroglycerin to reduce ventricular end-diastolic pressure mitigates the tendency of propranolol to increase end-diastolic pressure.
   c. Propranolol should not be used for Prinzmetal's (variant) angina, which is caused by coronary vasospasm.

4. **Adverse effects**
   a. Propranolol can worsen CHF and can precipitate bronchospasm in patients with bronchial asthma (see II E 1 e).
   b. Bradycardia and hypotension can occur.
   c. Renal plasma flow and glomerular filtration rate may be reduced.

C. Ca^{2+}-Channel blockers selectively inhibit Ca^{2+} influx into heart muscle (i.e., they block the slow inward channel for Ca^{2+}) and inhibit Ca^{2+} influx into vascular smooth muscle. They do not change the serum Ca^{2+} concentration.

1. **Classification**
   a. Nifedipine, nicardipine, and amlodipine are **dihydropyridines**.
   b. Verapamil
   c. Diltiazem

2. **Pharmacokinetics**
   a. Verapamil, diltiazem, nifedipine, and nicardipine are rapidly and almost fully absorbed after oral administration. Amlodipine is slowly absorbed.
   b. **Peak blood levels**
      (1) Nifedipine: 30 minutes
      (2) Diltiazem: 1 hour
      (3) Verapamil: 1–2 hours

(4) Nicardipine: 8–9 hours

(5) Amlodipine: 6–12 hours

   c. All five drugs are highly bound by serum proteins.

   d. Verapamil undergoes extensive first-pass biotransformation in the liver. All five drugs are excreted as metabolites in the urine.

3. Pharmacologic effects

   a. Cardiovascular effects. By their inhibition of Ca^{2+} influx into myocardial and vascular smooth muscle cells, Ca^{2+}-channel blockers have diverse effects on the cardiovascular system.

      (1) Verapamil and diltiazem are more likely than the dihydropyridines to suppress cardiac contractility and slow cardiac conduction.

      (2) The dihydropyridines are more potent vasodilators than verapamil and diltiazem.

   b. Extracardiac effects. Verapamil produces nonspecific sympathetic antagonism and has a local anesthetic effect.

4. Route of administration. Ca^{2+}-channel blockers may be given orally; for use in medical emergencies, verapamil is also available in intravenous form.

5. Therapeutic uses

   a. Use in angina. Ca^{2+}-channel blockers are useful in the treatment of both Prinzmetal's angina and classic exertional angina. Nifedipine appears to be the most effective for Prinzmetal's angina.

   b. Other uses

      (1) Verapamil, diltiazem, nicardipine, and amlodipine have been approved for use in **hypertension** (see IV D).

      (2) Verapamil is used to treat certain cardiac **arrhythmias** (see II H 1).

      (3) The Ca^{2+}-channel blockers are being studied for their value in migraine treatment.

6. Adverse effects

   a. The Ca^{2+}-channel blockers, perhaps especially when used in combination with β-adrenergic blocking agents, can produce or aggravate the following:

      (1) Hypotension

      (2) A-V block

      (3) CHF

      (4) Asystole

   b. Most of the adverse effects are mild; dizziness and peripheral edema are among the more common adverse effects.

   c. Treatment with verapamil increases serum levels of digitalis during the first week of therapy and, thus, can cause digitalis toxicity.

   d. Nicardipine can produce a negative effect on cardiac contractility when administered intravenously to patients with CHF.

   e. Unlike other dihydropyridines, amlodipine does not cause reflex tachycardia.

D. | **Other vasodilators**

1. Nylidrin

   a. Nylidrin is an **adrenergic vasodilator**. It acts primarily on the vascular bed of skeletal muscle by β-receptor stimulation.

   b. Because it is a cardiac stimulant, nylidrin is **contraindicated in progressive angina pectoris, acute myocardial infarction,** and **paroxysmal tachycardia**.

   c. The efficacy of nylidrin in increasing the blood supply in vasospastic disorders has not been proven.

2. Dipyridamole

   a. By inhibiting the uptake of adenosine into erythrocytes and other tissues, dipyridamole allows metabolically released adenosine, which is a coronary vasodilator, to accumulate in the plasma. The drug decreases coronary vascular resistance and increases coronary blood flow and coronary sinus oxygen saturation. (Dipyridamole also inhibits in vitro platelet aggregation and can be used to prevent the formation of thromboemboli in patients with prosthetic cardiac valves.)

    b. Dipyridamole has not been proven to be superior to placebo treatment for angina; it does not prevent the appearance of electrocardiographic signs of myocardial ischemia during exercise tolerance tests.

IV. DRUGS USED IN THE TREATMENT OF HYPERTENSION

A. **General considerations**

    1. Because the cause of essential hypertension is still unknown, drug therapy for this condition is empiric and often rather nonspecific. Inadequate treatment of hypertension can result in significant complications (Table 5-8).

    2. Traditionally, the first choice for the **initial treatment of chronic hypertension** has been a thiazide-type diuretic or a β-adrenergic receptor blocker. Some physicians prefer to start therapy with an ACE inhibitor or a Ca^{2+}-channel blocker. If the first agent is ineffective or poorly tolerated, another agent is substituted. If more than one agent is needed, a diuretic is added (Table 5-9).

    3. In **hypertensive emergencies,** parenteral therapy is indicated, usually with nitroprusside or diazoxide; intravenous labetalol or sublingual nifedipine is also suitable. Oral therapy should be started as soon as possible because parenteral therapy is not suitable for long-term management of hypertension.

B. **Diuretic agents** (see Chapter 6) are useful antihypertensive drugs when employed alone, as well as when used in combination therapy, in which they potentiate the action of other hypotensive drugs. Although the exact mechanism of their antihypertensive action is unknown, it is believed to result from their ability to produce a negative Na^+ balance.

    1. The **thiazides** are the most frequently used diuretics. Their early hypotensive effect is related to a reduction in blood volume; their long-term effect is related to a reduction in peripheral vascular resistance. Metolazone and indapamide may be effective in patients with impaired renal function.

    2. **Loop diuretics** produce greater diuresis than the thiazides, but they have a weaker antihypertensive effect and can cause severe electrolyte imbalance. Because they retain their effectiveness in the presence of impaired renal function, they are useful when renal function is so impaired that the thiazides can no longer promote sodium excretion.

    3. **Potassium-sparing diuretics** have modest hypotensive and diuretic effects and are useful in combination with a thiazide diuretic, whose effects they potentiate and where they minimize K^+ loss. Spironolactone is useful in treating patients whose hypertension results from mineralocorticoid excess (see Chapter 6 IX B).

C. **β-Adrenergic blocking agents** have become increasingly important as antihypertensive agents. They are discussed in Chapter 2 III B.

    1. These agents are useful both alone and in combination antihypertensive therapy. As a first-line course of therapy, β blockers are generally less effective than thiazides in black and elderly patients.

TABLE 5-8. Blood Pressure–Related Complications

Left ventricular hypertrophy	Strokes
Congestive heart failure	Dissecting aortic aneurysm
Transient ischemic attacks	Chronic renal failure

TABLE 5-9. Classes of Antihypertensive Medications

Class	Specific Agents
Diuretics	
Thiazide	Hydrochlorothiazide, chlorthalidone
Loop	Furosemide, ethacrynic acid, bumetanide
Potassium-sparing	Spironolactone, triamterene, amiloride
β Blockers	
Nonselective	Propranolol, timolol, nadolol, pindolol*, penbutolol*, carteolol*
Cardioselective	Metoprolol, acebutolol*, atenolol
Ca^{2+}-Channel blockers	
Dihydropyridines	Amlodipine, felodipine, isradipine, nifedipine, nicardipine
Other	Verapamil, diltiazem
Vasodilators	
Arteriolar (direct)	Hydralazine, minoxidil, diazoxide
Nonselective	Nitroprusside
α Blockers	Prazosin, terazosin
Centrally acting	Clonidine, methyldopa, guanabenz, guanfacine
Peripherally acting	Reserpine, guanethidine, guanadrel
ACE inhibitors	Captopril, enalapril, lisinopril, benazepril, fosinopril, quinapril, ramipril

ACE = angiotensin-converting enzyme.
*Possess intrinsic sympathomimetic activity as well. These drugs decrease blood pressure with less of a decrease in cardiac output or heart rate at rest. They are also unlikely to cause serum lipid abnormalities.

2. Their mechanism of action in hypertension is not known, but several consequences of β-adrenergic blockade probably play a role. For example:
   a. The β blockers reduce cardiac output.
   b. They also inhibit renin secretion.

3. **Sympathetic selectivity.** The various β blockers all appear to be equally effective for the treatment of hypertension. However, they vary in their selectivity for adrenoreceptors (see Chapter 2 III B).
   a. Cardioselective β blockers have a greater effect on $β_1$ adrenoreceptors than non-selective β blockers.
   b. Labetalol is a nonselective β blocker but possesses intrinsic sympathomimetic activity and blocks vascular postsynaptic α-adrenergic receptors.

4. **Adverse effects** (see Chapter 2 III B)
   a. The β-adrenergic receptor antagonists can exacerbate CHF, asthma, and chronic obstructive pulmonary disease.
   b. They can mask symptoms of hypoglycemia in individuals with diabetes mellitus.
   c. They can increase serum triglycerides and decrease high-density lipoprotein (HDL) cholesterol (Table 5-10).
   d. Labetalol, when used chronically, causes more frequent orthostatic hypotension and sexual dysfunction than do other β blockers.
   e. Patients taking β blockers who have allergic conditions may develop more serious anaphylactic reactions to allergens.

D. **Ca^{2+}-Channel blockers** (see III C) are rapidly becoming important antihypertensive agents by virtue of their vasodilating effects. Unlike β blockers, Ca^{2+}-channel blockers do not affect serum lipid concentrations or cause sexual dysfunction. Diuretics may enhance the efficacy of Ca^{2+}-channel blockers.

1. **Mechanism of action.** Amlodipine, diltiazem, verapamil, felodipine, isradipine, nifedipine, and nicardipine increase vasodilation and decrease peripheral resistance.

TABLE 5-10. Effects of β and α Antagonists on Serum Lipids

	LDL	HDL	Trig	Lipoprotein Lipase	LCAT
β Blockers	↑	↓	↑↑	↓	↓
α Blockers	↓	↑↑	→	↑	↑

LDL = low-density lipoprotein; HDL = high-density lipoprotein; Trig = triglycerides; LCAT = lecithin:cholesterol acyltransferase; ↑ = increased; ↓ = decreased;
→ = no change.

2. **Pharmacologic effects**
   a. Verapamil, amlodipine, and diltiazem cause little change in heart rate, whereas
   the dehydropyridines produce an initial increase, which is reflex-mediated.
   b. Diltiazem and verapamil depress A-V conduction and should not be used with
   β blockers.

3. **Adverse effects.** Verapamil can cause severe constipation.

E. **Arteriolar (direct) vasodilators**

1. **General considerations.** This group of antihypertensive drugs **directly relaxes arteriolar
   smooth muscle** and, thus, decreases peripheral vascular resistance and arterial blood
   pressure.
   a. The beneficial effect of these drugs on peripheral vascular resistance can be partially
   negated by the increased reflex sympathetic activity they produce, which can result
   in increased heart rate, stroke volume, and cardiac output.
   b. These drugs also can increase plasma renin activity as a result of increased reflex
   sympathetic discharge, causing a **pressor effect**.
   c. Finally, this group of drugs often causes salt and water retention and, thus, expansion
   of the extracellular fluid and plasma volume. Therefore, arteriolar vasodilators
   should be **used in conjunction with diuretic and β-adrenergic blocking therapy**.

2. **Hydralazine.** This phthalazine derivative has a greater effect on arterioles than on veins
   (which minimizes the incidence of postural hypotension). It may reduce diastolic more
   than systolic blood pressure.
   a. **Pharmacokinetics**
      (1) Hydralazine is well absorbed orally.
      (2) It is subject to extensive first-pass hepatic metabolism after oral administration.
      (3) It is extensively metabolized by several pathways, including acetylation, the rate
      of which is subject to genetic variation among individuals.
      (4) Its duration of effect ranges from 2–6 hours.
      (5) Tolerance develops after 24 months of therapy.
   b. **Therapeutic uses**
      (1) Hydralazine is used to treat **moderate to severe hypertension**.
      (2) It has also been used in the treatment of acute and chronic **CHF**.
   c. **Route of administration.** Hydralazine can be given orally or intramuscularly. For
   long-term treatment, hydralazine is administered orally.
      (1) Oral hydralazine is combined with a β blocker to prevent tachycardia and
      increased renin secretion resulting from reflex sympathetic stimulation.
      (2) Oral hydralazine is combined with a diuretic agent to prevent salt and water
      retention.
   d. **Adverse effects**
      (1) Headache, anorexia, nausea, dizziness, and sweating occur frequently but tend
      to diminish as hydralazine is administered over a period of time.
      (2) Hydralazine can worsen coronary artery disease because of the myocardial stim-
      ulation it produces.

(3) Hydralazine can cause a reversible lupus-like syndrome, especially when more than 400 mg/d are administered to slow acetylators of the drug (usually white patients).

3. **Minoxidil**
   a. **Pharmacokinetics**
      (1) Minoxidil is at least 90% absorbed after oral administration.
      (2) Approximately 90% of the drug is excreted as metabolites in the urine.
      (3) Although the plasma half-life averages approximately 4 hours, the duration of action may be significantly longer, because it is affected by hepatic blood flow and function.
   b. **Pharmacologic effects**
      (1) Minoxidil, a piperidinopyrimidine derivative, directly relaxes arteriolar smooth muscle.
      (2) It decreases peripheral vascular resistance more than hydralazine does.
      (3) It decreases renal vascular resistance while preserving renal blood flow and the glomerular filtration rate.
   c. **Therapeutic uses**
      (1) Minoxidil is indicated for the treatment of **severe hypertension** that does not respond adequately to more conventional antihypertensive therapy.
      (2) It may be particularly useful for **severe hypertension coupled with renal functional impairment**.
   d. **Route of administration.** Minoxidil is administered orally in single or divided doses. Like hydralazine, minoxidil should be used in combination with a β-adrenergic blocking agent and a diuretic to avert increased sympathetic activity and salt and water retention.
   e. **Adverse effects**
      (1) Like hydralazine, minoxidil can produce side effects related to increased reflex sympathetic stimulation and to salt and water retention.
      (2) Pericardial effusion and tamponade can occur, especially in patients with inadequate renal function.
      (3) Hirsutism occurs for unknown reasons; it is not associated with virilism or other endocrine abnormalities.

4. **Diazoxide** is chemically similar to the thiazide diuretics, but it causes salt and water retention rather than diuresis.
   a. **Pharmacokinetics**
      (1) Diazoxide is used as an antihypertensive drug in intravenous form only.
      (2) It has a rapid onset of action (3–5 minutes), and a given amount injected quickly produces a greater antihypertensive effect than the same amount injected slowly.
      (3) The plasma half-life averages 28 hours, but the antihypertensive effects usually last only 4–12 hours.
   b. **Pharmacologic effects**
      (1) Diazoxide exerts its vasodilator effect principally on arterioles and has little effect on capacitance vessels.
      (2) It causes a fall in both systolic and diastolic pressure, accompanied by an increase in both heart rate and cardiac output.
      (3) The drug relaxes other smooth muscle in addition to vascular muscle.
      (4) It inhibits the release of insulin.
   c. **Therapeutic uses.** Intravenous diazoxide is one of two major drugs used for **hypertensive emergencies** (see IV F 1 c). (Diazoxide is also used **orally to treat hypoglycemia** that is caused by hyperinsulinemia.)
   d. **Route of administration.** Diazoxide is given by rapid injection into a peripheral vein. Administration is started with a bolus dose, which can be repeated at 5–15-minute intervals until the desired effect on blood pressure is attained.
   e. **Adverse effects**
      (1) Diazoxide can cause severe hypotension.

(2) Its reflex sympathetic stimulation can cause angina and worsen myocardial ischemia.

(3) Diazoxide inhibits the release of insulin from the pancreas and can produce hyperglycemia.

(4) It can produce edema that is caused by significant retention of salt and water.

F. **Arterial and venous vasodilators.** These drugs reduce both arterial resistance and venous tone and markedly decrease arterial blood pressure.

1. **Sodium nitroprusside**
   a. **Pharmacokinetics**
      (1) Onset of action occurs within 1 minute of intravenous administration, and effects cease within 5 minutes of stopping an infusion.
      (2) The drug is rapidly inactivated by hepatic enzymes, first to cyanide and then to thiocyanate.
   b. **Pharmacologic effects**
      (1) Nitroprusside acts directly on arterial and venous smooth muscle but has little effect on other smooth muscle.
      (2) It decreases blood pressure in both the supine and upright positions.
      (3) The increased venous capacitance that it produces results in decreased cardiac preload and, thus, decreases myocardial oxygen demand for a given output.
      (4) Renal blood flow is maintained with nitroprusside, and renin secretion is increased.
   c. **Therapeutic uses**
      (1) Nitroprusside, like diazoxide, is used for short-term, rapid reduction of blood pressure in **hypertensive emergencies**. It is preferable to diazoxide for treating hypertensive emergencies in patients with coronary insufficiency or pulmonary edema because, in contrast to diazoxide, it reduces cardiac preload (by increasing venous capacitance) and, thus, myocardial oxygen demand.
      (2) Nitroprusside can also be used to produce controlled hypotension to **minimize bleeding** during surgery.
      (3) Nitroprusside **can improve left ventricular function** (lower ventricular filling pressure) in patients with acute myocardial infarction and has beneficial hemodynamic effects in the **treatment of acute CHF**.
   d. **Route of administration**
      (1) Na^+ nitroprusside is administered only as an intravenous infusion with sterile 5% dextrose in water. Once prepared, the solution must be protected from light and used within 4 hours.
      (2) Blood pressure must be monitored continuously while the drug is being given.
   e. **Adverse effects**
      (1) Hypotension, nausea, diaphoresis, headache, restlessness, palpitations, and retrosternal pain can occur secondary to excessive, rapid vasodilation.
      (2) The rate of conversion of nitroprusside from its metabolite cyanide to thiocyanate depends on the availability of sulfur (usually as thiosulfate). Rarely, when high doses of nitroprusside are administered for a prolonged period and sulfur stores are low, cyanide toxicity can occur.
      (3) Because thiocyanate is cleared slowly by the kidneys, it can accumulate during prolonged nitroprusside therapy, especially in patients with poor renal function. A plasma thiocyanate, concentration of greater than 10 mg/dl can cause weakness, nausea, muscle spasms, and psychosis, as well as hypothyroidism caused by interference with iodine transport.

2. **Prazosin.** This quinazoline derivative is a selective postsynaptic α_1-adrenergic receptor blocking agent that causes vasodilation of both the arteries and veins.
   a. **Pharmacokinetics**
      (1) Its plasma concentration peaks in about 3 hours. Plasma half-life is usually 2–3 hours but can be prolonged by CHF.
      (2) Prazosin is extensively metabolized, may undergo significant first-pass metabolism, has a bioavailability of about 60%, and is probably excreted in the feces and bile.

b. Pharmacologic effects

(1) Prazosin reduces peripheral vascular resistance and lowers arterial blood pressure in both supine and erect patients.

(2) Unlike nonselective α-adrenergic blockers, prazosin does not usually produce reflex tachycardia.

(3) Unlike β blockers, prazosin does not adversely affect insulin sensitivity or blood lipids (see Table 5-10).

(4) It does not increase plasma renin activity.

(5) Prazosin seems to produce minimal changes in cardiac output, renal blood flow, and glomerular filtration rate.

c. Therapeutic uses

(1) Prazosin is used to treat **mild to moderate hypertension**. It may be more effective in conjunction with a diuretic or an α-adrenergic blocking agent than when used alone.

(2) It is also used in the treatment of acute **CHF**.

d. Route of administration. Prazosin is given orally, two or three times daily.

e. Adverse effects

(1) Dizziness, headache, drowsiness, and palpitations can occur but often disappear with continued therapy and rarely cause discontinuation of the drug.

(2) The initial dose of prazosin, especially if larger than 1 mg, can induce postural hypotension and syncope, probably as a result of decreased venous return to the heart. It is, therefore, best to give the initial dose at bedtime.

(3) Tests for antinuclear factor may become positive with prazosin therapy.

3. **Terazosin** has a longer half-life (12 hours) and longer duration of action (24 hours) than does prazosin but is otherwise similar to prazosin. Terazosin is used to treat **benign prostatic hyperplasia** as well as **hypertension**.

a. Mechanism of action. Terazosin is a postsynaptic α-adrenoreceptor blocker that rapidly relaxes smooth muscle tone in the arteries, bladder neck, prostate capsule, and prostatic urethra.

b. Pharmacokinetics

(1) **Absorption.** Terazosin is rapidly and completely absorbed from the gastrointestinal tract. Food delays, but does not decrease, absorption.

(2) **Fate.** Terazosin is metabolized in the liver.

(3) **Excretion.** Terazosin is excreted mainly in bile and partially in urine.

c. Therapeutic uses

(1) Terazosin rapidly improves urine flow and decreases symptoms of obstruction in **benign prostatic hyperplasia**.

(2) It is used to treat **hypertension**.

d. Adverse effects

(1) **Orthostatic hypotension** and **syncope** may occur, especially with the first dose. Bedtime administration is recommended.

(2) Other adverse effects associated with α-adrenergic blockers may occur, including nasal congestion and impotence.

G. | **Centrally acting sympatholytic agents**

1. **Clonidine, guanabenz,** and **guanfacine** act centrally on the vasomotor centers of the brain predominantly by stimulating **α₂-adrenergic receptors**. The result is decreased sympathetic outflow from the CNS.

a. Pharmacokinetics

(1) The antihypertensive effects of clonidine and guanabenz develop within 30–60 minutes of oral administration, peak in 2–4 hours, and last for approximately 8 hours; therefore, they require twice-daily administration.

(2) Guanfacine has a longer half-life, permitting once-daily dosing.

b. Pharmacologic effects

(1) α₂-Adrenergic agonists lower arterial pressure and reduce secretion of renin.

(2) **Clonidine and guanabenz** tend to decrease cardiac output and leave peripheral vascular resistance unchanged.

(3) **Guanfacine** has little effect on cardiac output and decreases peripheral vascular resistance.

c. **Therapeutic uses**

(1) **Clonidine** can be used to treat **mild hypertension or moderate to severe hypertension**.

    (a) It can be used as a single agent or in combination with other antihypertensive agents.

    (b) It cannot be administered to patients taking tricyclic antidepressants because these drugs block clonidine's hypotensive effect. Clonidine may worsen depression.

(2) **Guanabenz** is similar to clonidine in effectiveness and adverse effects.

(3) **Guanfacine** lowers blood pressure without affecting cardiac output.

d. **Route of administration**

(1) **Clonidine**

    (a) **Clonidine** is often administered orally in two unequal doses with the larger one given at bedtime to minimize problems resulting from its sedative effects.

    (b) Clonidine is also available as a transdermal patch, which is applied once weekly.

(2) **Guanabenz** is administered orally in two equal doses.

(3) **Guanfacine** is administered orally once daily.

(4) **Concomitant diuretic administration** is often recommended, because of the retention of sodium and water that can occur with α_2-adrenergic agonists.

e. **Adverse effects**

(1) Dry mouth, drowsiness, and sedation are the most frequent problems and may require discontinuation of clonidine or guanabenz.

(2) Rebound hypertensive crises can result from abrupt cessation of clonidine tablets or patches when the drug is used as a single agent. Rebound hypertension is seen less frequently after the abrupt discontinuation of guanfacine therapy.

2. **Methyldopa**

a. **Mechanism of action**

(1) Methyldopa is an effective inhibitor of dopa decarboxylase and was initially thought to act as an antihypertensive agent by decreasing stores of norepinephrine in the sympathetic nervous system. However, its primary mode of action is via a central effect.

(2) Methyldopa is metabolized by decarboxylation and β-hydroxylation in adrenergic neurons of the CNS. The metabolite, α-methylnorepinephrine, stimulates α-adrenergic receptors in the brain, inhibiting sympathetic outflow. This effect on the CNS is believed to be the principal mechanism by which methyldopa exerts its antihypertensive effect.

(3) Methyldopa reduces renal vascular resistance, possibly as a result of an α-methylnorepinephrine being a weaker vasoconstrictor than norepinephrine in renal beds, and is thought to exert other direct actions on peripheral adrenergic neurons that contribute to its antihypertensive effect.

b. **Pharmacokinetics**

(1) Methyldopa is poorly absorbed (< 25%) after oral administration and may be subject to first-pass intestinal metabolism.

(2) Its peak effect is exerted 4–6 hours after administration, and its effect may last up to 24 hours.

(3) Methyldopa is excreted largely by the kidneys.

c. **Pharmacologic effects**

(1) Methyldopa decreases blood pressure and peripheral arteriolar resistance.

(2) It has little effect on cardiac output, renal blood flow, or glomerular filtration rate.

(3) It does not abolish sympathetic reflexes.

    d. Therapeutic uses. Methyldopa is used orally to treat mild or moderate to severe hypertension, usually in combination with a diuretic. Adverse effects limit its usefulness.

    e. Route of administration. Methyldopa is given orally or by slow intravenous infusion.

    f. Adverse effects

      (1) Sedation is common and, although it may decrease with continued administration of methyldopa, mental acuity may remain decreased.

      (2) Methyldopa can produce "drug fever" that mimics sepsis, with chills and high fever. Febrile episodes may be accompanied by alterations in liver function, which on rare occasions terminate in hepatic necrosis.

      (3) A positive direct Coombs' test develops in as many as 25% of patients taking methyldopa for more than 6 months. Hemolytic anemia, usually reversible on discontinuation of the drug, occurs in a small percentage of these patients.

      (4) Edema caused by salt and water retention can develop if a diuretic is not administered.

      (5) Rebound hypertension can follow the sudden withdrawal of methyldopa but occurs less frequently than with clonidine.

      (6) Orthostatic hypotension occurs more frequently than with clonidine but less frequently than with guanethidine.

      (7) Lactation can occur in either sex, and impotence can occur in some men.

H. **Agents that block postganglionic adrenergic neurons** (see Chapter 2 III C). This group of drugs selectively inhibits sympathetic neuron function through interference with chemical mediation at ganglionic nerve endings; one or more mechanisms may be involved.

  1. Reserpine

    a. Mechanism of action

      (1) Reserpine, a rauwolfia alkaloid, depletes catecholamine and serotonin stores in the peripheral and central nervous systems and causes impaired sympathetic nerve discharge (see Chapter 2 III C 1).

        (a) It interferes with intracellular storage of catecholamines by inhibiting the binding of norepinephrine to neurosecretory vesicles at the vesicle membrane, both centrally and peripherally.

        (b) Norepinephrine that diffuses from the storage site is degraded intracellularly by monoamine oxidase (MAO).

      (2) Reserpine decreases the synthesis of norepinephrine and increases its turnover rate.

    b. Pharmacokinetics

      (1) With oral administration, reserpine usually takes several days to several weeks to reach a maximum effect.

      (2) Hydrolysis of the ester linkage and demethylation are likely mechanisms for breaking down reserpine.

      (3) Reserpine is concentrated in tissues with a high lipid content.

    c. Pharmacologic effects

      (1) Reserpine decreases blood pressure, usually decreases heart rate and cardiac output, and may decrease peripheral vascular resistance.

      (2) In usual therapeutic doses, reserpine only partially inhibits cardiovascular reflexes.

      (3) Reserpine exerts central actions that produce sedation.

    d. Therapeutic uses. Reserpine is used principally in low oral doses in combination with other antihypertensive agents (e.g., a thiazide diuretic and vasodilator) to control **moderate hypertension**.

    e. Route of administration. Reserpine is usually given orally but is also available for parenteral administration.

    f. Adverse effects

      (1) Reserpine regularly causes sedation and can cause episodes of severe depression, which probably result from a reduction of biogenic amine levels in subcortical areas of the brain. Reserpine, therefore, should not be administered to patients prone to depression.

(2) Because reserpine decreases sympathetic activity, unopposed parasympathetic activity can result in bradycardia, nasal congestion, and increased gastrointestinal activity. It is contraindicated for patients with active peptic ulcers.

2. Guanethidine
  a. Mechanism of action
  (1) Guanethidine acts presynaptically to inhibit the release of neurotransmitter from peripheral adrenergic neurons, thus reducing the response to sympathetic nerve activation. Acutely, it produces sympathetic blockade before any appreciable decrease in norepinephrine stores has occurred; with chronic administration, it impairs the release of neurotransmitter from peripheral adrenergic neurons (see Chapter 2 III C 2).
    (a) For guanethidine to exert an antihypertensive effect, it must be taken up and stored in adrenergic nerve terminals in a manner similar to norepinephrine uptake.
    (b) Agents that prevent this uptake, such as cocaine and tricyclic antidepressants, inhibit the therapeutic effect of guanethidine.
  (2) Unlike reserpine, guanethidine can inhibit the pressor action of indirect-acting amines such as tyramine.
  (3) As with reserpine, the norepinephrine released by guanethidine is deaminated intraneuronally by MAO but to a lesser degree than with reserpine.
  (4) Although guanethidine displaces norepinephrine from storage granules and is subsequently released as a "false" neurotransmitter in response to stimulation of sympathetic nerves, this does not seem to be a primary mechanism of action.
  (5) The drug does not cross the blood–brain barrier like reserpine, and thus, it does not affect serotonin and norepinephrine stores in the CNS.
  (6) It is believed to decrease plasma renin activity.
  b. Pharmacokinetics
  (1) Absorption of guanethidine after oral administration varies among patients and is low (3%–30%).
  (2) The drug has a long duration of action.
  (3) Guanethidine is thought to be metabolized by hepatic enzymes and is excreted with its metabolites in the urine.
  c. Pharmacologic effects
  (1) Initially, guanethidine displaces and releases enough unchanged norepinephrine to cause mild, transient hypertension and cardiac stimulation.
  (2) Hypotension and bradycardia follow. Because guanethidine depresses vasoconstrictor reflexes, blood pressure is reduced significantly more when the patient is erect than when lying down. Venous return and cardiac output are decreased.
  (3) Guanethidine has a direct inhibitory effect on skeletal muscle contraction.
  (4) It increases the sensitivity of tissues to catecholamines.
  d. Therapeutic uses. Guanethidine is used in the treatment of **moderate to severe hypertension,** usually in combination with a thiazide diuretic or a diuretic and a vasodilator.
  e. Route of administration. Guanethidine is given orally. The dose can be increased at intervals of not less than 5 days until either the desired effect is attained or untoward effects develop.
  f. Adverse effects
  (1) Significant orthostatic hypotension and syncope frequently occur, especially during exercise, when patients first arise in the morning, during hot weather, and when patients ingest alcohol.
  (2) Salt and water retention occur but can be prevented or treated with a mild diuretic.
  (3) Gastrointestinal hyperactivity occurs, probably as a result of the parasympathetic predominance that follows sympathetic blockade.
  (4) Muscular aching and weakness can occur.

3. Guanadrel (see Chapter 2 III C 3) is similar to guanethidine but has a much shorter duration of action.

I. **Drugs that interfere with the renin–angiotensin system** (see Chapter 8 V C). The kidneys synthesize renin, which acts on a plasma globulin substrate to produce angiotensin I. This, in turn, is converted (by a peptidyl dipeptidase) to angiotensin II, a potent vasoconstrictor. Drugs in this exert an antihypertensive effect by interfering with either the formation or the utilization of angiotensin II.

1. **ACE inhibitors** include **captopril, enalapril, lisinopril, benazepril, fosinopril, quinapril,** and **ramipril** (see Chapter 8 V C 2).
   a. **Chemistry**
      (1) Enalapril is a prodrug that is hydrolyzed in the liver to the active compound enalaprilate. It differs structurally from captopril in that it lacks a sulfhydryl group.
      (2) Lisinopril is the lysine analog of enalaprilate.
      (3) Benazepril, fosinopril, ramipril, and quinapril, like enalapril, are prodrugs that are converted to active forms in the gut and liver. All lack the sulfhydryl group of captopril.
   b. **Mechanism of action**
      (1) ACE inhibitors are specific competitive inhibitors of peptidyl dipeptidase, the enzyme that converts angiotensin I to angiotensin II.
         (a) Angiotensin II is a potent direct vasoconstrictor. Thus, the drugs inhibit vaso-constriction.
         (b) Angiotensin II stimulates the secretion of aldosterone, which promotes salt and water retention. Thus, the drugs inhibit salt and water retention and slightly increase serum K^+ levels.
      (2) Because peptidyl dipeptidase is necessary to catalyze the degradation of bradykinin, the ACE inhibitors may increase the concentration of bradykinin, which is a potent vasodilator.
      (3) The ACE inhibitors also exert an antihypertensive effect in low-renin hyperten-sion; the mechanism of action in this case is not explained.
   c. **Pharmacokinetics**
      (1) **Captopril** is rapidly absorbed after oral administration and reaches peak blood levels within 1 hour. Approximately 95% of a dose is eliminated by the kidneys within 24 hours.
      (2) **Enalapril** is more potent than captopril, and its duration of action is more than 24 hours, twice as long as that of captopril. Because of its hepatic conversion and activation, enalapril does not reach clinically active levels for 2–4 hours, but it has a half-life of 11 hours.
      (3) **Lisinopril** is absorbed more slowly than enalapril and has a slower onset of action.
      (4) **Benazepril** and **ramipril** are excreted in urine and may require dosage adjust-ment when renal function is impaired.
      (5) **Fosinopril** is excreted in the bile in urine and does not require dosage adjust-ment in patients with impaired renal function.
      (6) **Quinapril** is a prodrug that is rapidly converted to its active form in the small intestine and liver.
   d. **Pharmacologic effects.** The cardiovascular effects of ACE inhibitors include a reduc-tion in total peripheral resistance and mean arterial blood pressure, and either no change or an increase in cardiac output.
   e. **Route of administration**
      (1) **Captopril** is given orally, 1 hour before meals. The initial dose can be increased at 1- to 2-week intervals.
      (2) **Enalapril, benazepril, fosinopril, quinapril,** and **ramipril** are given orally once or twice a day.
      (3) **Lisinopril** is given orally once a day.
   f. **Therapeutic uses**
      (1) **ACE inhibitors** are increasingly used for the treatment of **mild to moderate hypertension** because they are without the side effects associated with adrener-gic blockers.
         (a) ACE inhibitors are effective for low-renin, as well as high-renin, hypertension.

       (b) They are effective when used alone but are often administered with a thiazide diuretic, in which case the antihypertensive effects appear to be additive. An ACE inhibitor can also be given with a β blocker, but in this case, the antihypertensive effect appears to be less than additive.

    (2) ACE inhibitors also relieve chronic CHF and afterload.

    (3) These agents may be less effective than a diuretic for hypertension in black patients.

  g. Adverse effects

    (1) Proteinuria can occur, especially in patients with compromised renal function. Monitoring of urinary protein levels is recommended.

    (2) ACE inhibitors are contraindicated in patients with bilateral renal artery stenosis because acute renal failure may ensue.

    (3) Hypotension has followed the first dose of ACE inhibitors in Na^+-depleted patients.

    (4) Dry cough is common and bronchospasm may occur.

    (5) Neutropenia can occur; and, in patients who have impaired renal function or serious autoimmune disease (e.g., systemic lupus erythematosus), captopril should be used with caution. Neutropenia is rare with enalapril or lisinopril.

    (6) Approximately 10% of patients treated with captopril develop reversible skin rashes, alterations in taste, proteinuria, and leukopenia. The incidence is lower (1.5%) with enalapril and lisinopril because they lack a sulfhydryl group.

    (7) Headache, dizziness, and fatigue are the most common side effects associated with enalapril.

    (8) Hyperkalemia has been reported.

    (9) Rarely, angioedema occurs.

2. Drugs that block receptors for angiotensin (see Chapter 8 V C 1). **Saralasin,** an angiotensin II analog, exemplifies the drugs that interfere with the renin–angiotensin system by this mechanism.

  a. These drugs can be given only by intravenous infusion.

  b. They are primarily used diagnostically to detect a renal cause of hypertension.

V. DRUGS USED IN THE TREATMENT OF CORONARY ARTERY THROMBOSIS

(see Chapter 7 V C). More than 80% of patients with acute transmural myocardial infarction demonstrate thrombotic coronary artery occlusion within 6 hours of symptoms. **Streptokinase, urokinase, and tissue-type plasminogen activator (t-PA)** are available for intravenous administration in the treatment of coronary artery thrombosis associated with myocardial infarction.

A. Mechanism of action

1. Streptokinase, urokinase, and t-PA all **facilitate the conversion of plasminogen to plasmin**. Plasmin is fibrinolytic.

2. Because t-PA is more selective than the kinases, it has a high affinity for fibrin and induces the degradation of plasminogen to plasmin only in the presence of fibrin. Theoretically, it is less likely to have systemic effects on clotting.

B. Pharmacokinetics. The plasma half-life of t-PA is 5 minutes, compared to 16 minutes for urokinase and 23 minutes for streptokinase.

C. Therapeutic uses

1. Clinical studies comparing t-PA to streptokinase indicate the following:

  a. Both t-PA and streptokinase have comparable efficacy in the reduction of mortality and improvement of left ventricular function.

b. Streptokinase appears most effective when given less than 3 hours after the onset of symptoms.

2. Route of administration. Thrombolytic therapy is begun as soon as possible after the onset of symptoms of myocardial infarction.
a. Streptokinase is given by intravenous or intracoronary infusion.
b. Urokinase is infused into the occluded coronary artery.
c. t-PA is given by intravenous administration only.

D. Adverse effects and contraindications

1. Serious bleeding can occur; most important, gastrointestinal and intracranial hemorrhage are possible.

2. Streptokinase can cause anaphylaxis.

3. With any thrombolytic agent, cardiac arrhythmias can occur upon reperfusion of the occluded vessels.

4. Contraindications to the use of thrombolytic agents include internal bleeding, cerebral vascular accident, recent intracranial or intraspinal trauma, recent surgery, known bleeding diathesis, or severe uncontrolled hypertension.

5. Any condition in which bleeding would be a significant hazard is a relative contraindication and calls for a careful risk–benefit analysis before using thrombolytic therapy.

VI. DRUGS USED IN THE TREATMENT OF HYPERLIPIDEMIA

A. General considerations

1. Classes of lipoproteins and transport pathways
a. Exogenous pathways
(1) Chylomicrons are formed from dietary triglycerides and cholesterol.
(2) In adipose tissue and muscle, the enzyme **lipoprotein lipase** removes the triglycerides, leaving **chylomicron remnants** containing intact cholesterol esters.
(3) When chylomicron remnants reach the liver, they are taken up by hepatocytes and then cleaved, releasing **free cholesterol**.
(4) The cholesterol can be:
(a) Stored in hepatocytes as cholesterol esters
(b) Released in bile as cholesterol or as bile acids
(c) Used to form membranes or endogenous lipoproteins
b. Endogenous pathways
(1) Very low-density lipoprotein (VLDL) is formed in the liver from triglycerides and cholesterol, generally as a result of high caloric intake.
(2) VLDL is released into the plasma, where lipoprotein lipase cleaves the triglycerides from VLDL.
(3) The hydrolysis of VLDL produces **intermediate-density lipoprotein (IDL)**. The metabolic fate of IDL is twofold:
(a) Some IDL particles are taken up by the liver via endocytosis and then cleaved to produce free cholesterol. This receptor-mediated action is via the **low-density lipoprotein (LDL) receptor**.
(b) Some IDL particles remain in the circulation, where triglycerides are removed so that IDL is eventually metabolized to LDL.
(4) LDL is involved in the transport of endogenous cholesterol ester to the liver or to extrahepatic tissues. LDL constitutes 60%–70% of plasma cholesterol

levels. Metabolic demand for cholesterol (for synthesis of bile acids, steroids, or membranes) is met by increased synthesis of LDL receptors, which promote endocytosis and release of free cholesterol.

(5) **Apolipoproteins** are protein constituents of lipoproteins. **Apolipoprotein B** is the main structural protein of LDL and VLDL. High concentrations of apolipoprotein B are associated with an increased risk of coronary artery disease.

(6) **High-density lipoprotein (HDL)** is involved in the transport of cholesterol from peripheral cells back to the liver. HDL absorbs free cholesterol released during cell turnover. This cholesterol is esterified by the enzyme **lecithin:cholesterol acyltransferase,** and the cholesterol esters are transferred to VLDL or IDL particles.

c. **Nonspecific pathways**

(1) When plasma lipoprotein concentrations are high, macrophages and other scavenger cells take part in lipoprotein degradation.

(2) This leads to cholesterol deposits in macrophages or arterial walls (**atheromas**) and of tendons and skin (**xanthomas**).

2. **Hyperlipoproteinemias**

a. **Causes**

(1) **Primary hyperlipoproteinemias** may be single-gene congenital defects or polygenic (multifactorial).

(2) **Secondary hyperlipoproteinemia** may occur in diabetes, hypothyroidism, alcoholism, biliary cirrhosis, or renal disease, or in women taking oral contraceptives.

b. **Use of drug therapy**

(1) In persons with hyperlipoproteinemia, lowering the serum lipid concentration reduces the risk of atherosclerosis and its consequences. Specifically, a reduction in plasma LDL can reduce the risk of coronary artery disease.

(2) Some types of hypertriglyceridemia can cause life-threatening pancreatitis. Reduction of serum lipids has been demonstrated to be beneficial.

(3) Drug therapy is usually tried after dietary fat restriction, reduction of atherosclerosis risk factors, and moderate exercise programs have failed to lower serum lipids to an acceptable level.

(4) Bile acid sequestrants, niacin, β-hydroxy-β-methylglutaryl coenzyme A (HMG CoA) reductase inhibitors, and fibric acid derivatives demonstrably lower the risk of coronary artery disease; only niacin has been shown to reduce overall mortality.

B. **Antihyperlipidemic agents** (Table 5-11)

1. **Bile acid sequestrants (cholestyramine, colestipol)**

a. **Mechanism of action and pharmacologic effects**

(1) Cholestyramine and colestipol are resins that bind bile acids in the intestine, forming insoluble complexes, which are then excreted in the feces.

(2) The loss of bile acids leads to an increased conversion of cholesterol into bile acids.

(3) There is also a compensatory increase in hepatic LDL receptors.

(4) The net effect is a reduction in serum LDL and cholesterol levels.

b. **Therapeutic uses**

(1) The earliest use of bile acid sequestrants was to control pruritus in patients with cholestasis and elevated plasma bile acids.

(2) These agents are now also used to reduce elevated LDL levels.

(3) Patients with heterozygous familial hypercholesterolemia or polygenic hypercholesterolemia can be expected to respond.

(4) The bile acid sequestrants are not effective for treating patients with elevated chylomicrons, VLDL, or IDL; in addition, these agents elevate triglyceride levels.

TABLE 5-11. Antihyperlipidemic Agents

Drug	Effects	Therapeutic Uses	
		Lipoprotein State	**Clinical Condition**
Bile acid sequestrants (cholestyramine, colestipol)	↓ LDL ↑ HDL	High LDL	Heterozygous familial and polygenic hypercholesterolemias
HMG CoA reductase inhibitors (lovastatin, pravastatin, mevastatin)	↓ LDL	High LDL	Hypercholesterolemias with risk of myocardial infarction; diabetes and nephrosis-related hypercholesterolemias
Niacin (nicotinic acid)	↓ LDL ↓ VLDL ↑ HDL	Low HDL; high VLDL; high LDL	All hyperlipoproteinemias except lipoprotein lipase deficiency
Fibric acid derivatives (clofibrate, gemfibrozil)	↓↑ LDL ↑ HDL	Low HDL, high VLDL, high IDL (clofibrate); also high LDL (gemfibrozil)	Familial type III hyperlipoproteinemia (both derivatives); hypertriglyceridemia with or without hypercholesterolemia, type V hyperlipoproteinemia (gemfibrozil)

HMG CoA = β-hydroxy-β-methylglutaryl coenzyme A; LDL = low-density lipoprotein; HDL = high-density lipoprotein; VLDL = very low-density lipoprotein; IDL = intermediate-density lipoprotein; ↑ = increased; ↓ = decreased.

c. Adverse effects
  (1) Because bile acid sequestrants are not absorbed, they have no adverse systemic effects.
  (2) The most common untoward effects are gastrointestinal discomfort and constipation.
  (3) The resins may cause or aggravate steatorrhea.
  (4) These agents may bind other drugs (e.g., fat-soluble vitamins, chlorothiazide, anticoagulants, digitalis, glycosides), impeding their absorption.

2. HMG CoA reductase inhibitors (**lovastatin, pravastatin, simvastatin, mevastatin**)
  a. Mechanism of action and pharmacologic effects
    (1) 3-HMG CoA reductase is the rate-limiting enzyme in cholesterol biosynthesis.
    (2) Drugs that inhibit HMG CoA reductase are highly effective in lowering serum LDL-cholesterol levels.
      (a) HMG CoA reductase inhibitors block the hepatic synthesis of cholesterol.
      (b) This block leads to a compensatory reduction of serum LDL.
      (c) There is also a compensatory increase in synthesis of HMG CoA reductase so that inhibition of cholesterol synthesis is not complete.
    (3) These drugs reduce serum levels of LDL, LDL-cholesterol, VLDL-cholesterol, and triglycerides.
      (a) The decrease in LDL appears to result from an increase in hepatic LDL receptors, which causes an increase in receptor-mediated clearance of LDL and IDL.
      (b) HDL-cholesterol is elevated.
  b. Therapeutic uses. HMG CoA reductase inhibitors are:
    (1) Indicated for patients with hypercholesterolemia who are at high risk of myocardial infarction
    (2) Specifically indicated for types IIa and IIb hyperlipoproteinemia in which IDL and total cholesterol are elevated
    (3) Useful in secondary hyperlipoproteinemia resulting from diabetes mellitus or nephrotic syndrome
    (4) Useful in patients with combined elevated cholesterol and triglycerides

c. **Adverse effects**
   (1) Serum hepatic transaminases are elevated in 2% of patients and muscle creatine phosphokinase levels are elevated in 11%.
   (2) Gastrointestinal reactions include flatulence and diarrhea.
   (3) Periodic slit-lamp examinations are suggested before and during therapy, because ocular opacities have been noted in dogs.
   (4) When combined with another lipid-lowering drug or with cyclosporine, HMG CoA reductase inhibitor therapy can cause myopathies, sometimes progressing to rhabdomyolysis and renal failure.

3. **Niacin (nicotinic acid)**
   a. **Mechanism of action and pharmacologic effects**
      (1) In large doses, niacin reduces serum triglycerides by lowering VLDL, usually within 1–4 days.
      (2) The reduction of VLDL, in turn, reduces IDL and LDL.
      (3) Niacin usually produces a mild to moderate increase in HDL.
      (4) Niacin does not significantly affect either total body production or biliary excretion of cholesterol.
   b. **Therapeutic uses**
      (1) Niacin is helpful in controlling a wide range of hyperlipidemias.
      (2) It is particularly useful for type V hyperlipoproteinemia, characterized by severe hypertriglyceridemia and elevated chylomicrons.
      (3) It is not useful in familial lipoprotein lipase deficiency.
   c. **Adverse effects** can be minimized by taking the drug with meals and increasing the dosage gradually.
      (1) Niacin produces prostaglandin-mediated intense flushing and itching.
      (2) Gastrointestinal distress is common, and peptic ulceration has occurred.
      (3) Hepatic dysfunction can occur with high-dose regimens.
      (4) Glucose intolerance and hyperuricemia can occur.

4. **Fibric acid derivatives (clofibrate, gemfibrozil)**
   a. **Mechanism of action and pharmacologic effects**
      (1) The mechanism of action has not yet been fully established, but it is known that fibric acid derivatives increase the activity of lipoprotein lipase, the enzyme that degrades chylomicrons and VLDL.
      (2) **Pharmacologic effects.** The fibric acid derivatives decrease synthesis of apolipoprotein B and lower serum VLDL levels, thus reducing serum triglycerides.
         (a) With **clofibrate,** the net effect on serum cholesterol in most patients is minimal. However, serum cholesterol is significantly reduced in patients with familial type III hyperlipoproteinemia. Clofibrate has no effect on chylomicron levels or on HDL levels.
         (b) **Gemfibrozil** lowers plasma VLDL-cholesterol levels, lowers LDL-cholesterol to a lesser degree, and raises HDL-cholesterol.
   b. **Therapeutic uses**
      (1) Fibric acid derivatives are indicated for patients with familial type III hyperlipoproteinemia, in which VLDL and IDL levels are increased.
      (2) Gemfibrozil is useful for hypertriglyceridemia, whether or not accompanied by hypercholesterolemia.
      (3) Gemfibrozil is also useful in type V hyperlipoproteinemia in which both chylomicron and triglyceride levels are increased.
      (4) Neither clofibrate nor gemfibrozil is useful in type I hyperlipoproteinemia with elevated chylomicrons or triglycerides but normal VLDL levels.
   c. **Adverse effects.** Fibric acid derivatives are generally well tolerated. The most common unwanted effects are mild gastrointestinal reactions, including cholelithiasis.

5. **Lipophilic antioxidants (probucol)**
   a. **Mechanism of action and pharmacologic effects.** The mechanism of action is unclear but appears to involve inhibition of the oxidation of LDL and reduction of its uptake by macrophages.

(1) Effect on serum lipids
  (a) Probucol reduces total serum cholesterol; it lowers HDL-cholesterol more than LDL-cholesterol.
  (b) Probucol has little or no effect on VLDL or triglycerides.
(2) Effect on cholesterol deposits
  (a) Probucol induces marked regression of xanthomas.
  (b) In rabbits, a marked reduction in atheromatous deposits has been found.
b. Therapeutic uses. Probucol is generally combined with another type of lipid-lowering drug for the treatment of general hypercholesterolemia.
c. Adverse effects
  (1) Gastrointestinal reactions are the most common untoward effects.
  (2) Probucol is stored in body tissue for up to 6 months.

DIRECTIONS: Each of the numbered items or incomplete statements in this section is followed by answers or by completions of the statement. Select the ONE lettered answer or completion that is BEST in each case.

1. A 67-year-old man with a history of recurrent ventricular tachycardia presents with joint and muscle pain, fatigue (which proves to be the result of hemolytic anemia), and a skin rash. He is taking several "heart pills." A likely cause of his signs and symptoms is

(A) digoxin
(B) procainamide
(C) disopyramide
(D) minoxidil
(E) reserpine

2. Which antihyperlipidemic agent would reduce circulating cholesterol levels by binding to cholesterol in the gastrointestinal tract?

(A) Cholestyramine
(B) Clofibrate
(C) Gemfibrozil
(D) Lovastatin
(E) Nicotinic acid

DIRECTIONS: Each of the numbered items or incomplete statements in this section is negatively phrased, as indicated by a capitalized word such as NOT, LEAST, or EXCEPT. Select the ONE lettered answer or completion that is BEST in each case.

3. Actions of digoxin on the heart include all of the following EXCEPT

(A) increased force of systolic contraction
(B) prolonged atrioventricular (A-V) nodal conduction time
(C) a decrease in ventricular size of the failing heart
(D) a positive chronotropic effect in the failing heart
(E) an increase in the effective refractory period (ERP) of the atria

4. All of the following lipid-reducing agents are correctly matched with their pharmacologic mechanism of action EXCEPT

(A) cholestyramine—bile acid sequestrant
(B) probucol—enhanced low-density lipoprotein (LDL) clearance by nonreceptor mechanisms
(C) clofibrate—coenzyme A reductase inhibitor
(D) gemfibrozil—increases the activity of lipoprotein lipase
(E) lovastatin—inhibits the early stage of cholesterol biosynthesis

5. The antiarrhythmic agent tocainide has all of the following properties EXCEPT

(A) it can be used for ventricular arrhythmias
(B) it can be given orally
(C) it is also a local anesthetic
(D) it lengthens the action potential
(E) it is a class IB antiarrhythmic agent

6. All of the following measures can be used in the treatment of digoxin-induced arrhythmias EXCEPT

(A) stopping digoxin administration
(B) electrical conversion
(C) phenytoin administration
(D) lidocaine administration
(E) digoxin-specific antibody fragment

7. All of the following statements regarding nitroglycerin are true EXCEPT

(A) tablets should be stored in a dark glass container
(B) headache is a common early side effect
(C) transdermal administration is effective when administered daily for 24 hours
(D) it can be given intravenously in medical emergencies
(E) the nitrates are broken down in the liver by a glutathione-dependent organic reductase

8. Correct statements about the adverse effects of antihypertensive agents include all of the following EXCEPT

(A) hydralazine can induce a lupus-like syndrome
(B) diazoxide inhibits the release of insulin from the pancreas
(C) clonidine can cause fluid retention that often requires concurrent diuretic therapy
(D) reserpine augments sympathetic effects because of decreased parasympathetic activity
(E) captopril can cause cough and bronchospasm

9. A patient enters the emergency room with substernal chest pain that has lasted 1 hour. Within the next hour, the diagnosis of an acute transmural myocardial infarction is made. All of the following statements regarding the use of a thrombolytic agent in this situation are true EXCEPT

(A) tissue-type plasminogen activator (t-PA) would facilitate the conversion of plasminogen to plasmin
(B) t-PA has a shorter half-life than streptokinase
(C) t-PA administration is more likely to benefit this patient's chances of survival than streptokinase
(D) streptokinase appears more effective when given less than 3 hours after the onset of symptoms
(E) all thrombolytic agents can cause cardiac arrhythmias upon reperfusion

---

DIRECTIONS: Each set of matching questions in this section consists of a list of four to twenty-six lettered options (some of which may be in figures) followed by several items. For each numbered item, select the ONE lettered option that is most closely associated with it. To avoid spending too much time on matching sets with large numbers of options, it is generally advisable to begin each set by reading the list of options. Then, for each item in the set, try to generate the correct answer and locate it in the option list, rather than evaluating each option individually. Each lettered option may be selected once, more than once, or not at all.

Questions 10–13

Match each statement with the agent it describes.

(A) Digoxin
(B) Captopril
(C) Furosemide
(D) Propranolol
(E) Lidocaine

10. When added to digoxin and furosemide, this agent increases the survival rate among patients with mild to severe congestive heart failure (CHF).

11. When used chronically in the presence of compromised renal function, this agent can cause atrioventricular (A-V) dissociation and block.

12. This agent would be most effective for treating the ventricular tachyarrhythmias associated with digoxin.

13. This agent would be absolutely contraindicated in the presence of A-V block.

Questions 14–16

Match each arrhythmia with the appropriate treatment.

(A) Digoxin
(B) Atropine
(C) Lidocaine
(D) Propranolol
(E) Epinephrine

14.

15.

16.

Questions 17–20

A 50-year-old man has a blood pressure of 170/98. This blood pressure is confirmed over the following week. A complete physical examination and diagnostic work-up are unremarkable, except for mild wheezing. There is a family history of essential hypertension. Match each description with the appropriate agent.

(A) Verapamil
(B) Hydrochlorothiazide
(C) Methyldopa
(D) Enalapril
(E) Propranolol

17. Administration of this drug to the patient results in hypokalemia.

18. The patient is next administered a drug that results in complaints of increased wheezing.

19. The next drug administered leads to complaints of an annoying cough.

20. The patient is administered a drug that results in good control of blood pressure without side effects. Because it depresses atrioventricular (A-V) conduction, the use of β blockers is contraindicated when using this drug.

1. The answer is B *[II B 2 f (4)]*. Procainamide can produce a syndrome that resembles systemic lupus erythematosus, the signs and symptoms of which are similar to this patient's presenting problems. These untoward effects are caused by hypersensitivity to procainamide and are reversible once the drug is discontinued.

2. The answer is A *[VI B 1, 3, 4]*. Cholestyramine is a resin that binds bile acid in the intestine, thereby preventing its reabsorption. The reduction in bile acid leads to an increase in 7-α-hydroxylase, which, in turn, leads to an increased hepatic conversion of cholesterol into bile acids. Nicotinic acid and clofibrate alter the metabolism, not the transport, of cholesterol. Nicotinic acid depresses the synthesis of very low-density lipoprotein (VLDL), which indirectly depresses low-density lipoprotein (LDL) levels. Clofibrate and gemfibrozil reduce VLDL but may raise serum LDL. Lovastatin is a coenzyme A reductase inhibitor, which competitively inhibits the early stage of cholesterol biosynthesis.

3. The answer is D *[I B 3 b (3)]*. Digoxin increases the force of systolic contraction, prolongs atrioventricular (A-V) nodal conduction time, decreases ventricular size in the failing heart, and increases the effective refractory period (ERP) of the atria. It tends to slow the heart rate, especially in the failing heart (a negative chronotropic effect). By improving cardiac output, digoxin produces a decrease in sympathetic activity.

4. The answer is C *[VI B 1 a, 2 a, 4 a, 5 a]*. Probucol reduces total serum cholesterol by increasing the rate of degradation of low-density lipoprotein (LDL) and inhibition of the early stages of cholesterol synthesis. Clofibrate, like gemfibrozil, is fibric acid derivative that possibly increases the activity of lipoprotein lipase, the enzyme that degrades chylomicrons and very low-density lipoprotein (VLDL). Lovastatin and pravastatin are 3-hydroxy-3-methylglutaryl coenzyme A reductase inhibitors. They competitively inhibit the early stage of cholesterol biosynthesis. Cholestyramine is a resin that binds bile acids in the intestines, which are then excreted in the feces.

5. The answer is D *[II C 3 a–d]*. In arrhythmias, tocainide shortens, not lengthens, the action potential; it also shortens the effective refractory period (ERP). Tocainide is a lidocaine analog and a class IB antiarrhythmic agent. It closely resembles lidocaine in its effects; but unlike lidocaine, it can be used orally for arrhythmias. Tocainide is used to suppress ventricular arrhythmias; it is also a local anesthetic.

6. The answer is B *[I B 7 a, d, e, i, j]*. Electrical conversion can be hazardous because it can precipitate ventricular fibrillation. The use of phenytoin and lidocaine for various digoxin-induced arrhythmias is considered appropriate therapy. Digoxin and K+-depleting diuretics should be discontinued.

7. The answer is C *[III A 3 b, 4 b (1), 5 a–c]*. Transdermal nitroglycerin patches become ineffective if they are left in place for 24 hours and reapplied daily, even if the dosage is increased. Nitroglycerin patches delivering 10 mg or more remain effective if removed for 12 hours daily. Nitroglycerin can be given intravenously in medical emergencies. Nitroglycerin tablets should be stored in a dark glass container so that they do not lose potency. Headache is a common early side effect, resulting from vasodilation of cerebral vessels produced by nitrates. Nitrates are broken down in the liver by a glutathione-dependent organic nitrate reductase.

8. The answer is D *[IV E 2 d (3), 4 e (3), G 1 e, H 1 f (2), I 1 g (4)]*. Reserpine augments parasympathetic effects because of decreased sympathetic activity; this may result in bradycardia, increased gastrointestinal activity, and miosis. Hydralazine can induce a lupus-like syndrome. Diazoxide inhibits the release of insulin from the pancreas. Clonidine can cause fluid retention that often requires concurrent diuretic therapy. Captopril can cause cough and bronchospasm.

9. The answer is C *[V A–D]*. Both tissue-type plasminogen activator (t-PA) and streptokinase appear to reduce mortality equally when administered after the diagnosis of an acute transmural myocardial infarction. However, streptokinase appears to be most effective when given less than 3 hours after the onset of symptoms. t-PA facilitates the conversion of plasminogen to plasmin and has a shorter half-life than streptokinase. All thrombolytic agents can cause cardiac arrhythmias upon reperfusion.

10–13. The answers are: 10-B *[I C 3 b]*, **11-A** *[I B 6 e (6)]*, **12-E** *[I B 7 e]*, **13-D** *[II E 1 b (1)]*. Angiotensin-converting enzyme (ACE) inhibitors such as captopril are used as first-line agents in the treatment of congestive heart failure (CHF). Adding ACE inhibitors to a therapeutic regimen that includes digoxin and a diuretic such as furosemide increases the survival rate in patients with mild to severe CHF.

Digoxin has a low margin of safety. Intoxication is often precipitated by depletion of serum K^+ as a result of diuretic use or decreased renal function. Cardiac effects from intoxication include premature ventricular contractions (PVCs), ventricular tachycardia and fibrillation, atrioventricular (A-V) dissociation and block, sinus arrhythmia and sinoatrial (S-A) block, and paroxysmal atrial tachycardia, often with A-V block.

Lidocaine is effective for treating ventricular tachyarrhythmias associated with digoxin toxicity.

Because of its β-blocking activity, propranolol substantially increases the effective refractory period of the A-V node. Therefore, propranolol would be contraindicated in the presence of A-V block.

14–16. The answers are: 14-B *[Chapter 2 VI A 1]*, **15-C** *[II C 1 d]*, **16-A** *[I B 2 a, 5 b]*. The arrhythmia shown is sinus bradycardia. It would most effectively be treated with atropine, which competes reversibly with acetylcholine (ACh) at muscarinic receptors, slowing the heart rate.

Premature ventricular contractions (PVCs) dominate this abnormal electrocardiogram. PVCs are most effectively treated with lidocaine.

The arrhythmia shown is atrial fibrillation, which can be treated effectively with digoxin. Although it does not suppress the abnormal foci, digoxin decreases conduction through the atrioventricular (A-V) node, preventing ventricular irritability and the generation of a ventricular arrhythmia.

17–20. The answers are: 17-B *[IV A 2, B]*, **18-E** *[IV C 4 a]*, **19-D** *[IV I 1 g (4)]*, **20-A** *[IV D]*. Thiazide diuretics (e.g., hydrochlorothiazide) cause a loss of Na^+, water, and K^+. With chronic use of thiazide diuretics, potassium supplementation is necessary.

Propranolol is a nonselective β blocker that can exacerbate asthma and chronic obstructive pulmonary disease.

Enalapril is an angiotensin-converting enzyme (ACE) inhibitor that commonly causes a dry cough. Angioedema is a rarer adverse effect of enalapril.

Ca^{2+}-channel blockers such as verapamil are becoming important antihypertensive drugs because of their vasodilating effects. Verapamil and diltiazem depress A-V conduction and should not be used with β blockers.

Chapter 6
Diuretic Agents

I. **GENERAL CONSIDERATIONS.** Diuretics are drugs that promote a net loss of sodium ions (Na+) and water from the body, the net result being an increase in urine flow.

A. **Classification.** Diuretics are classified by structure and mechanism of action into eight groups listed below. Agents in the first four groups are seldom or no longer used, but their mode of action or their role in the history of diuretics is important.

1. Xanthine diuretics
2. Mercurial diuretics (e.g., mercaptomerin)
3. Carbonic anhydrase inhibitors (e.g., acetazolamide)
4. Acidifying salts [e.g., ammonium chloride (NH_4Cl)]
5. Thiazide diuretics (e.g., chlorothiazide, hydrochlorothiazide)
6. Loop (high-ceiling) diuretics (e.g., furosemide, ethacrynic acid, bumetanide, torsemide)
7. Osmotic diuretics (e.g., mannitol, urea, isosorbide)
8. Potassium (K+)-sparing diuretics (e.g., triamterene, amiloride, spironolactone)

B. **Mechanisms of action**

1. **Renal.** The general mechanisms of diuresis are shown in Figure 6-1.
2. **Nonrenal.** Some drugs increase urine flow by nonrenal mechanisms (e.g., by increasing cardiac output in a patient with congestive heart failure or by reducing prostatic hyperplasia), but these drugs are not generally regarded as diuretics.

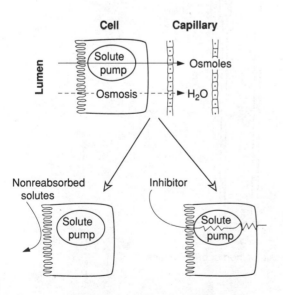

FIGURE 6-1. Renal mechanisms of diuresis. Diuretics increase urine flow by interfering with ionic transport to promote sodium and water loss. (*A*) Impermeant luminal solutes. Osmotic diuretics are freely filterable at the glomerulus and are relatively inert. They undergo limited reabsorption by the renal tubule. (*B*) Inhibitors of solute transport. Loop diuretics, thiazides, mercurials, carbonic anhydrase inhibitors, and potassium (K+)-sparing diuretics act directly on the kidney to increase the excretion of sodium chloride and water. With the exception of K+-sparing diuretics, they also increase the excretion of potassium. (Redrawn and modified with permission from Smith TW and Braunwald E: The management of heart failure. In *Heart Disease: A Textbook of Cardiovascular Medicine,* 2nd ed. Edited by Braunwald E. Philadelphia, WB Saunders, 1984, p 527.)

C. **Sites of action.** Although a diuretic can act on several areas of the nephron, the major sites of action for the diuretics are shown in Figure 6-2.

D. **Therapeutic uses**

1. Diuretics are frequently used for the **clinical management of disorders involving abnormal fluid distribution,** such as **edema,** or for **hypertension.**

2. They are **used to reduce the toxicity of ingested or administered substances.** For example, mannitol, an osmotic diuretic, reduces the renal toxicity of the antitumor agent cisplatin, and acetazolamide, a carbonic anhydrase inhibitor, is used to alkalinize the urine and increase salicylate elimination.

FIGURE 6-2. Major sites of action of the diuretics.

E. Efficacy

1. The efficacy of the different classes of diuretics varies significantly. The xanthine diuretics are the least effective and the loop diuretics are the most effective.

2. The establishment of a net negative Na$^+$ balance, particularly with the less efficacious diuretics, can also depend on limiting the Na$^+$ intake.

3. Prolonged use of some diuretics (e.g., mercurials, carbonic anhydrase inhibitors) results in refractoriness or a reduction in efficacy. These agents are self-limiting and not frequently used.

F. **Adverse effects.** Reduction in serum K$^+$ levels (**hypokalemia**) is one of the most important adverse effects of many diuretics. A summary of the adverse effects of important diuretics is presented in Table 6-1.

II. XANTHINE DIURETICS

A. Mechanism of action

1. By increasing cardiac output, xanthine diuretics increase renal plasma flow, promoting a higher glomerular filtration rate.

2. They also appear to inhibit Na$^+$ reabsorption in the proximal convoluted tubule.

B. **Therapeutic uses.** Xanthines are rarely used as diuretics, but the diuretic action may be seen with xanthines used as bronchodilators (e.g., aminophylline) or In caffeine products (e.g., tea, coffee, soda).

C. **Adverse effects.** Xanthine diuretics may cause the following:

1. Central nervous system (CNS) stimulation

2. Gastrointestinal upset, including vomiting and consequent dehydration

3. Cardiovascular toxicity, including palpitations, hypotension, and circulatory collapse

TABLE 6-1. Adverse Effects of Diuretics

Diuretic	Hyperglycemia	Hyperuricemia	Hypokalemia	Ototoxicity	Calcium Excretion
Thiazide	+	+	+	−	↓
Ethacrynic acid	+	+	+	+	↑
Furosemide	+	+	+	+	↑
Bumetanide	+	+	+	+	↑
Torsemide	+	+	+	+	↑
Mercurials	−	−	−	−	−*
Acetazolamide	−	−	+	−	−*
Indapamide	+	+	+	−	↓

+ = side effect; − = no side effect; ↑ = increase; ↓ = decrease.
*No effect.

III. MERCURIAL DIURETICS

A. Mechanism of action

1. The major effect of organomercurial agents is to inhibit active chloride (Cl^-) transport in the ascending limb of the loop of Henle.

2. In an **acidic environment,** the mercuric ion (Hg^{2+}) dissociates and binds to sulfhydryl enzymes, inactivating them.
   a. As a result, reabsorption of Na^+ is diminished and the excretion of Na^+ and Cl^- is increased.
   b. More Cl^- than Na^+ is lost; thus, to maintain electrical neutrality, cations such as hydrogen (H^+) and, to a lesser degree, K^+ are also lost.
   c. Because excess Cl^- is excreted, bicarbonate (HCO_3^-) remains to maintain balanced anions, and the resulting metabolic picture is a **hypochloremic alkalosis**.

3. In an **alkaline environment,** Hg^{2+} does not dissociate from the mercurial diuretics to take an active form; thus, patients become **refractory** to the mercurials in about 1 week. However, an acidifying agent, such as NH_4Cl, can be combined with the mercurial agent to create a metabolic acidosis, offsetting the metabolic alkalosis and combating refractoriness.

B. Route of administration.
Mercurial diuretics are poorly absorbed by the oral route and, thus, are administered **parenterally**. **Mercaptomerin** is administered daily, intramuscularly or subcutaneously.

C. Therapeutic uses.
The mercurial diuretics are seldom used because they must be given parenterally and because of their adverse effects. Because the mercurial diuretics do not disrupt K^+ balance as much as many of the other diuretics, they occasionally are used in congestive heart failure, cirrhosis, and portal obstruction.

D. Adverse effects include the following:

1. Systemic mercury poisoning

2. Cardiac toxicity (ventricular fibrillation can follow rapid intravenous administration, possibly because the mercurial agent binds to sulfhydryl enzymes in cardiac muscle)

3. Hypersensitivity reactions

4. Aggravation of acute nephritis or renal insufficiency

IV. CARBONIC ANHYDRASE INHIBITORS

A. Mechanism of action

1. Carbonic anhydrase inhibitors inhibit the carbonic anhydrase enzyme predominantly at the proximal convoluted tubules, reducing the number of hydrogen ions available for Na^+–H^+ exchange. Carbon dioxide (CO_2) reabsorption from the glomerular filtrate is suppressed, and HCO_3^- excretion is increased.
   a. Because of decreased Na^+ reabsorption, the Na^+–K^+ exchange in the distal convoluted tubule increases, causing a loss of K^+ in the urine.
   b. Increased urinary amounts of Na^+, K^+, and HCO_3^- result in an alkaline urine.

2. To maintain ionic balance, Cl^- is retained by the kidney, resulting in a hyperchloremic acidosis. The acidosis eventually induces a refractory state (i.e., decreased diuresis).

B. | **Route of administration**

1. As a diuretic, **acetazolamide** is given orally once daily or every other day.

2. For use in glaucoma, it is given orally 2–4 times daily.

C. | **Therapeutic uses**

1. Carbonic anhydrase inhibitors are weak diuretics and have largely been replaced by the thiazide diuretics. Historically, however, they are important.

2. They are still used with moderate success for the following purposes:
   a. In **glaucoma,** to reduce the rate of aqueous humor formation
   b. In **petit mal epilepsy,** in which they act as an anticonvulsant and decrease the rate of spinal fluid formation (the mechanism of action of this therapeutic effect is unclear)
   c. To **alkalinize the urine**
      (1) In the treatment of salicylate or barbiturate poisoning
      (2) In combination with HCO_3^- to maintain electrolyte balance

D. | **Adverse effects** with carbonic anhydrase inhibitors are few.

1. They are aromatic sulfonamides, which can cause blood dyscrasias and allergic skin reactions, but these are rare.

2. Drowsiness and paresthesias can occur with large doses but these conditions are reversible.

3. They inhibit iodide uptake by the thyroid but are not therapeutic as agents used to treat goiters.

V. | ACIDIFYING SALTS

A. | **Mechanism of action**

1. Acidifying salts such as NH_4Cl lower the pH in the extracellular fluid and urine.
   a. The ammonium (NH_4) in NH_4Cl is metabolized by the liver to urea, resulting in the net formation of H^+.
   b. H^+ then is buffered by HCO_3^-, and CO_2 is formed.
   c. Cl^- from the NH_4Cl replaces HCO_3^-, leading to acidosis.
   d. An excess of Cl^- also occurs in the tubular lumen and takes Na^+ along with it to maintain electrical neutrality.
   e. The glutaminase system becomes activated, producing ammonia (NH_3).
   f. The kidney secretes H^+ in exchange for Na^+, and Cl^- is excreted in combination with NH_4^+.

2. Ultimately, the amount of NH_4Cl ingested is equal to the amount excreted by the kidney, and a refractory state is produced.

B. | **Route of administration.** NH_4Cl is administered as enteric-coated tablets given orally 4–6 times per day for 2 days.

C. | **Therapeutic uses**

1. As a primary diuretic, NH_4Cl is effective for only 1–2 days; thus, it is seldom used.

2. The drug has been used to augment the effect of mercurial and loop diuretics by maintaining an available source of Cl^- in the blood to compensate for diuretic-induced alkalosis.

D. **Adverse effects** include the following:

1. Gastric irritation

2. Uncompensated acidosis that occurs when renal function is impaired

3. Exacerbation of hepatic failure

VI. THIAZIDE DIURETICS (BENZOTHIADIAZIDES AND SULFONAMIDE DIURETICS)

A. **Chemistry** (Figure 6-3)

1. **Thiazide diuretics** (e.g., **chlorothiazide, hydrochlorothiazide**) have a sulfonamyl group, which enables them to inhibit carbonic anhydrase activity. These agents vary widely in this ability, however, and inhibition of carbonic anhydrase is not their primary mechanism of action.

2. **Sulfonamide diuretics.** Certain other diuretics—**indapamide, chlorthalidone, quinethazone,** and **metolazone**—are pharmacologically similar to the thiazides, but the nature of their heterocyclic ring makes them chemically different from the thiazides.

B. **Mechanism of action.** Thiazide diuretics inhibit Cl^- reabsorption, particularly in the distal portion of the ascending limb of the loop of Henle and the very early portion of the distal tubule. Refractoriness does not occur.

C. **Pharmacologic effects**

1. Renal excretion of Na^+, Cl^-, HCO_3^-, and K^+ is increased.

A

FIGURE 6-3. (*A*) Hydrochlorothiazide, a thiazide diuretic, and (*B*) chlorthalidone, a sulfonamide diuretic. These agents are pharmacologically similar but chemically different.

B

2. The initial hypotensive effect of the thiazide diuretics is a result of a reduction in blood volume, and a continued hypotensive effect occurs because of direct relaxation of arteriolar smooth muscle.

D. **Route of administration**

1. **Thiazides.** There are many analogs, but the two most important prototypes are chlorothiazide and hydrochlorothiazide, which are administered orally 1–2 times daily.

2. **Sulfonamides.** Because of their long duration of action (24 hours), sulfonamides are administered orally once daily.

E. **Therapeutic uses**

1. Thiazide diuretics are used to treat **chronic edema,** usually associated with cardiac decompensation. A diuretic response occurs in 2–3 hours and lasts for about 1 day.

2. Thiazides are used in the treatment of **essential hypertension**.

3. They sometimes are effective in the treatment of **nephrosis**.

4. They are occasionally used for the **palliation of nephrogenic and pituitary** [antidiuretic hormone (ADH)-sensitive] **diabetes insipidus**. By decreasing the urinary volume through their natriuretic action, these drugs may enhance the action of ADH.

5. They are used in the management of **hypercalciuria**.

F. **Adverse effects**

1. Electrolyte abnormalities such as **hypokalemia** can occur; thus, K+ supplementation is recommended. **Particular caution is needed when a thiazide is administered in combination with a digitalis preparation for the treatment of congestive heart failure.** If digitalis is administered in the presence of hypokalemia, digitalis intoxication and serious cardiac arrhythmias can result.

2. **Hyperuricemia** may result from an inhibition of renal tubular secretion of uric acid. Because thiazides are excreted by glomerular filtration and tubular secretion, the thiazides compete with uric acid for tubular secretion.

3. **Hyperglycemia** can occur, aggravating preexisting diabetes mellitus. Thiazides may interfere with the conversion of proinsulin to insulin.

4. **Hypercalcemia** and **hypophosphatemia** have occurred in a few patients on prolonged thiazide therapy, because thiazide diuretics may reduce urinary calcium excretion. Suppression of parathyroid hormone and reduction in intestinal calcium absorption may occur.

5. Thiazide diuretics occasionally may **aggravate renal or hepatic insufficiency**.

6. **Lassitude, weakness,** and **vertigo** can occur **with large doses**.

7. **Thiazide-induced pancreatitis** has been reported.

8. Several reports have implicated thiazides in **increasing lipid and lipoprotein changes** that could enhance **atherogenesis**.

VII. LOOP (HIGH-CEILING) DIURETICS

A. **Mechanism of action**

1. **Inhibition of electrolyte absorption.** Loop diuretics inhibit electrolyte reabsorption in the **thick ascending limb of the loop of Henle**. Because they act at the luminal surface of the nephron, they must reach the urine to exert a diuretic effect.

FIGURE 6-4. Furosemide, a loop diuretic, is a structural derivative of the thiazides.

   2. Inhibition of carbonic anhydrase
   a. Furosemide (Figure 6-4), **bumetanide,** and **torsemide are weak inhibitors of carbonic anhydrase,** probably as a result of the substituted sulfonamide side chain.
   b. Ethacrynic acid lacks a sulfonamyl group and **does not inhibit carbonic anhydrase.**

B. Pharmacologic effects

   1. Cl⁻ excretion is greater than Na⁺ excretion. Hypochloremic alkalosis can occur, but it does not produce a refractory state.

   2. These diuretics increase renal blood flow without increasing the glomerular filtration rate.

   3. Large doses promote uric acid excretion.

C. Route of administration

   1. Furosemide, bumetanide, and **torsemide** are usually administered orally in a single dose once or twice daily. Both also can be administered intramuscularly or (more frequently) intravenously.

   2. Ethacrynic acid is administered orally or intravenously once or twice daily. One of the main differences between furosemide and ethacrynic acid is that the former has a broader dose–response curve.

D. Therapeutic uses

   1. Loop diuretics are useful for the treatment of **acute episodes of pulmonary edema.**

   2. They are effective for **edema associated with congestive heart failure, cirrhosis,** and **renal disease.**

   3. Because of its potent edema-reducing ability, **furosemide** has been used to treat elevated **intracranial pressure.**

E. Adverse effects

   1. Fluid and electrolyte imbalances are the most commonly seen adverse effects. The loop diuretics frequently are administered to patients on digitalis so **hypokalemia** may be a particular problem.

   2. Hyperuricemia results because these diuretics are actively secreted by the renal and biliary secretory systems; thus, they block (by competition) renal uric acid secretion. Even though hyperuricemia is relatively common, it is benign.

   3. Transient deafness is a risk if a potentially ototoxic drug (e.g., an aminoglycoside antibiotic) is administered concomitantly. In such circumstances, another class of diuretic should be used.

   4. Patients who are allergic to sulfonamides may have **allergic reactions** to torsemide.

5. Transient granulocytopenia and **thrombocytopenia** have occurred.

6. Severe muscle pain and tenderness have been reported **in patients with renal failure**.

VIII. OSMOTIC DIURETICS

A. Mechanism of action

1. Osmotic diuretics are filtered at the glomerulus but are poorly reabsorbed because of their molecular size. The presence of these unresorbed solutes in the proximal tubule decreases reabsorption of Na^+ and water, resulting in a large volume of urine.

2. Mannitol causes an increase in renal medullary blood flow via a prostaglandin-mediated mechanism.

B. Pharmacologic effects. Osmotic diuretics do not markedly influence Na^+ and Cl^- excretion.

C. Route of administration

1. **Mannitol** is a six-carbon sugar alcohol that is administered intravenously because it is not absorbed well from the gastrointestinal tract. It is not metabolized.

2. **Urea** is the least used osmotic diuretic. It can be given orally, but, because of its bitter taste, it is generally administered intravenously.

3. **Isosorbide** is used orally for ophthalmologic emergencies such as acute angle-closure glaucoma.

D. Therapeutic uses

1. The osmotic diuretics are used to **reduce cerebrospinal fluid pressure**.

2. They transiently **reduce intraocular fluid pressure**.

3. They are used as an adjunct in the prevention or treatment of **oliguria** and **anuria**.

4. The osmotic diuretics, especially mannitol, are used **prophylactically for acute renal failure** in situations such as cardiovascular operations, treatment with nephrotoxic anticancer agents, severe traumatic injury, and management of hemolytic transfusion reactions.

E. Adverse effects

1. Because they do not penetrate cells and their mode of excretion is by glomerular filtration, osmotic diuretics increase blood volume, which can cause decompensation in patients with congestive heart failure.

2. When osmotic diuretics are used for the treatment of renal failure or cirrhotic disease, hyperosmolality and hyponatremia can occur.

IX. POTASSIUM (K^+)-SPARING DIURETICS

A. Triamterene and amiloride

1. **Mechanism of action**
   a. Triamterene and amiloride (Figure 6-5) inhibit active Na^+ reabsorption.

A

B

FIGURE 6-5. (*A*) Triamterene and (*B*) amiloride, potassium (K^+)-sparing diuretics.

(1) The increased excretion of Na^+ and Cl^- disrupts normal Na^+ transport and produces a net change in the electrogenic force across tubular membranes.

(2) This reduces the net driving force for K^+ secretion.

b. Triamterene and amiloride cause a moderate increase in Na^+, Cl^-, and HCO_3^- excretion.

c. Their action is independent of aldosterone.

2. **Route of administration**
   a. **Triamterene** is administered orally twice daily.
   b. **Amiloride** is administered orally once daily.

3. **Therapeutic uses.** Triamterene or amiloride is used in combination with other diuretic agents for the treatment of hypertension; this combined therapy augments the natriuretic effect while diminishing kaliuresis.

4. **Adverse effects**
   a. **Hyperkalemia** can occur; thus, K^+-sparing diuretics are not given in combination with one another and are contraindicated in hyperkalemic patients. Hyperkalemia is especially likely in patients with diabetes or in those with impaired renal function.
   b. **Reversible azotemia** is relatively common.
   c. **Gastrointestinal disturbances,** including nausea and vomiting, occur on occasion.
   d. **Leg cramps** may occur.
   e. **Dizziness** has been reported.
   f. Triamterene causes a slight **increase in serum acid** and, thus, should be used with caution in patients with gout.

B. **Spironolactone**

1. **Mechanism of action**
   a. Spironolactone, a competitive antagonist of the mineralocorticoid aldosterone, interferes with aldosterone-mediated Na^+–K^+ exchange, increasing Na^+ loss at the distal tubular site while decreasing K^+ loss.
   b. It is most effective when circulating aldosterone levels are high.

2. **Route of administration.** Spironolactone is usually given orally four times daily.

3. **Therapeutic uses**
   a. Spironolactone is often used as an adjunct to other diuretics to reduce the loss of K$^+$ in the management of refractory edema, such as that associated with Laënnec's cirrhosis.
   b. It also is used when adrenal gland tumors result in increased aldosterone levels.
   c. It can be used for edema resulting from congestive heart failure, although other diuretic agents are more effective.

4. **Adverse effects**
   a. **Hyperkalemia** can occur or be exacerbated, especially in patients with impaired renal function. Spironolactone is **contraindicated in patients with acute renal insufficiency or hyperkalemia** and is not given in combination with another K$^+$-sparing diuretic.
   b. **Gastrointestinal disturbances** include diarrhea.
   c. **Androgenic side effects** include menstrual irregularities and hirsutism.
   d. **CNS disturbances** include lethargy and mental confusion.

DIRECTIONS: The numbered item or incomplete statement in this section is followed by answers or by completions of the statement. Select the ONE lettered answer or completion that is BEST.

1. A patient with a history of glaucoma, epilepsy, and edema would be a candidate for treatment with which one of the following diuretics?

(A) Ethacrynic acid
(B) Chlorothiazide
(C) Furosemide
(D) Acetazolamide
(E) Spironolactone

DIRECTIONS: Each of the numbered items or incomplete statements in this section is negatively phrased, as indicated by a capitalized word such as NOT, LEAST, or EXCEPT. Select the ONE lettered answer or completion that is BEST in each case.

2. Furosemide is prescribed to treat significant edema in an elderly patient with severe, chronic heart failure. Shortly thereafter, the patient burns himself in the kitchen, and the physician prescribes gentamicin cream. The patient begins to feel better and breaks two doctor's appointments. Six weeks later, he returns for an office visit. Physical examination and laboratory parameters demonstrate significant adverse effects from the furosemide. These effects could include all of the following EXCEPT

(A) a fasting blood sugar level of 190 mg/dl
(B) an increased blood uric acid level
(C) decreased urinary excretion of calcium
(D) a serum potassium level of 2.8 mEq/L
(E) transient deafness

3. The potential for digitalis-induced cardiac arrhythmias is increased by each of the following diuretics EXCEPT

(A) ethacrynic acid
(B) chlorothiazide
(C) spironolactone
(D) furosemide
(E) mercaptomerin

4. The thiazide diuretics have a useful therapeutic effect in all of the following conditions EXCEPT

(A) chronic edema associated with cardiac decompensation
(B) antidiuretic hormone (ADH)-secreting pulmonary tumors
(C) hypercalciuria
(D) hypertension
(E) nephrosis

5. All of the following statements about mercurial diuretics are true EXCEPT

(A) their mercuric ion dissociates in an acidic environment
(B) they can induce a hypochloremic alkalosis
(C) they rarely produce a refractory state
(D) they must be given parenterally
(E) rapid intravenous administration can result in ventricular fibrillation

6. Properties of triamterene include all of the following EXCEPT

(A) it acts primarily in the distal nephron
(B) it inhibits the secretion of potassium
(C) it produces reversible azotemia relatively commonly
(D) it is weakly uricosuric
(E) it is a weak competitive antagonist of aldosterone

ANSWERS AND EXPLANATIONS

1. The answer is D *[IV C]*. The carbonic anhydrase inhibitor acetazolamide, although a weak diuretic, is useful in the treatment of glaucoma and petit mal epilepsy. The high-ceiling diuretics, namely ethacrynic acid and furosemide, the thiazide diuretic, chlorothiazide, and the potassium (K^+)-sparing diuretic, spironolactone, are not effective agents in the treatment of glaucoma or epilepsy, although they are more effective as diuretics.

2. The answer is C *[VII E]*. Loop (high-ceiling) diuretics (e.g., furosemide) increase, rather than decrease, urinary excretion of calcium. Electrolyte imbalances (e.g., hypokalemia) can occur. Because furosemide is actively secreted, it competes with renal uric acid secretion, resulting in hyperuricemia. Hyperglycemia can occur. Transient deafness may occur with the concomitant administration of aminoglycoside antibiotics, such as gentamicin.

3. The answer is C *[IX B]*. Reduction in serum potassium levels (hypokalemia) is a common adverse effect of most diuretics. Hypokalemia greatly increases the potential for digitalis-induced cardiac arrhythmias. The potassium (K^+)-sparing diuretics, such as spironolactone, do not produce hypokalemia and, thus, do not add to the toxic potential of digitalis.

4. The answer is B *[VI E]*. The thiazide diuretics are not useful in treating pulmonary tumors that secrete antidiuretic hormone (ADH). By decreasing the urinary volume (due to their natriuretic action), thiazide diuretics may enhance the action of ADH. Because of this effect, they have been used for the palliative treatment of diabetes insipidus.

5. The answer is C *[III A, D 2]*. With the use of mercurial diuretics, refractoriness does occur. Mercurial diuretics can produce a clinical metabolic picture of hypochloremic alkalosis. In an alkalotic environment, the mercuric ion will not dissociate from the drug into its active form; the result is that a refractory state soon develops, requiring use of an acidifying agent (e.g., ammonium chloride [NH_4Cl]) to reverse the alkalosis. Ventricular fibrillation is probably the result of binding to cardiac sulfhydryl enzymes.

6. The answer is E *[IX A; Figure 6-2]*. A potassium (K^+)-sparing diuretic, triamterene acts primarily in the distal nephron. The increased excretion of sodium and chloride induced by triamterene disrupts normal sodium transport and causes a net change in electrogenic forces across the tubular membranes. This reduces the net driving force for potassium secretion, resulting in decreased excretion of potassium. Triamterene also causes a slight increase in uric acid excretion. Triamterene is not a competitive antagonist of aldosterone. Unlike spironolactone, triamterene acts independently of aldosterone.

Chapter 7

Drugs Affecting Hematopoiesis and Hemostasis

I. DRUGS FOR IRON-DEFICIENCY ANEMIA

A. Physiology

1. The major portion of iron in body stores is found in **hemoglobin**.
   a. Molecular oxygen is bound reversibly by the iron in hemoglobin.
   b. The **ferric state of iron** (Fe^{3+}) **in methemoglobin** is less able to carry oxygen than the **ferrous form** (Fe^{2+}) **in hemoglobin**.

2. Inorganic iron in the ferrous form is most readily absorbed from the gastrointestinal tract.
   a. Men require a nutritional input of about 0.5–1 mg of iron per day.
   b. Menstruating women require up to 2 mg of iron per day.
   c. Although pregnant women (especially in the last two trimesters of pregnancy) require 5–6 mg of iron per day, there is little evidence that routine iron supplementation during pregnancy improves the clinical outcome of the mother, fetus, or newborn.

3. About 1 mg of iron is lost per day in the feces, sweat, and desquamated skin.
   a. Menstruating women can lose up to 30 mg of iron per menstrual period.
   b. Pregnant women can lose up to 500 mg of iron per full-term pregnancy.

4. About 1 g of iron is stored as **ferritin** and **hemosiderin** in the bone marrow, liver, and spleen. This stored iron is available for the synthesis of hemoglobin if blood is lost from the body.

5. Internal exchange of iron is mediated by a plasma transport protein, **transferrin**. Transferrin receptors on cell membranes mediate endocytosis of the transferrin–iron complex.

B. Pathophysiology of iron-deficiency anemia

1. **Symptoms.** Depletion of body iron can be associated with fatigability, anorexia, headache, and a characteristic hypochromic, microcytic anemia.

2. **Laboratory findings.** A low plasma iron level in iron-deficiency anemia is associated with an elevated total iron-binding capacity of plasma transferrin so that the ratio of serum iron to iron-binding capacity is less than 10%:

$$\frac{\text{Serum iron level}}{\text{Total iron-binding capacity}} < 10\%$$

In other words, the serum iron carrier, transferrin, is less than 10% saturated with iron. This ratio in normal individuals is 35% ± 15%.

3. **Diagnosis.** A definitive diagnosis of iron-deficiency anemia is made by confirming reduced bone marrow iron stores.

4. **Complications.** Severe iron deficiency can cause Plummer-Vinson syndrome, which is associated with dysphagia, hypopharyngeal webs, gastritis, and hypochlorhydria.

5. **Etiology.** Iron-deficiency anemia is often caused by significant blood loss. Underlying disorders should be sought.

C. **Oral iron**

1. **Preparations and therapeutic uses.** The different ferrous salt forms used in oral iron preparations have about the same bioavailability and are absorbed about three-fold better than ferric salt forms.
   a. **Ferrous sulfate,** containing about 20% elemental iron, is the drug of choice for iron-deficiency anemia.
   b. **Ferrous fumarate** contains 33% elemental iron. It is principally used in multivitamin–mineral mixtures.
   c. **Ferrous choline citrate** and **ferrous gluconate** both contain 12% elemental iron.

2. **Adverse effects** are related to the amount of soluble iron in the upper gastrointestinal tract.
   a. Nausea, heartburn, diarrhea, and constipation can all occur.
   b. Hemochromatosis is rare and is usually the result of an underlying disorder that augments the absorption of iron.

D. **Parenteral iron** is used in patients unable to take iron orally and in patients with malabsorption syndromes.

1. **Preparations. Iron dextran,** a complex of ferric hydroxide and low–molecular-weight dextran, is the preparation used parenterally. Each milliliter of iron dextran preparation contains 50 mg of elemental iron.

2. **Pharmacokinetics.** Reticuloendothelial cells phagocytize the iron dextran, splitting off the iron from the dextran molecule.

3. **Administration**
   a. Iron dextran delivered intramuscularly may become fixed (up to 50%) locally. This route is inappropriate unless the intravenous route is inaccessible.
   b. Because of serious local reactions, the **intravenous route is preferred**. A test dose is first given over a 5-minute period to test for anaphylaxis.

4. **Adverse effects**
   a. If given intramuscularly, iron dextran may cause local discomfort, discoloration, and potentially malignant skin changes.
   b. Headache, fever, arthralgias, and lymphadenopathy can occur.
   c. Anaphylactic reactions, although rare, can be fatal.

II. DRUGS FOR MEGALOBLASTIC ANEMIAS

A. **Etiology of megaloblastic anemia**

1. Megaloblastic anemia is almost always caused by deficiencies of vitamin B_{12} or folic acid. These vitamins are essential in DNA synthesis, and thus, the high cell turnover in hematopoiesis is dramatically affected by deficiencies.

2. The most helpful diagnostic tests are evaluations of serum folate and vitamin B_{12} levels, the Schilling test for urinary vitamin B_{12} excretion, and analysis of gastric function.

3. A characteristic morphologic feature is the abnormal macrocytic red blood cell.

B. **Folic acid**

1. **Daily requirements**
   a. Folic acid is found in a variety of foods, with its highest content found in yeast, liver, and green vegetables.
   b. The minimum daily adult dietary requirement is 50 µg, although pregnant or lactating women may need 100–200 µg per day.

2. **Physiology**
   a. Folic acid is completely absorbed in the proximal third of the small intestine.
   b. Folates present in food are in the reduced polyglutamate form. The mucosae of the duodenum and the upper jejunum contain dihydrofolate reductase, which methylates the reduced folate.
   c. Once absorbed, folate is transported to tissues where it is stored within cells as polyglutamate.
   d. Supplies are maintained by food intake and by the enterohepatic cycle.
   e. Folates and their cleavage products are mainly excreted through urine.
   f. Folic acid is a precursor of several coenzymes, and several derivatives of tetrahydrofolic acid are important in single carbon atom transfers, such as the synthesis of thymidylate from deoxyuridylate.

3. **Deficiency**
   a. Folate deficiency can result from:
      (1) Inadequate dietary supply
      (2) Disease involving the small intestine
      (3) Defects in the folate enterohepatic cycle (e.g., hepatic toxicity from alcoholism)
      (4) A low concentration of folate-binding proteins in plasma
      (5) Certain drugs (e.g., methotrexate, trimethoprim, anticoagulants, contraceptives)
      (6) Normal pregnancy, which produces an increased requirement for folate
   b. Folate deficiency can result in megaloblastic anemia.
      (1) The onset is more rapid than with a vitamin B_{12} deficiency.
      (2) There is **no neurologic abnormality associated with folate deficiency**.

4. **Therapeutic uses**
   a. The major therapeutic use for folic acid is in the therapy of folic acid deficiency.
   b. Leucovorin calcium (folinic acid) injection is used to circumvent the action of dihydrofolate reductase inhibitors, such as methotrexate. It is not used as a treatment for ordinary folate deficiency.

5. **Preparations and administration**
   a. Folic acid can be given orally (or parenterally) and usually cures an uncomplicated megaloblastic anemia resulting from folate deficiency.
   b. Folic acid injection contains the sodium salt and is principally used in acute illness. It is given by intramuscular, intravenous, or deep subcutaneous injection.

6. **Adverse effects**
   a. The oral form of folic acid is nontoxic at therapeutic doses, but large amounts may counteract the antiepileptic action of phenobarbital, phenytoin, and primidone.
   b. There have been rare allergic reactions to parenteral administration.

C. **Vitamin B_{12}** is essential for cell growth and for maintenance of normal myelin. It is also important for the normal metabolic functions of folate.

1. **Physiology**
   a. Vitamin B_{12} (cyanocobalamin) is a cobalt-containing compound that is synthesized by the bacterial flora in the colon. However, it cannot be absorbed there, and humans must obtain the vitamin from the dietary intake of meat and vegetables that possess B_{12}-forming bacteria.
   b. **Intrinsic factor,** a glycoprotein produced by the gastric parietal cells, is necessary for the gastrointestinal absorption of vitamin B_{12}.
      (1) Gastric acid releases the vitamin from proteins, allowing it to form a complex with intrinsic factor.
      (2) The vitamin B_{12}–intrinsic factor complex binds to ileal mucosal cell receptors, from where it is transported into the circulation.
   c. Once in the circulation, vitamin B_{12} is transported to the tissues by a plasma β-globulin, transcobalamin II.

d. The liver preferentially stores vitamin B_{12}. A portion of the stored vitamin is secreted into the bile each day and is normally reabsorbed in the ileum.

2. Deficiency
  a. Vitamin B_{12} deficiency can result from:
    (1) Inadequate secretion of intrinsic factor
    (2) Intestinal disorders, including ileal disease, gastric atrophy, or surgery
    (3) An insufficient dietary supply, although this is rarely the case
    (4) Congenital absence of transcobalamin II
    (5) Interference with the reabsorption of vitamin B_{12} excreted in the bile
  b. Vitamin B_{12} deficiency can result in:
    (1) Megaloblastic anemia; although this is most common, all blood cell lines can be affected, resulting in pancytopenia
    (2) Demyelination and cell death, which can produce irreversible damage to the central nervous system (CNS)

3. Therapeutic uses
  a. The most common therapeutic use for vitamin B_{12} is the treatment of pernicious anemia (addisonian anemia). This condition is usually caused by atrophy of the gastric mucosa with achlorhydria and failure to secrete intrinsic factor.
  b. Lifetime maintenance therapy with vitamin B_{12} is required.

4. Preparations and administration
  a. If the patient lacks intrinsic factor or has ileal disease, vitamin B_{12} must be administered parenterally. Cyanocobalamin injection, a bright red solution, is administered by the intramuscular or deep subcutaneous route, but never intravenously.
  b. Oral combinations of vitamin B_{12} with intrinsic factor usually produce unreliable absorption; therefore, this approach is not recommended.

5. Adverse effects from vitamin B_{12} administration are rare.

III. ERYTHROPOIETIN FOR ANEMIA ASSOCIATED WITH CHRONIC RENAL FAILURE

A. Physiology

1. Erythropoietin is a glycoprotein hormone produced by the kidneys and released in response to tissue hypoxemia. It is a primary regulator of erythropoiesis.

2. Erythropoietin stimulates the proliferation of immature erythroid progenitor cells. These cells give rise to marrow normoblasts, the immediate precursors of reticulocytes and mature red blood cells.

3. Erythropoietin has been produced by recombinant DNA technology as a 165-amino acid glycoprotein.
  a. It contains the identical amino acid sequence of isolated natural erythropoietin.
  b. Antibodies to erythropoietin have not been detected.

B. Pharmacokinetics

1. Erythropoietin is administered parenterally (intravenously or subcutaneously) because it is broken down in the gastrointestinal tract.

2. The half-life ranges from 5–13 hours when administered intravenously to patients in chronic renal failure.

3. The pharmacokinetics of erythropoietin are not affected by dialysis.

C. Therapeutic uses

1. Erythropoietin is indicated for the treatment of anemia associated with chronic renal failure, including patients on and off dialysis.

2. Erythropoietin elevates or maintains red blood cell levels, decreasing the need for transfusions.

3. Erythropoietin is not intended for patients needing immediate correction of severe anemia.

4. Recent data suggest that erythropoietin may also be useful for treating anemia in patients with AIDS who are being treated with zidovudine, but only in patients with low endogenous erythropoietin levels.

D. Adverse effects

1. Hypertension may occur.

2. Seizures may occur, especially during the first 90 days of treatment.

3. High doses of heparin may be needed for adequate anticoagulation during hemodialysis.

IV. COLONY-STIMULATING FACTORS (CSFs) FOR WHITE BLOOD CELL DEFICIENCY

A. Physiology

1. CSFs are **naturally occurring cytokine glycoproteins** that stimulate the proliferation, differentiation, and activity of neutrophils, monocytes, and macrophages.
   a. **Granulocyte CSF (G-CSF)** affects neutrophils.
   b. **Granulocyte-macrophage CSF (GM-CSF)** affects neutrophils, monocytes, and macrophages.

2. **Recombinant forms** of these glycoproteins have been formed by cloning the genes for the CSFs.
   a. **Filgrastim** is the **synthetic form of G-CSF.**
   b. **Sargramostim** is the **synthetic form of GM-CSF.**

B. Filgrastim and sargramostim

1. **Pharmacologic effects**
   a. When administered to patients with normal bone marrow function, an increase in the number of white blood cells occurs within 2–3 days.
   b. In patients with bone marrow suppression, a similar increase occurs within 7–14 days. When these agents are administered to AIDS patients following zidovudine therapy, the number of neutrophils increases but the incidence of opportunistic infections remains the same.

2. **Therapeutic uses**
   a. These agents are used for the short-term treatment of **patients with primary bone marrow deficiency states or dysfunction** (e.g., following cancer chemotherapy or bone marrow transplantation)
   b. In **patients with aplastic anemia,** administration of filgrastim and sargramostim increases the number of neutrophils and decreases infectious complications.

3. **Administration.** Filgrastim and sargramostim may be administered subcutaneously or intravenously.

4. Adverse effects
   a. Filgrastim can cause bone pain, splenomegaly, and abnormalities in uric acid concentrations and lactate dehydrogenase.
   b. Sargramostim can cause fluid accumulation, including pleural and pericardial effusions.

V. ANTICOAGULANTS FOR HEMOSTASIS

A. Heparin and enoxaparin

1. **Pharmacokinetics**
   a. Heparin is a highly negatively charged mucopolysaccharide that is prepared commercially from bovine lung and porcine intestinal mucosa. Because of its highly negative charge and large molecular size, it is **administered parenterally**.
   (1) Heparin displays dose-dependent half-life kinetics, although the half-life may be prolonged in cirrhotic patients or patients with renal dysfunction.
   (2) Heparin is metabolized in the liver by heparinase. The inactive products are excreted in the urine.
   b. Enoxaparin, a low–molecular-weight heparin, is formed by depolymerizing standard heparin. Enoxaparin is more bioavailable and has a longer half-life than standard heparin.

2. **Pharmacologic effects**
   a. Heparin
   (1) Heparin prolongs the clotting time of blood, both in vivo and in vitro, by preventing fibrin formation during the process of coagulation (Figure 7-1).
       (a) Heparin increases the activity of antithrombin III, which inhibits the conversion of prothrombin to thrombin by thromboplastin and directly inactivates thrombin.
       (b) Heparin inactivates Factors IXa, Xa, XIa, and XIIa.
   (2) Injected heparin causes the release of tissue-bound lipoprotein lipase, which hydrolyzes the triglycerides of chylomicrons and low-density lipoproteins bound to capillary endothelial cells. This produces a clearing effect on postprandial turbid lipemic plasma.
   (3) Heparin suppresses the rate of aldosterone secretion and increases the concentration of free thyroxine.
   (4) Heparin slows wound healing and probably also depresses cell-mediated immunity.
   b. Enoxaparin has relatively more anti-Factor Xa activity than heparin. Factor Xa converts prothrombin to thrombin.

3. **Therapeutic uses**
   a. Because heparin, enoxaparin, and the oral anticoagulants reduce the rate of fibrin formation, they are primarily used in the **prophylaxis of venous thrombosis**. Venous (red) thrombi consist of a fibrin network enmeshed with red blood cells and platelets.
   b. The anticoagulants are generally ineffective in the treatment of arterial (white) thrombi, made up of adhering platelets. Arterial thrombi are treated with the antithrombotics and thrombolytics (see V C).

4. **Preparations and administration**
   a. Heparin
   (1) The prophylactic treatment of venous thrombotic disease usually involves an intravenous bolus dose and continuous infusion.
   (2) In the preoperative use of heparin to prevent postoperative venous thrombosis and embolism, a low dose is given by subcutaneous injection, then additional intermittent subcutaneous injections are given.
   (3) Heparin therapy is monitored by the **partial thromboplastin time (PTT)**.

INTRINSIC SYSTEM

FIGURE 7-1. The coagulation cascade. Heparin inactivates factors XIIa, XIa, IXa, and Xa and increases the activity of antithrombin III (*shading*). Antithrombin III inhibits the conversion of prothrombin to thrombin and directly inactivates thrombin. *Open arrows* indicate conversion of a substrate or a reactant to a product. (Modified with permission from *NMS Hematology*. Baltimore, Williams & Wilkins, 1992, p 225.)

      (a) The test is done at any time during continuous infusion therapy; if the heparin is given intermittently, the PTT is measured before an injection.

      (b) During therapy, the PTT should be twice the control value.

      (c) Once the PTT is stable, daily monitoring is performed.

   (4) Intramuscular injections are contraindicated because they can cause painful hematomas.

  b. Enoxaparin is effective for preventing deep venous thrombosis after hip replacement (30 mg administered twice daily by subcutaneous injection for 7–10 days).

5. Adverse effects and contraindications

  a. Heparin

   (1) Hypersensitivity reactions can occur. A test dose should be given to patients with a prior allergic history.

   (2) Hemorrhage resulting from excessive blockade of fibrin formation and interference with normal hemostasis accounts for the primary toxicity of heparin. Bleeding should be reduced by careful control of dosage.

   (3) Osteoporosis may complicate prolonged heparin therapy.

   (4) Transient alopecia can occur.

   (5) Transient thrombocytopenia can occur in up to 25% of patients receiving heparin therapy, resulting from heparin-induced platelet aggregation; severe cases result from the formation of heparin-dependent antiplatelet antibodies.

   (6) Heparin is **contraindicated** in patients who are hypersensitive to the drug. Bacterial endocarditis, active tuberculosis, recent head trauma, neurosurgery, and recent major surgery are also contraindications to the use of heparin or other anticoagulants.

b. Enoxaparin. Because enoxaparin causes less inactivation of thrombin, less inhibition of platelets, and less vascular permeability than heparin, bleeding complications may be slightly lower than with heparin.

B. Warfarin

1. **Pharmacokinetics**
   a. Racemic warfarin (i.e., the mixture of the dextro- and levo-forms) is well-absorbed orally and reaches peak plasma concentrations in 1 hour.
   b. Warfarin is 99% bound to plasma albumin, which prevents its diffusion into red blood cells, cerebrospinal fluid, urine, and breast milk.
   c. Warfarin is metabolized in the liver, undergoes enterohepatic circulation, and then is excreted in the urine and feces.

2. **Pharmacologic effects**
   a. The coumarin-derived anticoagulants interfere with vitamin K–dependent synthesis of active coagulation Factors II (prothrombin), VII, IX, and X.
   b. The oral anticoagulants are effective only in vivo. Their therapeutic effect depends on the half-lives of Factors II, VII, IX, and X; thus, 8–12 hours are required for action.

3. **Preparations and administration**
   a. For warfarin sodium and warfarin potassium, the maintenance dose is determined by **one-stage prothrombin activity,** which should be about 1 1/2–2 1/2 times the control value. For more adults, this dosage is 5 mg/day. Once the prothrombin activity is stable, bimonthly checks are sufficient.
   b. Warfarin sodium is available in injectable form, but parenteral administration is seldom needed.

4. **Factors affecting activity**
   a. Conditions that **increase the response to anticoagulants** include:
      (1) Anything that can cause vitamin K deficiency, such as disease of the small bowel
      (2) Hypermetabolic states, such as hyperthyroidism
      (3) Debilitating states, such as congestive heart failure
      (4) Age: the older the patient, the greater the response to these anticoagulants
      (5) Impaired hepatic synthesis of clotting factors can lead to an increased hypoprothrombinemic response to oral anticoagulants during hepatic disease or in alcoholic individuals. Excessively reduced levels of prothrombin result in hemorrhage.
   b. Conditions that **decrease the response to anticoagulants** include pregnancy. During pregnancy, vitamin K–dependent factors are increased, resulting in a **decreased** responsiveness to oral anticoagulants. Because heparin does not cross the placenta, it is considered safe for the fetus.
   c. Table 7-1 lists the **drugs that increase or decrease the response** to oral anticoagulants.

5. **Therapeutic uses**
   a. These agents are widely used in the secondary prophylactic treatment of venous thrombosis and pulmonary embolism to prevent the recurrence or extension of venous thrombus formation.
   b. Because oral anticoagulants have no effect on platelets, they are not used in the treatment of thrombotic disease in the arterial system.

6. **Adverse effects**
   a. **Major bleeding** occurs in 2% of patients, whereas minor bleeding occurs in 5%.
   b. **Warfarin necrosis** is a painful erythematous patch on the skin that can progress to gangrene. This condition occurs most frequently in women, usually within 3–10 days of starting warfarin therapy. Thrombi occur in the vasculature of affected tissue.
   c. A **"purple toe" syndrome** can occur 3–8 weeks after starting warfarin therapy. It is caused by cholesterol emboli from atheromatous plaques, following bleeding into the plaques.
   d. Warfarin is **contraindicated in pregnancy** but not for the nursing mother, because it is not excreted in milk.

TABLE 7-1. Drug Interactions with Oral Anticoagulants

Drugs	Effect on Response to Anticoagulant	Mechanism
Acetylsalicylic acid	↑	↓ ADP release by platelets, impairing platelet aggregation
Barbiturates, glutethimide	↓	Induce drug microsomal metabolizing system
Cholestyramine	↓	↓ hypoprothrombinemia; ↑ plasma clearance of drug
Cimetidine	↑	Unknown
Clofibrate	↑	↓ platelet adhesiveness and ↑ turnover of vitamin K–dependent factors
Disulfiram, metronidazole, trimethoprim–sulfamethoxazole	↑	↑ hypoprothrombinemia by prolonging levowarfarin half-life
Phenobarbital	↓	↑ biotransformation of coumarin
Phenylbutazone, oxyphenbutazone	↑	Impair platelet aggregation; displace warfarin from albumin
Rifampin	↓	↓ blood concentration of drug

ADP = adenosine diphosphate; ↑ = increased; ↓ = decreased.

e. The risk of **subdural or intracerebral hematoma** is 10-fold higher in long-term patients older than 50 years of age.

7. Reversal of anticoagulant effects

　　a. Following discontinuation of oral anticoagulants, the one-stage prothrombin time (PT) gradually returns to normal. Oral administration of **vitamin K$_1$ (phytonadione)** enhances recovery.

　　b. For severe hemorrhage, phytonadione is given intravenously. The one-stage PT activity returns to normal within 6–12 hours, no matter how much coumarin anticoagulant is ingested. Phytonadione is administered slowly to avoid precipitating a hypotensive episode. Fresh frozen plasma or coagulation-factor concentrate may be needed when bleeding is severe.

C. | Antithrombotic and thrombolytic drugs

1. General considerations

　　a. Antithrombotic agents are those agents that prevent or reduce the formation of arterial platelet thrombi. The antithrombotic actions of **aspirin** and **sulfinpyrazone** are discussed in Chapter 9 II A 3 h and IV C 4, respectively, and those of **dipyridamole** in Chapter 5 III D 2.

　　b. Thrombolytic drugs [e.g., **streptokinase, anistreplase (eminase), recombinant tissue-type plasminogen activator (t-PA),** and **urokinase**] are used in acute, extensive thromboembolic disease, acting via the conversion of endogenous plasminogen to plasmin, a protease. The newly formed plasmin hydrolyzes fibrin in hemostatic plugs and degrades fibrinogen and Factors V and VII.

　　　　(1) Thrombotic coronary artery occlusion occurs in more than 80% of patients with acute transmural myocardial infarction. Recent data suggest that, when administered to patients after myocardial infarction, t-PA produces a greater reduction of mortality rates than streptokinase.

　　　　(2) The use of thrombolytic agents is contraindicated in the presence of recent stroke, craniotomy, head trauma, or brain tumor.

2. Preparations

a. Streptokinase is a purified preparation of a bacterial protein elaborated by group C β-hemolytic streptococci.

(1) Pharmacokinetics

(a) Streptokinase produces an activator complex that converts plasminogen to plasmin. The half-life of the activator complex is 80 minutes.

(b) The mechanism of elimination is unknown. The complex is inactivated in part by antistreptococcal antibodies.

(c) A loading dose of 25 mg (250,000) must be given to overcome plasma antibodies.

(2) Pharmacologic effects

(a) Streptokinase decreases fibrinogen levels for 24–36 hours.

(b) Plasma and blood viscosity and red blood cell aggregation are decreased.

(c) Intravenous administration reduces blood pressure, total peripheral resistance, and cardiac afterload.

(3) Therapeutic uses

(a) The primary use of streptokinase is for the management of acute myocardial infarction resulting from intracoronary thrombi. Fibrinolytics may be administered intravenously or by the intracoronary route.

(b) Reduction in acute mortality is 20%–30% and is time-dependent with the greatest recovery rate among patients treated within 1 hour of onset of chest pain.

(c) Left ventricular ejection fraction improves in 3%–6% of patients.

(d) Streptokinase is used for lysis of pulmonary emboli, deep venous thrombosis, and acute arterial thrombi and emboli not originating from the left side of the heart.

(e) It can be used to clear occluded arteriovenous cannulae.

(4) Adverse effects

(a) Systemic bleeding, particularly intracranial hemorrhage, occurs in 1% of patients. Gastrointestinal bleeding occurs in 5%–10% of patients.

(b) Hypotension may occur.

(c) Allergic reactions, ranging from minor bronchospasm to anaphylactic reactions, are common.

(d) Reperfusion atrial or ventricular dysrhythmias may occur.

b. Anistreplase (eminase) is a plasminogen activator approved for the intravenous treatment of coronary thrombosis. Anistreplase is an acylated inactive complex of streptokinase and human lys-plasminogen.

(1) Pharmacokinetics. Anistreplase has a half-life of 90 minutes. Slow hydrolysis of the acyl group accounts for its long half-life. It does not require a prolonged infusion.

(2) Pharmacologic effects

(a) After injection, the acyl group slowly hydrolyzes, producing an activator that converts plasminogen to plasmin, initiating fibrinolysis.

(b) Like streptokinase, anistreplase reduces acute mortality and improves the left ventricular ejection fraction.

(3) Therapeutic uses. Management of acute myocardial infarction consists of the intravenous administration of anistreplase to lyse intracoronary thrombi. Intravenous administration is more convenient because it does not require prolonged infusion.

(4) Adverse effects

(a) Bolus injections may produce systemic bleeding and hematoma formation at the catheter entry site (30%), intracranial hemorrhage (< 21%), and gastrointestinal bleeding (5%–10%).

(b) Hypotension, allergic reactions, and reperfusion dysrhythmias have been reported.

c. t-PA is a commercial formulation of a naturally occurring thrombolytic enzyme.

(1) Pharmacokinetics. t-PA is rapidly metabolized in the liver and excreted in the urine. The half-life is only 5 minutes. After 10 minutes, 80% of the dose is cleared from the blood.

    (2) Pharmacologic effects
       (a) t-PA selectively promotes the conversion of plasminogen to plasmin in the presence of fibrin.
       (b) t-PA binds to fibrin and activates bound plasminogen several hundred times more rapidly than circulating plasminogen.
    (3) Therapeutic uses and administration. Management of acute myocardial infarction resulting from intracoronary thrombi is the primary use of t-PA.
       (a) As with thrombolytics, treatment should be initiated as soon as possible after the onset of symptoms.
       (b) Heparin is generally given with t-PA to maintain patency of catheters and prevent reocclusion of coronary arteries.
    (4) Adverse effects
       (a) Bleeding complications include:
          (i) Hematomas at the catheterization site (40%)
          (ii) Intracranial hemorrhage (1%)
          (iii) Gastrointestinal bleeding (5%–10%)
       (b) Serious allergic reactions have not been reported.
       (c) Reperfusion dysrhythmias have been reported.
  d. Urokinase is an enzyme produced by the kidney and found in the urine.
    (1) Pharmacokinetics. Urokinase is administered intravenously and is cleared rapidly by the liver. The half-life is 20 minutes.
    (2) Pharmacologic effects. Urokinase converts endogenous plasminogen to the enzyme plasmin, which degrades fibrin clots, fibrinogen, and other plasma proteins.
    (3) Therapeutic uses
       (a) Urokinase is used in cases of acute massive pulmonary emboli.
       (b) Urokinase is used to restore patency to intravenous catheters.
       (c) Urokinase is used in cases of acute thrombi obstructing coronary arteries. (It has not been demonstrated that intracoronary administration during transmural myocardial infarction results in myocardial salvage or improved mortality.)
    (4) Adverse effects
       (a) Systemic bleeding, similar to that which occurs with use of streptokinase, results from poor plasminogen selectivity.
       (b) Allergic reactions are usually mild and rare.
       (c) Fever occurs in 2%–3% of treated patients.

D. **Other drugs affecting blood flow**

1. **Pentoxifylline,** a methylxanthine derivative, is used for the treatment of intermittent claudication resulting from occlusive arterial disease.
  a. Mechanism of action
    (1) Pentoxifylline is thought to increase the flexibility of erythrocytes, thereby easing their passage through the capillary microcirculation.
    (2) Serum fibrinogen is also reduced, and platelet aggregation is inhibited.
  b. Pentoxifylline is metabolized by the liver and is excreted by the kidney within 24 hours after an oral dose.
  c. Adverse effects include minor nausea, dizziness, and headache.

2. **Danazol,** a synthetic androgen, has been found to increase serum concentrations of clotting Factors VIII and IX, but long-term use in the treatment of hemophilias A and B has not proved efficacious. However, danazol has been associated with a rise in platelet count in patients with idiopathic thrombocytopenic purpura and with a rise in serum α_1-antitrypsin activity in those with α_1-antitrypsin deficiency.

STUDY QUESTIONS

DIRECTIONS: Each of the numbered items or incomplete statements in this section is negatively phrased, as indicated by a capitalized word such as NOT, LEAST, or EXCEPT. Select the ONE lettered answer or completion that is BEST in each case.

1. All of the following statements about iron-deficiency anemia are true EXCEPT

(A) menstruating women require about twice as much dietary iron as men do
(B) iron deficiency can lead to the Plummer-Vinson syndrome
(C) ferrous sulfate is the drug of choice for iron-deficiency anemia
(D) ferrous sulfate contains more than 90% elemental iron
(E) diarrhea or constipation can occur with ferrous sulfate use

2. Folate deficiency can result from all of the following EXCEPT

(A) inadequate secretion of intrinsic factor
(B) inadequate dietary supply
(C) disease involving the small intestine
(D) low concentration of folate-binding proteins in plasma
(E) defects in the folate enterohepatic cycle

3. Vitamin B_{12} has all of the following characteristics EXCEPT

(A) it is a cobalt-containing compound
(B) it is synthesized by the bacterial flora in the colon
(C) it is preferentially stored in the bone marrow
(D) it is obtained from the dietary intake of animal products
(E) it is required for myelin maintenance

4. Vitamin B_{12} deficiency can result from all of the following EXCEPT

(A) an insufficient dietary supply
(B) inadequate secretion of intrinsic factor
(C) ileal disease
(D) excessive transcobalamin II
(E) interference with the reabsorption of vitamin B_{12} excreted in the bile

5. A patient with chronic renal failure is given erythropoietin. Adverse effects that need monitoring include all of the following EXCEPT

(A) hypertension
(B) seizures
(C) antibody production of erythropoietin
(D) partial thromboplastin time (PTT)

6. All of the following statements regarding enoxaparin are true EXCEPT

(A) it has more anti-Factor Xa activity than standard heparin
(B) it is more bioavailable and has a shorter half-life than standard heparin
(C) bleeding complications are similar or slightly lower than those that occur with standard heparin
(D) it causes less inactivation of thrombin than standard heparin
(E) it causes less inhibition of platelets than standard heparin

7. Heparin administration would be contraindicated in all of the following situations EXCEPT

(A) active tuberculosis
(B) bacterial endocarditis
(C) certain types of surgery
(D) diffuse intravascular coagulopathy
(E) thrombocytopenia

8. The therapeutic effect of sodium warfarin depends on the half-lives of all of the following coagulation factors EXCEPT

(A) II
(B) V
(C) VII
(D) IX
(E) X

9. A patient with metastatic cancer is treated with high-dose cancer chemotherapy. A bone marrow deficiency state results. Filgrastim is administered. All of the following statements are true EXCEPT

(A) administration of filgrastim stimulates proliferation, differentiation, and functional activity of neutrophils
(B) a rise in white blood cell count is seen in 2–3 days in this patient
(C) administration can result in bone pain
(D) administration can result in splenomegaly
(E) this drug would also be beneficial for an AIDS patient

10. All of the following drugs, if given concomitantly with warfarin, would probably require a reduction in warfarin dosage EXCEPT

(A) aspirin
(B) barbiturates
(C) cimetidine
(D) disulfiram
(E) phenylbutazone

11. A patient comes to the emergency room complaining of significant chest pain. An electrocardiogram reveals an evolving myocardial infarction and tissue-type plasminogen activator (t-PA) therapy is initiated. All of the following statements are true EXCEPT

(A) t-PA treatment should begin as soon as possible
(B) heparin should be administered with the t-PA
(C) after 10 minutes, 80% of the dose can be found circulating in the blood
(D) a hematoma at the catheterization site is common
(E) intracranial hemorrhage is a rare but serious complication

DIRECTIONS: Each set of matching questions in this section consists of a list of four to twenty-six lettered options (some of which may be in figures) followed by several numbered items. For each numbered item, select the ONE lettered option that is most closely associated with it. To avoid spending too much time on matching sets with large numbers of options, it is generally advisable to begin each set by reading the list of options. Then, for each item in the set, try to generate the correct answer and locate it in the option list, rather than evaluating each option individually. Each lettered option may be selected once, more than once, or not at all.

Questions 12–14

The response to a dose of an oral anticoagulant is often changed by concomitant administration of other drugs. Match each mechanism to the appropriate drug.

(A) Phenobarbital
(B) Rifampin
(C) Clofibrate
(D) Acetylsalicylic acid

12. Impairs platelet aggregation, increasing the response to the oral anticoagulant

13. Induces the drug microsomal metabolism system, decreasing the response to the oral anticoagulant

14. Reduces platelet adhesiveness and increases turnover of vitamin K–dependent factors, increasing the response to the oral anticoagulant

Questions 15–17

Match each thrombolytic agent with the statement that most aptly describes it.

(A) Streptokinase
(B) Tissue-type plasminogen activator (t-PA)
(C) Urokinase
(D) Anistreplase

15. The acyl group is hydrolyzed slowly, accounting for the longer half-life

16. Least likely agent to cause serious allergic reactions

17. Enzyme produced by the kidney

1. The answer is D *[I A 2, B 4, C 1 a, 2].* Ferrous sulfate contains about 20% elemental iron. All of the other statements are true. Men require about 0.5–1 mg of iron daily, while menstruating women require up to 2 mg/day. The Plummer-Vinson syndrome is associated with severe iron deficiency and is characterized by dysphagia, hypopharyngeal webs, gastritis, and hypochlorhydria. Diarrhea or constipation, nausea, and heartburn can all occur with oral iron preparations.

2. The answer is A *[II B 3 a (1)–(4)].* Inadequate secretion of intrinsic factor can result in vitamin B_{12} deficiency. Folate deficiency can result from an inadequate dietary supply or disease, which would affect its absorption in the small intestine. Low concentrations of folate-binding proteins in plasma can result in folate deficiency. Hepatic toxicity from alcoholism can result in defects in the folate enterohepatic cycle.

3. The answer is C *[II C 1 a, d].* The liver, not the bone marrow, preferentially stores vitamin B_{12}. Vitamin B_{12} is a cobalt-containing compound that is synthesized by the bacterial flora in the colon. However, because it cannot be absorbed there, humans must obtain vitamin B_{12} from the dietary intake of animal products, some legumes, or vitamin supplements. A portion of the stored vitamin is secreted into the bile each day and is absorbed in the ileum. Vitamin B_{12} is essential for cell growth and for the maintenance of normal myelin. It is also important for the normal metabolic functions of folate.

4. The answer is D *[II C 2 a].* Congenital absence of transcobalamin II, the plasma β-globulin that transports vitamin B_{12}, can result in vitamin B_{12} deficiency. Because vitamin B_{12} is available in many dietary animal products, some legumes, and many vitamin supplements and because only minute amounts are required, vitamin B_{12} deficiency is highly unlikely to occur, except in strict vegetarians or in individuals with reabsorption defects, including those with ileal disease or with inadequate secretion of intrinsic factor.

5. The answer is C *[III D 1–4].* Antibodies to erythropoietin have not been detected. A patient with chronic renal failure who has been given erythropoietin should be monitored for hypertension and seizures. Increased

doses of heparin may be necessary for adequate anticoagulation.

6. The answer is B *[V A 1 b, 2 b, 5 b (2)].* Enoxaparin is more bioavailable but has a longer half-life than standard heparin. Enoxaparin is produced by depolymerizing standard heparin, creating lower molecular-weight fragments. Compared with standard heparin, enoxaparin has more anti-Factor Xa activity and causes less inactivation of thrombin and less inhibition of platelets. Bleeding complications are similar or slightly less than those associated with standard heparin.

7. The answer is D *[V A 5 f].* Heparin is an acceptable form of therapy for diffuse intravascular coagulopathy. Heparin is contraindicated when the patient has a low platelet count. Bacterial endocarditis, active tuberculosis, and certain types of surgery are also contraindications to heparin use.

8. The answer is B *[IV B 2 b].* Sodium warfarin is the prototype of the coumarin-derived anticoagulants. The therapeutic effect of this class of anticoagulants depends on the half-lives of Factors II, VII, IX, and X; thus, 8–12 hours are required for action. Factor V is unaffected.

9. The answer is B *[IV B 1 b, 2, 4].* When administered to patients with normal bone marrow function, filgrastim, a granulocyte colony-stimulating factor (G-CSF), produces a rise in white blood cell count in 2–3 days; but when it is given to individuals with bone marrow suppression, the rise doesn't occur until 7–14 days following administration. G-CSF stimulates proliferation, differentiation, and functional activity of neutrophils; a granulocyte–macrophage colony-stimulating factor (GM-CSF), such as sargramostim, would affect monocytes and macrophages as well. Administration of filgrastim may result in bone pain, splenomegaly, and abnormalities in uric acid concentrations and lactate dehydrogenase. Short-term treatment using filgrastim would also be appropriate for bone marrow transplant patients, AIDS patients, and patients with aplastic anemia.

10. The answer is B *[V B 4; Table 7-1].* Barbiturates and glutethimide reduce the response to warfarin and, thus, would probably require an increase in warfarin dosage because they induce the hepatic enzyme system that increases drug metabolism. Disulfiram, aspirin, phenylbutazone, and cimetidine increase the response to warfarin and other oral anticoagulants; thus, their use would probably require a reduction in warfarin dosage. Disulfiram affects warfarin activity by prolonging the half-life of levowarfarin; this effect increases hypoprothrombinemia. Aspirin and phenylbutazone both impair platelet aggregation. Cimetidine binds to cytochrome P-450, thereby diminishing the activity of the hepatic microsomal mixed-function oxidases.

11. The answer is C *[V C 2 c (1)–(4)]*. The half-life of tissue-type plasminogen activator (t-PA) is only 5 minutes, and after 10 minutes, 80% of the dose is cleared from the blood. t-PA treatment should be administered as soon as possible after onset of symptoms. Heparin is generally given with t-PA to maintain patency of catheters and prevent reocclusion of coronary arteries. Bleeding complications include hematomas at the catheterization site (40%), gastrointestinal bleeding (5%–10%), and intracranial hemorrhage (1%).

12–14. The answers are: 12-D *[Table 7-1]*, **13-A** *[Table 7-1]*, **14-C** *[Table 7-1]*. Acetylsalicylic acid decreases adenosine diphosphate

(ADP) release from platelets, resulting in impaired platelet aggregation and an increased response to orally administered oral anticoagulant.

Phenobarbital induces the drug microsomal metabolizing system, increasing the biotransformation of orally administered anticoagulant and decreasing its effective response.

Clofibrate decreases platelet adhesiveness and increases turnover of vitamin K–dependent factors, increasing response to orally administered anticoagulant.

15–17. The answers are: 15-D *[V C 2 b (1)]*, **16-B** *[V C 2 c (4)]*, **17-C** *[V C 2 d]*. Anistreplase is a plasminogen activator, which is an acylate inactive complex of streptokinase and human lys-plasminogen. Slow hydrolysis of the acyl group accounts for its long half-life.

Tissue-type plasminogen activator (t-PA) is a formulation of naturally occurring thrombolytic enzyme for which no serious allergic reactions have been reported. Streptokinase and anistreplase have the greatest chance of causing an allergic reaction.

Urokinase is an enzyme produced by the kidney and found in the urine. It converts endogenous plasminogen to the enzyme plasmin.

Chapter 8
Autacoids and Their Antagonists

I. INTRODUCTION

A. Definitions

1. **Autacoids** are circulating or locally acting hormone-like substances that originate from diffuse tissues.

2. **Autacoid antagonists** inhibit the synthesis or the receptor interactions of certain autacoids.

B. Physiologic roles

1. The two main functions of the autacoids are to **modulate local circulation** and to **influence the process of inflammation**.

2. Many autacoids have other physiologic and pathologic functions, which are not readily understood.

3. Some autacoid antagonists have therapeutic value.

C. Major classes. Autacoids can be divided into three categories on the basis of their structure:

1. **Decarboxylated amino acids** include histamine and serotonin.

2. **Polypeptides** include angiotensins, kinins, vasoactive intestinal polypeptide (VIP), and substance P.

3. **Eicosanoids** include prostaglandins (PGs), leukotrienes (LTs), and thromboxanes (TXs).

II. DECARBOXYLATED AMINO ACIDS

A. Histamine (Figure 8-1)

1. **Chemistry**
   a. **Biosynthesis.** Histamine is derived chiefly from dietary histidine, which is decarboxylated by *l*-histidine decarboxylase.

FIGURE 8-1. Histamine.

b. Metabolism. In humans, histamine is metabolized primarily by methylation to form 1-methylhistamine, which can undergo oxidation by monoamine oxidase (MAO) to form 1-methylimidazole acetic acid.

c. Storage sites. Histamine is stored in almost all mammalian tissues, although its concentration varies greatly.

   (1) The **principal sites of storage** are the **lungs, skin,** and **intestinal mucosa**.

      (a) Histamine that is stored in the **mucosal cells of the stomach** can be released by mechanical stimuli, such as food and vagal stimulation. The released gastric histamine regulates intestinal contraction and gastric secretion.

      (b) In **skin and lung tissue,** histamine is thought to be important in tissue growth and repair as well as in allergic responses.

      (c) In the central nervous system (CNS), a high concentration of histamine can be found in the **hypothalamus,** where it is thought to be released as a neurotransmitter.

   (2) Histamine is stored chiefly in **mast cells**. Although some nonmast cells can store the autacoid, in most such cells, histamine is synthesized but not stored.

2. Receptor classification. Three classes of receptors mediate the action of histamine.

   a. H_1 receptors are responsible for the contraction of bronchial and intestinal smooth muscle, vasodilation, increased capillary permeability, and pruritus.

      (1) The prototypical agonist is 2-methylhistamine.

      (2) Prototypical antagonists include pyrilamine, chlorpheniramine, and diphenhydramine.

   b. H_2 receptors principally regulate gastric acid secretion but can also cause vasodilation and inhibit neutrophil activation and T-cell cytotoxicity.

      (1) Prototypical agonists include 4-methylhistamine and impromidine.

      (2) Prototypical antagonists include cimetidine and ranitidine.

   c. H_3 receptor stimulation may have negative modulatory effects.

3. Mechanism of action

   a. Release. Histamine can be released from storage cells by either chemical or physical insults. The mechanism is thought to involve a high intracellular calcium (Ca^{2+}) concentration.

      (1) The **primary mechanism for histamine release is immunologic** during anaphylaxis and allergic reactions. Immunoglobulin E (IgE) antibody interacts with antigen on the surface of mast cells and basophils, which leads to histamine release without cell membrane disruption (immediate hypersensitivity reaction).

      (2) **Enzymes, venoms, organic bases** (e.g., morphine), and **polymers** (e.g., dextran) can liberate histamine without prior sensitization by disrupting the mast cell membrane.

      (3) **Tissue injury,** such as that caused by trauma or burns, can cause histamine release from storage sites.

   b. Inhibition of release can occur with high intracellular levels of cyclic adenosine 3´,5´-monophosphate (cAMP).

4. Pharmacologic effects

   a. Extravascular smooth muscle

      (1) The activation of H_1 receptors in smooth muscle results in **contraction**. In bronchial smooth muscle, this is seen in bronchoconstriction and decreased lung capacity; in gastrointestinal smooth muscle, this is seen in spasmodic contractions.

         (a) Activation of H_1 receptors indirectly leads to increased intracellular levels of free Ca^{2+}. The Ca^{2+}, in turn, helps to regulate contraction and secretion of histamine.

         (b) Contraction by H_1 receptors produces a rise in cyclic guanosine 3´,5´-monophosphate (cGMP) levels.

      (2) The activation of H_2 receptors produces relaxation of smooth muscle and a rise in cAMP levels.

b. Cardiovascular system

(1) Histamine induces vascular endothelium to release nitric oxide, which stimulates the production of guanylate cyclase. Increased levels of cGMP in vascular smooth muscle cause vasodilation.

(2) Histamine dilates the fine vessels of the microcirculation, an effect that involves activation of both H_1 and H_2 receptors.

(a) Capillary permeability is the characteristic effect of histamine on the fine vessels and results in edema.

(b) Decreased systemic blood pressure reflects capillary and arteriolar dilation.

(c) Vasodilation is most prominent in the skin of the upper body.

(d) Unilateral cluster headaches, or histamine headaches, result from the dilation of cranial blood vessels.

(3) Histamine produces positive inotropic and chronotropic effects, which are mediated by both H_1 and H_2 receptors.

(4) An intradermal injection of histamine results in the classic **triple response**:

(a) A **reddening** at the site of injection is caused by local vasodilation.

(b) A **wheal,** or disk of edema, is seen within 1–2 minutes after the histamine injection as the result of increased capillary permeability.

(c) A bright crimson **flare,** or halo, surrounding the wheal may be as large as 5 cm and may last for 10 minutes.

c. Exocrine glands

(1) When bound to H_2 receptors, histamine becomes a potent gastric secretagogue, causing the release of large quantities of highly acidic gastric juices, pepsin, and intrinsic factor.

(2) Histamine potentiates the release of gastric acid induced by gastrin and acetylcholine (ACh).

(3) Histamine can stimulate pancreatic and bronchiolar secretion, as well as lacrimation and salivation.

d. CNS. Although the brain contains histamine, little is known about histamine's physiologic role there. Histamine does not penetrate the blood–brain barrier.

5. Physiologic and pathologic roles

a. Gastric secretion. Histamine is a mediator of normal gastric secretion. It stimulates gastric acid and pepsin secretion by directly affecting parietal cell H_2 receptors.

b. Allergic reactions and anaphylactic shock. Histamine is one of several autacoids that participate in hypersensitivity reactions. Antigenic substances cause the release of histamine when they bind to IgE molecules located on a mast cell membrane.

c. Inflammation. Histamine may be responsible for the delayed vasodilation seen in inflammatory responses.

d. Tissue repair growth. A high histamine-synthesizing capacity is found in rapidly proliferating tissues, such as liver, bone marrow, and a variety of malignancies.

e. Neurotransmission. Histamine may be involved in the initiation of sensory impulses for pain and itching; high concentrations are also found in the hypothalamus.

f. Regulation of the microcirculation. Histamine plays a role in the regulation of the microcirculation through its vasoactive properties.

g. Immunoreactivity

(1) H_2-receptor activation elevates levels of intracellular cAMP, blocking T-cell–mediated cytotoxicity.

(2) H_2-receptor activation can also suppress lymphocyte proliferation and the release of cytokines.

(3) The activation of H_1 receptors on T lymphocytes inhibits suppressor cell function.

6. Preparations

a. Histamine phosphate is injected intravenously. It has been used as a diagnostic agent for testing gastric acid secretion, but side effects (see II A 8) have limited its use.

b. Betazole is an isomer of histamine with preferential effects on gastric secretion; it is 10 times more potent as a stimulator of gastric secretion than as a vasodilator. It is used as an alternative for histamine phosphate in tests of gastric function because it does not require premedication with an H_1- or H_2-receptor blocker.

    c. Pentagastrin is a pentapeptide that stimulates the secretion of gastric acid, pepsin, and intrinsic factor. The gastric secretory responses are similar to those induced by histamine or betazole. It is short acting and has few adverse effects.

    d. Impromidine stimulates the activity at H_2 receptors more than 10,000 times than at H_1 receptors.

7. Therapeutic uses

    a. Histamine and its analogues have **no well-established therapeutic uses**.

    b. They can, however, be used diagnostically.

        (1) Histamine and its analogues can be used to distinguish between pernicious anemia and other forms of anemia. The loss of the gastric parietal cells in pernicious anemia results from an inability to secrete gastric acid in response to histamine.

        (2) More selective H_2-receptor agonists, such as impromidine, can be used in tests of gastric acid secretion, as can pentagastrin, which is also used to test for achlorhydria.

8. Adverse effects

    a. The cardiovascular effects of histamine include vasodilation, which produces a decrease in blood pressure, flushing, and tachycardia.

    b. Skin temperature increases and headache and visual disturbances occur.

    c. Bronchoconstriction, dyspnea, and diarrhea are caused by smooth muscle stimulation.

    d. To reduce the effects of histamine in patients not in shock, epinephrine, because of its fast action, is preferred over an antihistamine.

B. **Serotonin** (5-hydroxytryptamine, 5-HT; Figure 8-2)

1. Chemistry

    a. Biosynthesis. Serotonin is primarily derived from dietary tryptophan, which is first hydroxylated and then decarboxylated to form 5-hydroxytryptamine (serotonin).

    b. Metabolism, distribution, and function

        (1) Serotonin is initially deaminated by MAO to form 5-hydroxyindoleacetaldehyde and is then rapidly oxidized to the major metabolite 5-hydroxyindoleacetic acid.

        (2) Approximately 90% of the body's serotonin is found in the enterochromaffin and enterochromaffin-like cells of the gastrointestinal tract. The function of this serotonin is uncertain.

        (3) Serotonin is also found in platelets, where its function has not been established, and in the CNS, where it is believed to be involved with the regulation of temperature, sleep, aggression, pain, and mood. As a component of the pineal gland, serotonin functions as a precursor of melatonin, a hormone that may influence endocrine function.

        (4) Carcinoid tumors synthesize large quantities of serotonin.

2. Pharmacologic effects. Serotonin, like histamine, shows wide species variations; human pharmacology is given here.

    a. Serotonin **constricts most arteries and veins,** especially in the renal and splanchnic beds, and **dilates the blood vessels in skeletal muscle**.

    b. Serotonin produces positive inotropic and chronotropic effects on the heart, but these effects may be masked by reflex responses.

FIGURE 8-2. Serotonin.

   c. The effects of a serotonin injection are complex.
     (1) Initially, a brief depressor phase is seen, which is the result of a transient reflex response to serotonin and vagus nerve stimulation.
     (2) This phase is followed by an increase in blood pressure, which results from an increase in cardiac output and a reduction in peripheral resistance.
     (3) Finally, a prolonged depressor action results from the dilation of blood vessels in skeletal muscles.

3. Therapeutic uses. Serotonin has no therapeutic use.

III. POLYPEPTIDES

A. Angiotensins

1. Chemistry. Figure 8-3 illustrates the formation of angiotensin II and the relationship of the renin–angiotensin system to the kinin system (see III B).

2. Mechanism of action
   a. Angiotensin II acts through specific cell surface receptors located on target tissues.
   b. The precise mechanism responsible for the ultimate pharmacologic effects of angiotensin II is unknown, but both PGs and cyclic nucleotides have been implicated.

3. Pharmacologic effects
   a. One of the major functions of the **renin–angiotensin system** is to regulate blood pressure.
     (1) Renin, a juxtaglomerular enzyme, controls the formation of angiotensin II.
     (2) Angiotensin II is one of the most potent vasoconstrictors; it is 40 times more potent than norepinephrine.
     (3) Angiotensin II produces **positive inotropic and chronotropic effects** through central and peripheral sympathetic stimulation.
   b. In addition to its centrally mediated hypertensive effect, blood-borne angiotensin II has a centrally mediated dipsogenic action.

FIGURE 8-3. The precursor for all angiotensins is angiotensinogen, a plasma α-globulin. Renin metabolizes angiotensinogen to form the decapeptide angiotensin I. Angiotensin-converting enzyme (ACE), a peptidyl dipeptidase found in large quantities on capillary endothelial cells, hydrolyzes angiotensin I to form the pharmacologically active peptide angiotensin II. Angiotensin II is metabolized by an aminopeptidase to form a less active autacoid, angiotensin III. Other routes of metabolism have been observed but appear less important. ACE also inactivates bradykinin. (Reprinted with permission from NMS *Physiology, 3e.* Baltimore, Williams & Wilkins, 1994, p 347.)

    c. Angiotensin II also stimulates sympathetic ganglion cells and enhances ganglionic transmission. This may be mediated by increased biosynthesis of norepinephrine, decreased reuptake of norepinephrine, or increased release of the neurotransmitter.

    d. Angiotensin II stimulates the synthesis and secretion of aldosterone, but this has little effect on blood pressure.

    e. Angiotensin II can stimulate the secretion of antidiuretic hormone (ADH) when injected intraventricularly.

4. Therapeutic uses

    a. There are no approved clinical uses for angiotensin.

    b. Angiotensin II amide, given as an infusion, has produced a sustained pressor response, but its value in the treatment of patients in shock is controversial because the vasoconstriction that angiotensin produces can lead to decreased tissue and organ perfusion.

B. **Kinins**

1. Chemistry

    a. Like angiotensin, the kinins are vasodilating polypeptides.

    b. Two enzymes called **kallikreins** catalyze the formation of the plasma kinins **bradykinin,** a nonapeptide, and **kallidin** (lysyl-bradykinin), a decapeptide, from α_2-globulin precursors called **kininogens**.

        (1) High–molecular-weight (HMW) kininogen is the precursor of **bradykinin**.

            (a) The formation of bradykinin is catalyzed by plasma kallikrein.

            (b) Plasma kallikrein is formed from prekallikrein in a reaction catalyzed by either activated Hageman factor or plasmin.

        (2) Low–molecular-weight (LMW) kininogen is the precursor of **kallidin**. The formation of kallidin is catalyzed by tissue kallikrein or by kininogens formed by complement-mediated cell lysis.

    c. Kinin synthesis and degradation show extensive **interactions** with other biochemical processes.

        (1) Hageman factor can activate prekallikrein.

        (2) Prekallikrein and HMW kininogen both activate Hageman factor.

        (3) Complement activation creates products that inhibit plasma kallikrein but promote tissue kallikrein.

        (4) Bradykinin is inactivated by angiotensin-converting enzyme (ACE), the same peptidyl dipeptidase that converts angiotensin I to angiotensin II (see Figure 8-3).

2. Mechanism of action. Although the mechanism of action of kinins is not well understood, some responses may be mediated by PGs resulting from the stimulation of phospholipase A_2 (see IV A 1 b).

3. Pharmacologic effects

    a. Kinins are powerful **algesic agents;** the algetic action is mediated by a direct stimulation of nerve endings.

    b. Kinins are potent **vasodilators**. They act directly on smooth muscles of fine resistance vessels and also cause the classic triple response seen with histamine [see II A 4 b (4)].

    c. In contrast to their actions on the fine resistance vessels, plasma kinins cause **constriction** of large arteries and most large and small veins.

        (1) Kinins dilate the fetal pulmonary artery and affect the neonatal circulation by promoting closure of the ductus arteriosus and constriction of the umbilical vessels.

        (2) Kinins are capable of constricting most nonvascular smooth muscle (e.g., bronchiolar, gastrointestinal).

4. Therapeutic uses. No therapeutic use exists for kinins.

C. **Vasoactive intestinal polypeptide (VIP)**

1. VIP derives its name from the original site of isolation, but it is prevalent in both central and peripheral nerves, including those serving the pancreas.

2. VIP is a potent vasodilator and a pancreatic secretagogue.

D. Substance P

1. An undecapeptide, substance P produces vasodilation, contraction of various smooth muscles, including intestinal muscle, salivary secretion, and diuresis.

2. Substance P causes depolarization of central and peripheral nervous system neurons, an action that is believed to be responsible for many of its effects. Stimulation of the preganglionic sympathetic nerve to the adrenal medulla results in a release of substance P and ACh.

3. Substance P is thought to be a neurotransmitter and is found in enterochromaffin cells. It is secreted by enterochromaffin tumors, thus playing a role in the carcinoid syndrome.

IV. EICOSANOIDS

A. General considerations

1. Chemistry (Figure 8-4)
  a. The eicosanoids—**PGs, TXs,** and **LTs**—are derived from unsaturated 20-carbon essential fatty acids, primarily **arachidonic acid,** which is a component of membrane phospholipids.
  b. The release of arachidonic acid from lipid storage sites by phospholipases, most notably **phospholipase A_2,** can be initiated by a variety of physical, chemical, hormonal, and neurochemical stimuli.
  c. Arachidonic acid metabolism follows several oxidative **pathways.**
    (1) The **cyclooxygenase** (PG synthetase) **pathway** leads to the PGs and TXs.
    (2) The **5-lipoxygenase pathway** leads to the LTs.
    (3) Other lipoxygenase pathways lead to 12- and 15-hydroperoxy and hydroxy derivatives of eicosatetraenoic acid (12-HPETE and 12-HETE, 15-HPETE and 15-HETE).

2. Nomenclature and structure
  a. The **eicosanoids** are so named because of their 20-carbon fatty acid derivation (from the Greek *eikosi,* "twenty"). Arachidonic acid is 5,8,11,14-eicosatetraenoic acid.
  b. The **PGs** are named because early researchers identified them in seminal fluid.
  c. The **LTs,** first found in **leuko**cytes, are conjugated **trienes**.
  d. The **TXs** are synthesized in platelets (**thrombo**cytes) and contain an **oxane** ring rather than the cyclopentane ring of the prostaglandins.
  e. Numeric subscripts denote the number of double bonds in the alkyl side chain, which derives from the fatty acid precursor. **Greek-letter subscripts** refer to the type of substituent at C_9 of the cyclopentane ring.

3. The eicosanoids are ubiquitous substances. They are generally not stored but are synthesized de novo.
  a. Most are rapidly inactivated and, thus, have short-lived biologic activities.
  b. For example, 95% of PGE_2 is inactivated in the first pass through the lungs.

B. Prostaglandins (PGs)

1. Pharmacologic effects
  a. PGG and **PGH** cause platelet aggregation and are potent vasoconstrictors.
  b. PGD has mixed actions on smooth muscle, constricting interpulmonary veins and relaxing renal vasculature.
  c. PGE causes smooth muscle relaxation and vasodilation. It promotes edema via plasma extrusion. It inhibits platelet aggregation. It is a secretagogue for various hormones; for example, it is luteotropic (i.e., it increases luteal progesterone secretion). At low doses, PGE_2 causes uterine contractions.

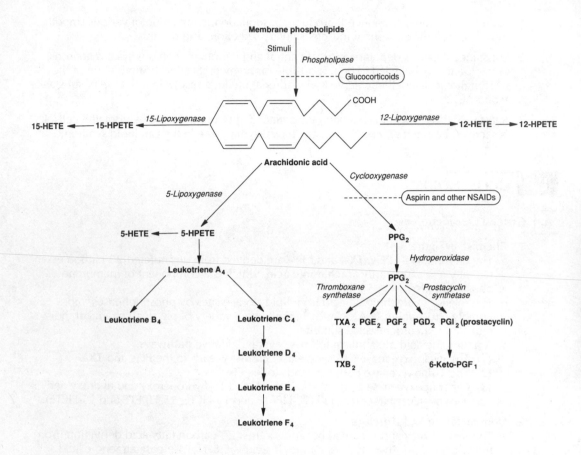

FIGURE 8-4. Major steps in the synthesis of eicosanoids and sites of inhibition by various agents. *HETE* and *HPETE* = hydroxy and hydroperoxy derivatives of eicosatetraenoic acid; *NSAIDs* = nonsteroidal anti-inflammatory drugs; *PG* = prostaglandin; *TX* = thromboxane. (Adapted from Zipser RD, Laffi G: Prostaglandins, thromboxanes, and leukotrienes in clinical medicine. *West J Med* 143:485–497, 1985.)

   d. PGF causes smooth muscle contraction and vasoconstriction. It is luteolytic (i.e., it causes the corpus luteum to regress and to stop producing progesterone).
   e. PGI inhibits platelet aggregation, inhibits gastric and intestinal secretions, and promotes vascular and bronchial smooth muscle relaxation.
   f. Several prostaglandins serve as mediators of the inflammatory response:
      (1) Heat: PGE_1, PGE_2
      (2) Vasodilation and redness: PGE_1, PGE_2, PGD_2, PGA_2
      (3) Edema: PGE, PGI_1, PGI_2 (by potentiating bradykinin effects)
      (4) Pain: PGI_2 (hyperalgesia for 30 minutes), PGE_1, PGE_2 (hyperalgesia for 2 hours)

2. Preparations
   a. Alprostadil (PGE_1) is available for use in infants with congenital heart defects to maintain a patent ductus arteriosus until definitive surgery can be performed.
   b. Carboprost (15-methyl $PGF_{2\alpha}$) induces second-trimester abortion. It is a more powerful uterine contractor than oxytocin. The methyl group prevents oxidation.
   c. Dinoprost ($PGF_{2\alpha}$) **tromethamine** is used intra-amniotically to induce abortion, usually in pregnancy of longer than 15 weeks.

d. **Dinoprostone** (PGE$_2$) is used in suppository form to induce abortion in pregnancies of less than 28 weeks. It is also used to induce full-term labor.

e. **Doxaprost,** a PGE analogue, may be useful for preventing bronchospasm. PGEs are more potent than isoproterenol as a bronchial relaxant, but they irritate the respiratory mucosa.

f. **Misoprostol** (PGE$_2$) and numerous PG analogues (arbaprostil, enprostil, enisoprost, deprostil, rioprostil, trimoprostil) inhibit gastric acid secretion; this may be the mechanism of the gastrointestinal damage that follows exposure to nonsteroidal anti-inflammatory drugs (NSAIDs).

   (1) Misoprostol is rapidly absorbed and metabolized in the liver and excreted in the urine. It has a half-life of less than 30 minutes.

   (2) Dose-related diarrhea can occur in as many as 40% of patients taking misoprostol.

   (3) Misoprostol is contraindicated during pregnancy. It causes bleeding in 40% of women and, in a lower percentage, partial or complete expulsion of the products of conception.

C. **Thromboxane A$_2$ (TXA$_2$) and prostacyclin (PGI$_2$)**

1. **Pharmacologic effects**

   a. **TXA$_2$** is synthesized in platelets.

      (1) It is a potent stimulator of platelet aggregation.

      (2) It is similar to angiotensin II in its vasoconstrictor effects.

      (3) It is also a bronchoconstrictor.

   b. **PGI$_2$** is synthesized in intact vascular endothelium.

      (1) PGI$_2$ is a vasodilator and bronchodilator.

      (2) It inhibits TXA$_2$ production and platelet aggregation by a mechanism that involves cAMP.

   c. PGI$_2$ synthesis is believed to prevent platelet aggregation and adherence and, therefore, to help prevent thrombus formation.

   d. When a vessel wall is damaged, a hemostatic plug forms because TXA$_2$ is released and PGI$_2$ synthesis is reduced.

2. **Therapeutic uses.** PGI$_2$ is being studied for its ability to inhibit platelet aggregation and for its vasodilating effects. It has been used as a heparin substitute in procedures involving extracorporeal circulation, such as hemodialysis and cardiopulmonary bypass surgery.

3. **TX antagonists**

   a. **TX synthetase inhibitors** may prevent thrombus formation in thromboembolic disorders. Agents in this category include **nictindole, imidazole** and its derivatives (**dazoxiben, anagrelide, trifenagrel**), and **hydralazine**.

   b. **Dipyridamole** (see Chapter 5 III D 2) increases cAMP, thereby potentiating the actions of PGI$_2$.

   c. **Pinane-thromboxane A$_2$,** a TXA$_2$ analogue, prevents platelet aggregation and vasoconstriction. At high concentrations, it may be a TXA$_2$ inhibitor.

   d. The antithrombotic actions of **aspirin** and **sulfinpyrazone** are discussed in Chapter 9 II A 3 e (5) and IV C 4, respectively.

D. **Leukotrienes (LTs)**

1. **Chemistry** (see Figure 8-4). LT synthesis takes place chiefly in leukocytes.

   a. Signals that induce leukotriene generation include:

      (1) Anti-IgE antibody in mast cells

      (2) Phagocytosis and immune complexes in macrophages

      (3) Platelet-activating factors, released by basophils and mast cells

      (4) 12-HPETE, a platelet-derived lipoxygenase product

   b. The enzymes 5-lipoxygenase and LT synthetase produce the common intermediate **LTA$_4$,** which has two possible **pathways.**

      (1) To LTB$_4$

      (2) Via glutathione-S-transferase, to LTC$_4$, LTD$_4$, and LTE$_4$, the **slow-reacting substance of anaphylaxis (SRS-A)**

2. **Pharmacologic effects**
   a. **LTC_4, LTD_4, and LTE_4 (SRS-A)**
      (1) These leukotrienes are potent vasoconstrictors; their relative potency is $LTD_4 > LTC_4 > LTE_4 >$ histamine.
      (2) They are also potent bronchoconstrictors.
      (3) They increase the permeability of postcapillary venules.
      (4) They increase mucus secretion.
   b. **LTB_4** is chemotactic and chemokinetic. It causes leukocytes to adhere to the vascular endothelium and to extravasate.
   c. **Interactions**
      (1) LTC_4 and LTD_4 enhance the production of PGE, PGI, and TXA.
      (2) PGE and PGD enhance the chemotactic effects of LTB_4.
      (3) PGE potentiates the vascular permeability induced by LTC_4 and LTD_4.

3. **LT receptor antagonists** are a new class of experimental agents that may prove useful in bronchial asthma, pulmonary fibrosis, bronchitis, and bronchiectasis, renal endotoxic shock, myocardial infarction, coronary artery disease, and inflammatory diseases.

V. AUTACOID ANTAGONISTS

A. **Histamine antagonists** fall into **two categories,** depending on whether they block H_1 or H_2 receptors.

1. **H_1-receptor antagonists** are the classic **antihistamine agents**.
   a. **Mechanism of action.** H_1-receptor antagonists block the histamine effect on:
      (1) Bronchial smooth muscle
      (2) Intestinal smooth muscle
      (3) Small blood vessels
      (4) Sensory impulses for itching
   b. **Structure and classification**
      (1) H_1-receptor antagonists are substituted ethylamines (Figure 8-5).
      (2) The major classes, their substituents at X in Figure 8-5, and typical drugs of each class are shown in Table 8-1.
   c. **Pharmacokinetics**
      (1) H_1-receptor antagonists are rapidly and almost completely absorbed from the gastrointestinal tract, allowing effective oral administration.
      (2) The time to peak plasma concentration and the duration of effect are listed in Table 8-2. Because of their higher tissue concentrations or active metabolites, the effects of H_1-receptor antagonists may persist even when plasma concentrations are undetectable.
      (3) Most H_1-receptor antagonists are metabolized by hydroxylation.
   d. **Pharmacologic effects**
      (1) **Sedation** is a common effect. There is little correlation between antihistamine potency and degree of sedation. Alcohol consumption greatly increases sedation.
      (2) The **anticholinergic properties** of H_1-receptor antagonists are useful in the treatment of motion sickness.
      (3) The **local anesthetic and antipruritic effects** of the H_1-receptor antagonists result from their ability to prevent histamine-induced itching and pain in the skin and mucous membranes.
   e. **Therapeutic uses***
      (1) H_1-receptor antagonists are useful in the **symptomatic treatment of patients with allergic conditions**.

---

*H_1-receptor antagonists are ineffectual in patients with bronchial asthma. Prophylaxis of asthma is accomplished with **cromolyn sodium,** which is neither an antihistamine nor a bronchodilator agent. Cromolyn sodium inhibits the release of histamine and other autacoids from mast cells in the lung.

FIGURE 8-5. Structure of the nucleus of H_1-receptor antagonists (H_1 blockers). X can be nitrogen, carbon, or an ether moiety (see Table 8-1). R_1 and R_2 are cyclic structures.

    (a) Disorders that respond to H_1 blockers include urticaria and seasonal rhinitis and conjunctivitis. **Levocabastine,** a topical ophthalmic H_1-receptor antagonist, has no structural relationship to any other antihistamine. It appears to be safe and effective for prevention and treatment of seasonal allergic conjunctivitis.

    (b) H_1 blockers are effective for alleviating drug reactions caused by allergic phenomena.

    (c) H_1 blockers have an adjuvant role in preventing systemic anaphylaxis.

  (2) H_1-receptor antagonists are used in **cough preparations**.

  (3) They are used **prophylactically for motion sickness and** for **vestibular disturbances** such as Ménière's disease. The ethanolamines and piperazines are especially useful in the treatment of patients with motion sickness.

  (4) H_1 blockers are used as **somnifacients**.

  (5) H_1-receptor antagonists can be used topically as well as orally for treating **urticaria** and **pruritus**.

  f. Preparations. Examples of the classic antihistamine agents are listed in Table 8-1.

  g. Adverse effects

    (1) First-generation H_1-receptor antagonists have a high therapeutic index. Acute toxicity is rare.

      (a) Overdosage may cause acute poisoning, especially in children. The principal symptoms reflect **CNS stimulation** [e.g., **hallucinations, excitement, ataxia, and convulsions** (which precede **death**)].

      (b) Therapeutic doses

        (i) Sedation (to the extent that it may interfere with the patient's daily activities) is the most common adverse effect. This effect can be avoided by reducing the dose or changing the antihistaminic agent.

        (ii) Tinnitus, lassitude, and **nervousness** may occur.

        (iii) Nausea, vomiting, or other gastric distress can occur; administration of the agent with meals can minimize these effects.

        (iv) Allergic manifestations may occur when the drug is administered topically.

        (v) Rarely, piperazine compounds are teratogenic.

TABLE 8-1. Classes of Antihistamine Agents (H_1-Receptor Antagonists)

Class	Substituent at X^*	Examples
Ethylenediamines	N	Tripelennamine (Pyribenzamine) Pyrilamine (Neo-Antergan)
Phenothiazines	N	Promethazine (Phenergan)
Alkylamines	C	Chlorpheniramine (Chlor-Trimeton)
Piperazines	C—N	Cyclizine (Marezine) Meclizine (Antivert, Bonine)
Ethanolamines	C—O	Diphenhydramine (Benadryl) Dimenhydrinate (Dramamine) Carbinoxamine (Clistin)
Other		Terfenadine (Seldane) Astemizole (Hismanal) Levocabastine (Livostin)

C = carbon; N = nitrogen; O = oxygen.
*See Figure 8-5.

TABLE 8-2. Pharmacokinetics of H_1-Receptor Antagonists

	Time to Peak Plasma Level (hr)	Half-life (hr)
First-generation		
Chlorpheniramine	3	28
Hydroxyzine	2	20
Diphenhydramine	2	9
Second-generation		
Terfenadine	3	17
Astemizole	0.5	24
Loratadine	1	11
Acrivastine	1	1.5

   (2) **Second-generation H_1-receptor antagonists**
      (a) **Overdosage** or **concomitant administration with macrolide antibiotics or with ketoconazole or itraconazole,** which inhibit the cytochrome P-450 system, may **prolong the QT interval** [i.e., cause **torsades de pointes**).
         (i) Terfenadine, but not its metabolite, blocks the outward potassium current of ventricular myocytes.
         (ii) No adverse effects of loratadine or acrivastine on the QT interval have been reported.
      (b) **Therapeutic doses.** The selectivity of the second-generation antagonists for H_1 receptors reduces CNS toxicity. This effect may result from the inability of these agents to cross the outer membranes of the endothelial cells lining the brain capillaries.

2. **H_2-receptor antagonists** (Figure 8-6) inhibit gastric acid secretion. They have no significant action at H_1 receptors.
   a. **Cimetidine,** the prototype of the H_2-receptor blockers, is a substituted imidazole compound that acts as a competitive antagonist at H_2 receptors.
      (1) **Pharmacokinetics.** Cimetidine is well absorbed when administered orally, and it is rapidly excreted by the kidney. It undergoes extensive first-pass biotransformation.
      (2) **Pharmacologic effects.** Cimetidine inhibits all phases of physiologic secretion of gastric acid.
         (a) The principal effect of cimetidine is to inhibit histamine-stimulated gastric acid secretion.
         (b) Cimetidine also inhibits gastric acid secretion induced by gastrin and acetylcholine.
      (3) **Therapeutic uses.** The major therapeutic use of cimetidine is in the treatment of **duodenal and gastric ulcers** and **gastric hypersecretory states** (e.g., **Zollinger-Ellison syndrome**).
      (4) **Adverse effects.** Generally, cimetidine is well tolerated.
         (a) High doses in elderly patients, especially those with some degree of renal dysfunction, have resulted in CNS disturbances (e.g., confusion).
         (b) Rarely, a weak antiandrogenic effect has been observed with very high doses, resulting in gynecomastia in men and galactorrhea in women.
         (c) Cimetidine reduces liver blood flow and, thus, can markedly decrease the hepatic clearance of drugs whose metabolism is dependent on liver blood flow (e.g., propranolol).
         (d) Because cimetidine reversibly inhibits the cytochrome P-450 hepatic enzyme system, a number of drug interactions have been observed. Warfarin, phenytoin, theophylline, propranolol, diazepam, and phenobarbital can accumulate.
   b. **Ranitidine** has a substituted furan ring. It is 4–12 times more potent than cimetidine.
      (1) **Therapeutic uses.** Ranitidine is approved for treatment of **gastroesophageal reflux disease** as well as **gastric** and **duodenal** ulcers.

FIGURE 8-6. Structures of H_2-receptor antagonists.

(2) Adverse effects
- **(a)** Ranitidine does not significantly affect the cytochrome P-450 hepatic enzyme system, but it does reduce liver blood flow.
- **(b)** Adverse CNS effects and drug interactions have been reported.
- **(c)** The risk of untoward antiandrogenic effects from ranitidine use appears to be minimal.

c. Famotidine is a thiazole derivative.
- **(1)** Although famotidine is most potent on a weight basis, its efficacy in patients with peptic ulcer disease is similar to that of other agents.
- **(2)** Famotidine has a longer half-life than cimetidine or ranitidine (3 hours versus 2 hours).
- **(3)** Pharmacodynamics and adverse reactions are similar to those of ranitidine.

d. Nizatidine, like famotidine, is a thiazole derivative.
- **(1)** Nizatidine has the highest bioavailability and shortest half-life (1.6 hours) of the available H_2-receptor antagonists.
- **(2)** Nizatidine, like all of the available H_2-receptor antagonists, is principally excreted in the urine. Renal elimination involves both glomerular filtration and tubular secretion.
- **(3)** Pharmacodynamics and adverse reactions are similar to those of ranitidine.

B. | **Serotonin antagonists** are of two general classes: ergot alkaloid derivatives and phenothiazine derivatives.

1. Methysergide
a. Chemistry
- **(1)** Methysergide is a semisynthetic ergot alkaloid congener that lacks any intrinsic vasoconstrictor or oxytocic activity.
- **(2)** Methysergide is a competitive antagonist of serotonin, inhibiting its vasoconstrictor and pressor effects.

b. Therapeutic uses. Methysergide is useful for the **prophylactic treatment of migraine** and other vascular headaches, but the mechanism for this action is unknown.

c. Adverse effects
- **(1)** The major adverse effects of methysergide are gastrointestinal irritation and CNS effects, such as insomnia, restlessness, nervousness, and unsteadiness.
- **(2)** Fibrotic changes in retroperitoneal, pleuropulmonary, and cardiac tissues are rare side effects that occur after prolonged, uninterrupted use.

2. Cyproheptadine
a. Chemistry
- **(1)** Cyproheptadine is a phenothiazine that also blocks H_1 receptors.
- **(2)** Cyproheptadine has weak anticholinergic activity and possesses mild central depressant properties.
- **(3)** Cyproheptadine is a competitive antagonist of serotonin, blocking its vascular effects.

b. Therapeutic uses. Cyproheptadine is used mainly to treat **pruritic dermatoses**.
c. Adverse effects are usually mild; dry mouth and drowsiness are the most common.

C. | **Antagonists of the renin–angiotensin system.** There are two major classes of substances that can inhibit the renin–angiotensin system: angiotensin II antagonists and inhibitors of the enzyme peptidyl dipeptidase.

1. Angiotensin II antagonists
- **a.** The prototypical agent is **saralasin,** a competitive inhibitor of angiotensin II receptors.
- **b.** In normal individuals, the angiotensin II–receptor antagonists have partial agonist activity, resulting in both mild pressor response and increased secretion of aldosterone.
- **c.** In patients with malignant hypertension who are sodium (Na^+)-depleted, saralasin and congeners produce profound hypotension and decreased secretion of aldosterone.

2. **Inhibitors of peptidyl dipeptidase**
   a. **Captopril** (the prototype), **enalapril, lisinopril,** and other agents of this class block the enzymatic conversion of angiotensin I to angiotensin II. Because the responsible enzyme, a peptidyl dipeptidase, is an **ACE,** drugs of this class are known as **ACE inhibitors**.
      (1) These agents are not angiotensin II antagonists, nor do they possess agonist activity.
      (2) ACE inhibitors reduce systemic blood pressure in patients with increased angiotensin I levels but not in normal individuals who are in sodium balance.
      (3) When administered orally, these agents reduce blood pressure in hypertensive patients with high, normal, or low plasma renin levels.
      (4) Many hypertensive patients with normal renin levels respond to captopril, which suggests that other factors affecting the renin–angiotensin system (e.g., sodium depletion) may have a role in hypertension.
   b. ACE inhibitors also increase the actions of bradykinin, which is inactivated by peptidyl dipeptidase.
   c. ACE inhibitors can depress the secretion of aldosterone by lowering angiotensin II production.

D. **Eicosanoid antagonists.** The sites of action of the major classes of eicosanoid antagonists are shown in Figure 8-4.

1. **Glucocorticoids** inhibit the release of arachidonic acid in a number of tissues and, thus, block the production of all eicosanoids in these tissues.
   a. The effect is caused by the inhibition of phospholipase A_2 by glycoproteins that are collectively known as **lipocortins** and produced by the steroids. One such substance is the polypeptide **macrocortin**.
   b. The consequent reduction of LT synthesis may be responsible for the efficacy of glucocorticoids in allergic disorders, such as asthma, and in inflammatory diseases.

2. **NSAIDs,** discussed in Chapter 9, inhibit cyclooxygenase activity and, thus, inhibit the synthesis of both PGs and TXs.
   a. The anti-inflammatory, analgesic, and antipyretic effects of NSAIDs are attributable to the inhibition of PGs, especially PGE_2.
   b. The NSAIDs vary in their cyclooxygenase-inhibiting effects because of varying effects in different tissues. For example, aspirin strongly inhibits TXA_2 but is a weaker inhibitor of PG synthesis than many newer NSAIDs.
   c. It is possible that NSAIDs promote LT synthesis by diverting arachidonic acid metabolism away from the cyclooxygenase pathway and into the lipoxygenase pathways. This might be the cause of allergic reactions occasionally seen with aspirin or other NSAIDs.

3. **Inhibitors of more specific sites** in the arachidonic acid pathways are discussed in IV C 3 and IV D 3.

VI. OTHER AGENTS FOR THE TREATMENT OF PEPTIC ULCERS

A. **Sucralfate** is a complex substance formed from a sulfated disaccharide and polyaluminum hydroxide. It polymerizes when the pH falls below 4.

1. The condensed polymer forms a gel, which adheres to the base of a duodenal ulcer crater.

2. When sucralfate is administered before meals, it is effective for treatment of duodenal ulcer disease. Omeprazole and H_2-receptor antagonists provide better pain relief.

3. Adverse reactions are minimal because sucralfate is not systemically absorbed.

B. **H⁺-K⁺-ATPase inhibitors. Omeprazole** is the prototype of the benzimidazole sulfoxide prodrugs that diffuse across the gastric parietal cell cytoplasm where they are protonated. Omeprazole binds to parietal H⁺-K⁺-ATPase, inhibiting secretion of hydrogen ions into the gastric lumen.

1. Omeprazole is unstable in acid and is formulated in gelatin capsules. It is metabolized in the liver and excreted in the bile and urine.

2. By irreversibly inhibiting parietal H⁺-K⁺-ATPase and preventing the secretion of hydrogen ions into the gastric lumen, the drug appears to be more effective than ranitidine for treatment of gastroesophageal reflux and Zollinger-Ellison syndrome. Omeprazole relieves pain and heals peptic ulcers more rapidly than H_2-receptor antagonists.

3. Omeprazole inhibits the oxidative metabolism of phenytoin, diazepam, and other drugs.

C. **Misoprostol** is less effective than an H_2-receptor antagonist for acute treatment of peptic ulcers but it can prevent gastric ulcers in patients on chronic NSAID therapy.

D. **Antibacterial agents.** Many peptic ulcers not caused by NSAID therapy are thought to be associated with infection of the gastric mucosa by *Helicobacter pylori*. The antibacterial drugs used most often are **bismuth, tetracycline, metronidazole, amoxicillin,** and **clarithromycin,** usually two or three together with an antisecretory drug. Eradication of *H. pylori* with these combinations has led to rapid healing of active peptic ulcer and low recurrence rates.

DIRECTIONS: Each of the numbered items or incomplete statements in this section is followed by answers or by completions of the statement. Select the ONE lettered answer or completion that is BEST in each case.

1. Which of the following effects might be observed in a patient who is accidentally given an overdose of histamine while being tested for achlorhydria?

(A) Severe localized blanching of the skin
(B) Decreased capillary permeability
(C) Bronchoconstriction
(D) Relaxation of gastrointestinal smooth muscle
(E) Gastric acid suppression

2. Many peptic ulcers are now thought to be associated with infection of the gastric mucosa by *Helicobacter pylori*. Which one of the following therapeutic regimens is most likely to rapidly heal the active peptic ulcers and minimize recurrence?

(A) Cimetidine and omeprazole
(B) Cefazolin and cimetidine
(C) Clarithromycin and omeprazole
(D) Bismuth and famotidine
(E) Clindamycin and nizatidine

3. A 50-year-old woman is being treated with ketoconazole for a fungal infection. After 5 days, she returns to her physician's office and complains of "feeling funny." Further discussion reveals that she had "borrowed" her daughter's terfenadine because her "hay fever" was "acting up." When the terfenadine failed to help her runny nose and itchy eyes, she tripled the dose. The physician performs an electrocardiogram (ECG). What might the ECG show?

(A) Sinus bradycardia
(B) Sinus tachycardia
(C) Atrial fibrillation
(D) A prolonged QT interval
(E) Atrial flutter

4. A young child who ingests a fatal dose of dimenhydrinate will most likely die from

(A) renal dysfunction
(B) general central nervous system (CNS) stimulation with convulsions
(C) bronchospasm and suffocation
(D) anaphylactic shock
(E) severe cardiac arrhythmia

5. Which topical ophthalmic H_2-receptor antagonist appears to be effective for the treatment of seasonal allergic conjunctivitis?

(A) Terfenadine
(B) Astemizole
(C) Acrivastine
(D) Levocabastine
(E) Loratadine

6. A patient with a history of gastric ulcers is diagnosed with rheumatoid arthritis. The patient will need to undergo chronic non-steroidal anti-inflammatory drug (NSAID) therapy for the arthritis. What drug could the physician prescribe along with the NSAID to minimize the risk of gastric ulcer formation in this patient?

(A) Cimetidine
(B) Omeprazole
(C) Misoprostol
(D) Ranitidine
(E) Famotidine

DIRECTIONS: Each of the numbered items or incomplete statements in this section is negatively phrased, as indicated by a capitalized word such as NOT, LEAST, or EXCEPT. Select the ONE lettered answer or completion that is BEST in each case.

7. Physiologic and pathologic roles for histamine include all of the following EXCEPT

(A) inhibition of gastric acid secretion
(B) participation in hypersensitivity reactions
(C) inactivation of sensory impulses for itching
(D) participation in the regulation of microcirculation
(E) delayed vasodilation in inflammatory responses

8. True statements concerning the classic antihistamines (H_1-receptor antagonists) include all of the following EXCEPT

(A) they block histamine receptors on bronchial and intestinal smooth muscle
(B) they are substituted ethylamines
(C) they may induce hepatic microsomal enzymes
(D) overdosage in children may cause death following generalized convulsions
(E) they effectively treat bronchial asthma

9. Specific leukotriene receptor antagonists that could selectively inhibit LTC_4, LTD_4, and LTE_4 would produce all of the following pharmacologic effects EXCEPT

(A) vasodilation
(B) bronchodilation
(C) decreased permeability of postcapillary venules
(D) increased mucus secretion

10. Prostaglandin I_2 (PGI_2) exhibits all of the following properties EXCEPT

(A) it is a vasodilator
(B) it is a bronchodilator
(C) it inhibits platelet aggregation
(D) it promotes thromboxane A_2 (TXA_2) production
(E) it inhibits gastric secretions

DIRECTIONS: Each group of items in this section consists of lettered options followed by a set of numbered items. For each item, select the ONE lettered option that is most closely associated with it. Each lettered option may be selected once, more than once, or not at all.

Questions 11–14

Match each of the following autacoid antagonists to the enzyme that it inhibits.

(A) Cyclooxygenase
(B) Peptidyl dipeptidase
(C) Phospholipase
(D) Thromboxane (TX) synthetase
(E) Cystathionine synthetase

11. Captopril

12. Hydralazine

13. Ibuprofen

14. Prednisolone

Questions 15–17

Match each agent with the statement that is most closely associated with it.

(A) Sucralfate
(B) Omeprazole
(C) Cimetidine
(D) Ranitidine

15. This agent is an H_2-receptor antagonist that does not significantly affect the cytochrome P-450 hepatic enzyme system.

16. This agent acts by binding to parietal cell H^+-K^+-ATPase.

17. This agent polymerizes when the pH falls below 4.

1. The answer is C *[II A 4 a (1), 8]*. Broncho-constriction would be the most prominent adverse effect. The overdose of histamine would increase capillary permeability, stimulate gastrointestinal smooth muscle, and stimulate gastric acid secretion. Vasodilation and increased skin temperature would also occur.

2. The answer is C *[VI B, D]*. Clarithromycin has been approved for the eradication of *Helicobacter pylori*. It is most often combined with an H^+-K^+-ATPase inhibitor (e.g., omeprazole) to promote rapid healing of active peptic ulcers and minimal recurrence. The other combinations (i.e., cimetidine and omeprazole, cefazolin and cimetidine, bismuth and famotidine, and clindamycin and nizatidine) would not be as effective against infections caused by *H. pylori*.

3. The answer is D *[V A 1 g (2) (a)]*. Over-dosage or concomitant administration of ter-fenadine, a second-generation H_1-receptor antagonist, and ketoconazole, an antifungal agent that inhibits the cytochrome P-450 system, may cause torsades de pointes (i.e., prolongation of the QT interval). This adverse effect is also seen with concomitant administration of terfenadine or astemizole and macrolide antibiotics. Lethal ventricular tachyarrhythmias have occurred, although this is rare.

4. The answer is B *[V A 1 g]*. Dimenhydrinate is a "classic" antihistaminic agent—an H_1-receptor antagonist. A toxic dose of dimen-hydrinate would result in generalized central nervous system (CNS) stimulation with convulsions. Renal dysfunction is not a side effect of H_1-receptor antagonists. Bronchospasm, suffocation, and cardiac arrhythmias are also not adverse effects seen with acute poisoning. Allergic manifestations may be observed with topical application of the drug, but these are not severe enough to constitute anaphylactic shock and would not be lethal.

5. The answer is D *[V A 1 e (1) (a)]*. Levocabastine has no structural relationship to any other antihistamine but appears safe and effective for the prevention and treatment of seasonal allergic conjunctivitis. Terfenadine, astemizole, loratadine, and acrivastine are second-generation systemically administered H_1-receptor antagonists.

6. The answer is C *[VI C]*. Misoprostol is less effective than an H_2-receptor antagonist (e.g., cimetidine, ranitidine, famotidine, nizatidine) for the acute treatment of peptic ulcers, but it is effective in preventing gastric ulcer formation in patients on chronic nonsteroidal anti-inflammatory drug (NSAID) therapy. Omeprazole, an H^+-K^+-ATPase blocker, heals gastric ulcers more rapidly than the H_2-receptor antagonists, but it cannot prevent ulcer formation.

7. The answer is A *[II A 5 a]*. Histamine stimulates gastric acid and pepsin secretion by directly affecting parietal cell H_2 receptors. All of the other roles listed in the question are true physiologic and pathologic roles for histamine.

8. The answer is E *[V A 1 a, b, c (3), e]*. H_1-receptor antagonists are useful in the symptomatic treatment of patients with allergic conditions, but they are ineffective in patients with bronchial asthma. The classic antihistamines are substituted ethylamines. They block histamine receptors on bronchial, intestinal, and microvascular smooth muscle. They may induce hepatic microsomal enzymes. Therapeutic doses produce central nervous system (CNS) depression, but convulsions and death can occur with toxic doses, especially in children.

9. The answer is D *[IV D 2]*. The leukotrienes LTC_4, LTD_4, and LTE_4 collectively are the slow-reacting substance of anaphylaxis and are associated with vasoconstriction, bronchoconstriction, increased permeability of postcapillary venules, and increased mucus secretion. Specific leukotriene receptor antagonists could potentially reverse these pharmacologic actions.

10. The answer is D *[IV C 1, 2]*. Prostaglandin I_2 (PGI_2, prostacyclin) inhibits thromboxane A_2 (TXA_2) production. TXA_2 stimulates platelet aggregation and causes vasoconstriction and bronchoconstriction, whereas PGI_2 has the opposite effects. PGI_2 has been studied for its clinical value in preventing thrombus formation because of its ability to prevent platelet aggregation and adherence. PGI_2 has also been used as a heparin substitute in extracorporeal circulation procedures. In addition to its effects on platelets, PGI_2 is also a vasodilator, bronchodilator, and inhibitor of gastric and intestinal secretions.

11–14. The answers are: 11-B *[V C 2]*, **12-D** *[IV C 3 a]*, **13-A** *[V D 2]*, **14-C** *[V D 1 a]*. Captopril belongs to the class of drugs known as angiotensin-converting enzyme (ACE) inhibitors because they inhibit peptidyl dipeptidase, the ACE that normally converts angiotensin I to angiotensin II. The autacoid angiotensin II is a potent vasoconstrictor that raises blood pressure; thus, ACE inhibitors are used clinically to treat hypertension.

Hydralazine inhibits thromboxane (TX) synthetase, the enzyme involved in the formation of TX from prostaglandin H (PGH). TXA_2 is, like angiotensin II, a potent vasoconstrictor, and hydralazine is used clinically as an antihypertensive vasodilator.

Ibuprofen is a nonsteroidal anti-inflammatory drug (NSAID). These agents act by inhibiting cyclooxygenase; thus, they inhibit the synthesis of both PGs and TXs. Several PGs serve as mediators of the inflammatory response. Some NSAIDs inhibit 15-lipoxygenase as well as cyclooxygenase, and aspirin, by inhibiting platelet cyclooxygenase, also interrupts the TX synthetase pathway.

Prednisolone and other glucocorticoids inhibit phospholipase in a number of tissues, thereby blocking all eicosanoid formation in these tissues. Thus, glucocorticoids block the synthesis of PGs, leukotrienes, and TXs, which probably explains their potent anti-inflammatory effects. Moreover, because leukotrienes play a role in hypersensitivity reactions, their suppression may explain the efficacy of glucocorticoids in allergic disorders.

15–17. The answers are: 15-D *[V A 2 a (4)]*, **16-B** *[VI B]*, **17-A** *[VI A]*. Cimetidine is the prototype of the H_2-receptor blockers. Cimetidine, unlike ranitidine, significantly inhibits the cytochrome P-450 hepatic enzyme system.

Omeprazole is the prototype of the benzimidazole sulfoxide prodrugs that diffuse across the gastric parietal cell cytoplasm, where they are pronated. By binding to H^+-K^+-ATPase, it inhibits the secretion of hydrogen ions into the gastric lumen.

Sucralfate is a complex substance formed from sulfated disaccharide and polyaluminum hydroxide. It polymerizes when the pH falls below 4. The polymer adheres to the base of the duodenal ulcer crater.

Chapter 9

Non-Narcotic Analgesics, Nonsteroidal Anti-Inflammatory Drugs, and Drugs Used in the Treatment of Gout

I. **INTRODUCTION.** This chapter discusses drugs that are anti-inflammatory, analgesic, and antipyretic; their mechanisms of action differ from those of anti-inflammatory steroids and narcotic analgesics. Agents that modify the progression of rheumatoid arthritis and agents used in the treatment of gout are also discussed.

A. **Nonsteroidal anti-inflammatory drugs (NSAIDs)** are either salicylates (e.g., aspirin) or nonsalicylates (e.g., ibuprofen).

1. **Mechanism of action.** Aspirin and most NSAIDs exert their anti-inflammatory and analgesic action via **inhibition of prostaglandin (PG) biosynthesis** (Figure 9-1).
   a. By inhibiting the **cyclooxygenase** enzyme, these agents inhibit the formation of PGE_2, PGI_2, and $PGF_{2\alpha}$, which are putative mediators of vasodilation, pain, and edema associated with inflammation (see Chapter 8 IV B 1 f).
   b. **Thromboxane A_2 (TXA_2)** formation is also inhibited, which is clinically evidenced by prolonged bleeding times (see II A 3 h). This reduced thrombus formation becomes clinically significant in the postmyocardial infarction patient; an aspirin regimen has been demonstrated to increase long-term survival.

2. **Commonly used NSAIDs** include:
   a. Aspirin and other salicylates (e.g., diflunisal)
   b. Acetaminophen
   c. Indomethacin and sulindac
   d. Mefenamic acid and meclofenamate
   e. Tolmetin
   f. Propionic acid derivatives (e.g., ibuprofen)
   g. Piroxicam
   h. Nabumetone
   i. Etodolac
   j. Phenylbutazone
   k. Diclofenac
   l. Ketorolac, the first injectable NSAID for analgesic use

B. **Disease-modifying antirheumatic drugs (DMARDs)** are typically used in conjunction with an NSAID regimen to treat rheumatoid arthritis. These include:

1. Gold compounds (e.g., aurothioglucose, gold sodium thiomalate, auranofin)

2. Methotrexate

3. Azathioprine and cyclophosphamide

4. Cyclosporine

5. Corticosteroids (injected intra-articularly)

6. Penicillamine

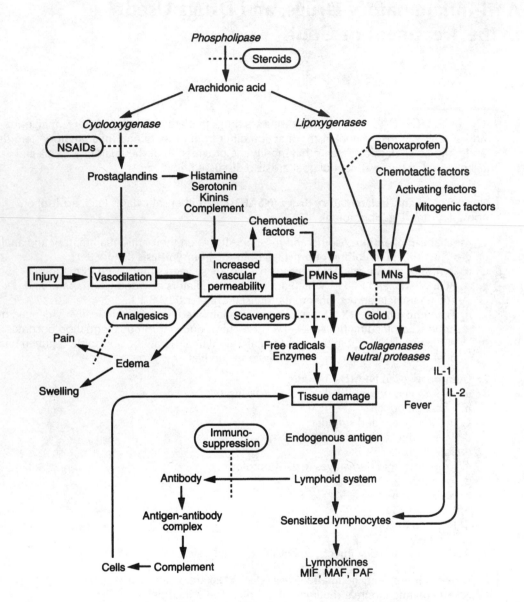

FIGURE 9-1. The events of the inflammatory response and mechanisms of anti-inflammatory agents. *IL-1* = interleukin-1; *IL-2* = interleukin-2; *MAF* = macrophage activating factor; *MIF* = migration inhibiting factor; *MNs* = macrophages; *NSAIDs* = nonsteroidal anti-inflammatory drugs; *PAF* = platelet activating factor; *PMNs* = polymorphonuclear leukocytes. [Adapted from Sedgwick AD, Willoughby DA: Initiation of the inflammatory response and its prevention. In *The Pharmacology of Inflammation (Handbook of Inflammation,* vol 5). Edited by Bonta IL, Bray MA, Parnham MJ. New York, Elsevier, 1985, p 40.]

7. Hydroxychloroquine

8. Sulfasalazine

9. Capsaicin

C. **Drugs used in the treatment of gout** are:

1. Probenecid

2. Sulfinpyrazone

3. Colchicine

4. Allopurinol

5. Phenylbutazone

II. NONSTEROIDAL ANTI-INFLAMMATORY DRUGS (NSAIDs)

A. **Aspirin (acetylsalicylic acid) and other salicylates**

1. **Chemistry.** Aspirin was first isolated in 1829 by Leroux from willow bark, yielding a bitter glycoside called **salicin,** a white crystalline substance (Figure 9-2). It is stable in dry air but hydrolyzes to salicylic and acetic acids in moist air.

2. **Pharmacokinetics**
   a. **Absorption**
      (1) **Oral absorption** of salicylates is fairly rapid, with appreciable blood levels appearing within 30 minutes and peaking at about 2 hours.
         (a) Upon oral administration of the salicylates, a portion is **rapidly absorbed from the stomach**.
         (b) **Most** of an orally ingested salicylate dose, however, is **absorbed from the upper portion of the small intestine**.
      (2) **Rectal absorption** of the salicylates is slow and unpredictable.
   b. **Distribution.** Once absorbed, the salicylates are distributed throughout the body by a pH-dependent passive diffusion process. Most of the salicylates bind avidly to serum proteins. Aspirin binds to a lesser extent.
   c. **Biotransformation** of salicylates occurs in the microsomal drug-metabolizing system, and the following metabolic products are seen in the urine: **salicyluric acid** (75%), **phenolic glucuronide** (10%), **acyl glucuronide** (5%), and **free salicylic acid** (10%).
   d. **Excretion.** Alkalinization of urine (pH 8) significantly increases the excretion of salicylates because of increased ionization and decreased reabsorption through the renal tubules.

3. **Pharmacologic effects**
   a. **Antipyretic action**
      (1) Aspirin is rapidly effective in febrile patients, yet has little effect on normal body temperature, suggesting that PGs have little influence on normal homeostatic mechanisms for body temperature.

FIGURE 9-2. Acetylsalicylic acid.

(2) The antipyretic action is centrally mediated; the central nervous system (CNS) action is thought to be due to inhibited PGE_2 synthesis from the hypothalamus in response to an endogenous pyrogen.

(3) Hyperpyrexia can occur in salicylate toxicity, but this is partially the result of an increase in oxygen consumption and metabolic rate.

b. Anti-inflammatory effects

(1) Salicylates, and NSAIDs in general, are anti-inflammatory due to the inhibition of PG synthesis (see Figure 9-1); however, there is a wide range of potency.

(2) The primary clinical application is in the treatment of **musculoskeletal disorders,** such as rheumatoid arthritis, osteoarthritis, and ankylosing spondylitis.

(3) Although these agents may provide symptomatic relief from pain or joint stiffness, occult joint damage may still occur to the point of necessitating an additional regimen of a DMARD.

c. Analgesic effects

(1) The analgesia is usually effective for low- to moderate-intensity pain; integumental pain is relieved better than is pain from hollow visceral areas.

(2) Relief of pain occurs through both **peripheral** and **central mechanisms.**

  (a) Peripherally, the salicylates inhibit the synthesis of PGs in inflamed tissues, thus preventing the sensitization of pain receptors to both mechanical and chemical stimuli.

  (b) Centrally, the analgesic site exists in close proximity to the antipyretic region in the hypothalamus. The analgesia produced by the salicylates is not associated with mental alterations, such as hypnosis or changes in sensation other than pain.

d. Respiratory effects

(1) Therapeutic doses. Salicylates stimulate respiration directly and indirectly; oxygen consumption and carbon dioxide production are increased, particularly in skeletal muscle.

  (a) This effect appears to be mediated by a salicylate-induced uncoupling of oxidative phosphorylation.

  (b) The increased carbon dioxide production stimulates respiration, but this is characterized by deep respirations rather than an increase in respiratory rate.

(2) High doses result in medullary stimulation, leading to hyperventilation and a respiratory alkalosis. Compensation rapidly occurs because the kidney is able to increase the excretion of bicarbonate, producing a **compensated respiratory alkalosis.**

(3) Toxic doses or very prolonged salicylate administration can depress the medulla, resulting in an **uncompensated respiratory acidosis.** Because renal bicarbonate excretion is elevated and the salicylates cause the accumulation of organic acids, a **metabolic acidosis** also results.

e. Cardiovascular effects

(1) Therapeutic doses of salicylates have no significant cardiovascular effect; however, the **prophylactic use** of aspirin to reduce thromboembolic events in coronary and cerebral circulation has increased. Studies have demonstrated that such use results in long-term survival and reduced frequency of second myocardial infarctions.

(2) High doses may cause peripheral vasodilation by exerting a direct effect on smooth muscle.

(3) Toxic doses depress circulation directly and by central vasomotor paralysis. Noncardiogenic pulmonary edema may occur in older patients on long-term salicylate therapy.

f. Gastrointestinal effects

(1) Salicylates can cause **epigastric distress, nausea,** and **vomiting** by irritating the gastric mucosal lining and stimulating the chemoreceptor trigger zone (CTZ) in the CNS.

(2) Salicylates, and NSAIDs in general, may cause a dose-related **gastric ulceration, bleeding, exacerbation of peptic ulcer symptoms,** and **erosive gastritis.**

(a) Salicylates inhibit the formation of PGI_2 (prostacyclin), which inhibits gastric acid secretion and has a cytoprotective effect, especially on gastric mucosal cells.

(b) Misoprostol (see Chapter 8 VI C) is useful for the prevention of NSAID-induced gastric ulcers.

(c) Salicylate-induced gastric bleeding is painless and may lead to an **iron deficiency anemia**.

g. Hepatic effects. Salicylate-related hepatic damage is usually anicteric, mild, and reversible after discontinuation of therapy. Salicylates can produce at least two forms of hepatic injury.

(1) One form is dose-dependent and usually occurs in patients with connective tissue disorders. Usually, asymptomatic, elevated plasma transaminase levels (i.e., serum glutamic-oxaloacetic transaminase and serum glutamate pyruvate transaminase) are the key indication of hepatic insult.

(2) A second form of salicylate-induced hepatic injury is more severe and associated with the encephalopathy seen in **Reye's syndrome**.

(a) This rare, and often fatal, disorder can occur with infection from varicella (chickenpox) virus and influenza virus.

(b) **Use of salicylates in children with chickenpox or influenza is contraindicated.**

h. Hematologic effects

(1) Aspirin has no effect on leukocyte count, hemoglobin, or hematocrit at therapeutic doses. There is, however, a **prolongation of bleeding time** with doses as small as 300 mg of aspirin. This dose irreversibly inhibits platelet function for the 7-day lifetime of the platelet.

(2) Because it can acetylate and inactivate cyclooxygenase, aspirin has important effects on the delicate balance between the initiation and the inhibition of **platelet aggregation**.

(a) Platelets are ordinarily nonadherent. However, vascular injury and exposure to subendothelial structures result in activation of the platelet cyclooxygenase enzyme system, leading to the production of TXA_2, via thromboxane synthetase. TXA_2 can induce platelet aggregation.

(b) Concurrently opposing this physiologic process is the cyclooxygenase and prostacyclin synthetase enzyme system of the vascular endothelium. Instead of thromboxane synthetase, vascular endothelial cells contain a prostacyclin synthetase, which converts the cyclooxygenase products PGG_2 and PGH_2 to PGI_2, a potent inhibitor of platelet clumping.

(c) It is thought that aspirin in appropriate doses can preferentially inhibit the platelet cyclooxygenase system, blocking the formation of TXA_2, thereby suppressing platelet clumping.

(d) By inhibiting initial platelet aggregation to subendothelial structures, aspirin also prevents the secondary release of adenosine diphosphate (ADP) from platelet granules, a process that normally occurs when platelets clump. ADP release ordinarily brings about additional waves of platelet aggregation, leading to thrombus formation. This effect persists 4–7 days after the drug has been discontinued.

(3) In doses greater than 6 g/d, aspirin may **reduce plasma prothrombin levels**.

(4) Because of its effects on the blood, aspirin should be avoided in patients with severe hepatic disease, hypoprothrombinemia, vitamin K deficiency, or hemophilia.

i. Renal effects

(1) Salicylates decrease renal blood flow, resulting in salt and water retention, which increases circulating plasma volume (by about 20%) in patients taking large doses.

(2) In patients with congestive heart failure, impaired renal function, or hypovolemia, salicylates can further exacerbate renal dysfunction.

(3) The vasodilatory effects of PGI_2 on renal blood flow (and now glomerular filtration rate) may be more critical during impaired renal function.

       (4) Salicylates also affect uric acid secretion, but the effect is dose-dependent: Low doses may decrease urate excretion whereas large doses may induce uricosuria.

       (5) Small doses of salicylates may be enough to block the uricosuric action of probenecid and other agents that decrease tubular reabsorption of uric acid. Salicylates should not be used concomitantly with uricosuric agents in the treatment of gout (see IV F 3).

  j. Metabolic effects

       (1) The salicylates uncouple oxidative phosphorylation.

       (2) Large doses of the salicylates can produce hyperglycemia and glycosuria and can deplete liver and muscle glycogen.

       (3) Aspirin, like other salicylates, can reduce lipogenesis by blocking the incorporation of acetates into fatty acids.

       (4) Toxic doses can cause significant nitrogen loss, characterized by aminoaciduria.

  k. Endocrine effects

       (1) The salicylates, in very large doses, can stimulate steroid secretion by the adrenal cortex. This effect is mediated through action on the hypothalamus.

       (2) Long-term salicylate therapy can decrease thyroidal uptake and clearance of iodine and can increase oxygen metabolism and the rate of disappearance of triiodothyronine (T_3) and thyroxine (T_4) from the circulation. These effects probably result from a competitive displacement of iodinated proteins from plasma proteins by salicylates.

       (3) Use of salicylates may prolong the gestational period during pregnancy. This may be due to a delay in the onset of labor caused by the inhibition of PG synthesis in the uterus; PGs are believed to be involved in eliciting uterine contractions.

4. Therapeutic uses

  a. The salicylates are used in restricted situations for the **symptomatic relief of fever**.

       (1) They have no effect on the underlying cause of a fever, and because the hyperthermic response in an illness may be a normal protective physiologic mechanism, they should not be used routinely or trivially for this purpose.

       (2) Because of an increased incidence of Reye's syndrome in children who previously were given aspirin for the relief of viral fevers, it is now recommended that a child with any fever be given acetaminophen instead, if medication is required.

  b. The salicylates are useful as **analgesics** for certain categories of pain (e.g., headache, arthritis, dysmenorrhea).

  c. The salicylates, by way of their anti-inflammatory action, provide relief of symptoms in **acute rheumatic fever**.

  d. The salicylates remain the standard, first-line drug in the therapy of **rheumatoid arthritis**.

       (1) Both the analgesic and the anti-inflammatory actions provide symptomatic relief in this disorder.

       (2) Relatively large doses are required, however, and these may not be well tolerated in some individuals, necessitating the use of other agents either alone or in combination with the salicylates.

  e. Because of aspirin's antiplatelet activity, some clinicians recommend small daily doses of aspirin for **prophylaxis of thromboembolism, stroke,** or **myocardial infarction**.

5. Preparations and administration

  a. Aspirin is available as tablets, capsules, and suppositories in a wide range of dosages.

       (1) Rectal administration may be required in infants or if oral administration is impossible.

       (2) **Buffered** or **enteric-coated aspirin** preparations may be better-tolerated.

  b. Nonacetylated salicylates, such as sodium salicylate, salsalate, and choline magnesium salicylate, appear to cause less gastric irritation and have less effect on platelet function than aspirin. Although they may be safer than acetylated salicylates for aspirin-sensitive patients, they may not be as effective.

  c. Diflunisal is a salicylate that can be taken twice daily. It has four times the potency of aspirin when used in the treatment of osteoarthritis or musculoskeletal pain.

d. Mesalamine (5-aminosalicylic acid) is used for inflammatory bowel disease; it has poor oral absorption and, thus, is used for its local effect in rectal preparations.

6. Salicylate intoxication (see Chapter 14 II C 3)

a. Mild intoxication from aspirin or other salicylates is referred to as **salicylism** and usually occurs with repeated administration of large doses. Characteristic findings include:

(1) Headache, mental confusion, lassitude, and drowsiness

(2) Tinnitus and difficulty in hearing

(3) Hyperthermia, sweating, thirst, hyperventilation, vomiting, and diarrhea

b. More severe salicylate intoxication can result in more severe CNS disturbances, including hallucinations, vertigo, or convulsions. In addition, skin eruptions and, more important, marked alterations in acid–base balance are observed.

c. Fatal intoxication can be produced in children by ingestion of as little as 10 g of aspirin or as little as 5 g of **methyl salicylate,** which is widely used as a counterirritant in liniments and has the characteristic odor and taste of wintergreen.

d. Treatment of salicylate poisoning includes:

(1) Inducing emesis with syrup of ipecac or administering gastric lavage

(2) Appropriate infusion measures to correct abnormal electrolyte balance and dehydration

(3) Alkalinization of the urine

(4) Dialysis as required

B. **Acetaminophen**

1. Chemistry. A para-aminophenol derivative, acetaminophen (Figure 9-3) is the major active metabolite of phenacetin.

2. Pharmacokinetics

a. Absorption. Acetaminophen is completely and rapidly absorbed from the gastrointestinal tract, with peak plasma levels reached within 30–60 minutes. The plasma half-life is about 2 hours.

b. Metabolism and excretion. About 3% is excreted unchanged in the urine, and 80%–90% is conjugated with glucuronic or sulfuric acid in the liver and then excreted in the urine within the first day.

(1) Small amounts of hydroxylated metabolites are ordinarily excreted.

(2) At high doses, one of these metabolites undergoes spontaneous dehydration to form N-acetyl-p-benzoquinone, the metabolite thought to be responsible for hepatotoxicity (see II B 6 b).

3. Pharmacologic effects

a. Analgesic and antipyretic effects. Acetaminophen is as effective as aspirin, is similar in potency, and, in single analgesic doses, has the same time–effect curve. However, acetaminophen has **no anti-inflammatory activity,** for reasons that are not completely understood. Acetaminophen appears to be an inhibitor of PG synthesis in the

NHCOCH$_3$

OH   **FIGURE 9-3.** Acetaminophen.

brain, thus accounting for its analgesic and antipyretic activity; but it is much less effective than aspirin as an inhibitor of the peripherally located PG biosynthetic enzyme system that plays such an important role in inflammation.

b. Acetaminophen exerts little or no pharmacologic effect on the cardiovascular, respiratory, or gastrointestinal systems, on acid–base regulation, or on platelet function.

4. **Therapeutic uses**
   a. Acetaminophen provides an effective **alternative when aspirin is contraindicated** (e.g., in patients with peptic ulcer or hemophilia) and **when the anti-inflammatory action of aspirin is not required**.
   b. Acetaminophen has virtually replaced the formerly popular phenacetin because of the renal toxicity ascribed to the latter drug. However, acetaminophen, the main metabolite of phenacetin, is also associated with renal toxicity in a dose-dependent manner.

5. **Preparations and administration.** Acetaminophen is available in tablet and liquid form and is administered orally.

6. **Adverse effects**
   a. At **therapeutic doses,** acetaminophen is well tolerated; however, adverse effects include:
      (1) Skin rash and drug fever (hyperpyrexia caused by an allergic reaction to the drug)
      (2) Rare instances of blood dyscrasias
      (3) Renal tubular necrosis and renal failure
      (4) Hypoglycemic coma
   b. An **overdose** of acetaminophen (about 15 g in an adult; about 4 g in a child) can result in severe hepatotoxicity, resulting in centrilobular hepatic necrosis. Doses greater than 20 g are potentially fatal.
      (1) The toxic metabolite of acetaminophen appears to be inactivated in the liver by glutathione.
      (2) It is thought that when glutathione stores are consumed, the N-acetyl-p-benzoquinone metabolite binds covalently to cellular constituents, producing hepatocellular damage.
      (3) Although clinical symptoms such as nausea and vomiting occur during the first 24 hours after toxic ingestion, signs of hepatic damage (e.g., enzyme abnormalities) may not occur for 2–6 days.
      (4) **Treatment** consists of:
         (a) Emptying the stomach and administering activated charcoal
         (b) Hemodialysis, if begun within the first 12 hours after ingestion
         (c) Administration of sulfhydryl compounds (e.g., acetylcysteine), which probably replenish hepatic stores of glutathione.

C. Indomethacin

1. **Chemistry.** Indomethacin is a methylated indole derivative.

2. **Pharmacokinetics**
   a. **Absorption** from the gastrointestinal tract is rapid and virtually complete, with peak plasma levels reached in approximately 2 hours. As with other drugs, absorption may be delayed when taken with meals.
   b. **Distribution**
      (1) Indomethacin is **90% bound to plasma proteins** and exhibits extensive tissue binding.
      (2) Concentration of indomethacin in **synovial fluid** is equal to plasma levels within 5 hours of administration.
   c. **Metabolism.** Indomethacin is largely inactivated by O-demethylation (approximately 50%) and glucuronidation (approximately 10%).

3. **Pharmacologic effects.** Indomethacin has prominent **anti-inflammatory, antipyretic,** and **analgesic** activity.
   a. Although indomethacin is a more potent anti-inflammatory agent than aspirin, the doses of indomethacin that are well tolerated by patients with rheumatoid arthritis do not show superior results compared with the salicylates.
   b. There is evidence for both a central and peripheral action.

4. **Therapeutic uses.** Because of its toxicity and side effects, indomethacin is not routinely used for analgesia or antipyresis.
   a. The major uses of indomethacin are in the treatment of **rheumatoid arthritis, ankylosing spondylitis, osteoarthritis,** and **acute gout**.
   b. It has also been used in the treatment of **patent ductus arteriosus** in neonates, and in the treatment of **Bartter's syndrome** (juxtaglomerular cell hyperplasia), characterized by hypokalemic alkalosis, hyperaldosteronism, and normal blood pressure despite high renin blood levels.

5. **Administration**
   a. Indomethacin usually is administered orally. It should be taken with meals to lessen gastric irritation.
   b. An intravenous solution is available for treating patent ductus arteriosus.

6. **Adverse effects.** Overall, 35%–50% of all patients receiving indomethacin report some adverse effect; approximately 20% must discontinue therapy. Most adverse effects are dose-related.
   a. **Gastrointestinal complaints** include:
      (1) Anorexia, nausea, and abdominal pain
      (2) Ulcers, sometimes with perforations and hemorrhage
      (3) Diarrhea, sometimes associated with ulcerative lesions of the lower gastrointestinal tract
      (4) Pain caused by decreased mesenteric blood flow
   b. **CNS effects,** which are the most frequently reported, include:
      (1) Severe frontal headache (25%–50%)
      (2) Dizziness and vertigo
      (3) Mental confusion
      (4) Severe depression, psychosis, hallucination, and suicide
   c. **Hematologic reactions,** such as neutropenia, thrombocytopenia, impaired platelet function, and, rarely, aplastic anemia
   d. **Hypersensitivity reactions,** such as rashes, itching, urticaria, and acute asthma (aspirin-sensitive patients may exhibit cross-reactions to indomethacin)
   e. Indomethacin is **contraindicated in:**
      (1) Pregnant or nursing women (indomethacin crosses the placenta freely, which can result in constriction of the fetal ductus arteriosus and oligohydramnios as a result of decreased fetal urine output)
      (2) Patients with psychiatric disorders
      (3) Patients with epilepsy
      (4) Patients with parkinsonism
      (5) Patients with renal disease
      (6) Patients with gastrointestinal ulcerative lesions
      (7) Machine operators

7. **Drug interactions**
   a. Indomethacin does not appear to alter the uricosuric effects of probenecid. It is routinely used in the treatment of gout.
   b. Indomethacin does not appear to modify the effect of oral anticoagulants, but concurrent administration could be hazardous because of increased potential for gastrointestinal bleeding.
   c. Indomethacin does antagonize the natriuretic and antihypertensive effects of furosemide, thiazide diuretics, β-adrenergic blocking agents, and angiotensin-converting enzyme (ACE) inhibitors.

D. **Sulindac**

1. **Chemistry.** Structurally, sulindac is an indene-derived NSAID and is closely related to indomethacin.

2. **Pharmacokinetics**
   a. **Absorption.** Approximately 90% of the drug is absorbed after oral administration, with peak plasma levels of sulindac and its sulfide metabolite occurring at 1 hour and 2 hours, respectively.
   b. **Distribution.** Sulindac and its major metabolites are all extensively bound to plasma proteins. The half-life of sulindac is approximately 7 hours, but the sulfide metabolite half-life is approximately 18 hours.
   c. **Excretion.** Urine and feces are principal routes of excretion.

3. **Pharmacologic effects**
   a. Sulindac is an **anti-inflammatory, analgesic,** and **antipyretic** drug with a relative strength of approximately half of indomethacin's potency.
   b. Sulindac is a **prodrug**. Its sulfide metabolite is more than 500 times more potent (than sulindac) as an inhibitor of cyclooxygenase.

4. **Therapeutic uses.** Sulindac is primarily used in the treatment of **osteoarthritis, rheumatoid arthritis, ankylosing spondylitis,** and **acute gout**.

5. **Administration.** Sulindac is given orally.

6. **Adverse effects.** Sulindac has a lower incidence of toxicity as compared with indomethacin.
   a. Gastrointestinal effects occur in about 20% of patients, although the reactions are generally mild.
   b. There are reports of cross-reactivity to sulindac in aspirin-sensitive patients. Skin rash and pruritus occur at approximately a 5% incidence.
   c. Platelet function may be impaired, and bleeding time is prolonged.
   d. Sulindac does not appear to be "renal-sparing" and should be used cautiously in patients with compromised renal function.

E. **Fenamates: mefenamic acid and meclofenamate**

1. **Chemistry**
   a. Mefenamic acid and meclofenamate are both N-substituted phenylanthranilic acids.
   b. Other chemical members of this family include flufenamic, tolfenamic, and etofenamic acids.

2. **Pharmacokinetics.** Peak plasma levels for meclofenamate and meclofenamic acid are reached at approximately 2 hours and 2–4 hours, respectively. Plasma half-lives for these drugs are about 2–4 hours, with more than 50% eliminated in the urine.

3. **Pharmacologic effects.** The fenamates are **anti-inflammatory, analgesic,** and **antipyretic**.

4. **Therapeutic uses**
   a. Mefenamic acid is primarily used as an analgesic in **rheumatoid arthritis, soft-tissue injury,** and **dysmenorrhea**. Toxicity limits its usefulness, and it appears to have no advantage over other analgesic agents.
   b. As anti-inflammatory agents, the fenamates have been used in short-term trials for **osteoarthritis** and **rheumatoid arthritis** but, again, offer no clear advantage over other NSAIDs.

5. **Adverse effects**
   a. The most commonly reported adverse effects involve the gastrointestinal system and include dyspepsia or general discomfort.
      (1) Diarrhea, which may be severe and associated with steatorrhea or bowel inflammation, is also common.

   (2) The fenamates are contraindicated in patients with a history of gastrointestinal disease.
   b. Hemolytic anemia is a serious side effect and may be of an autoimmune origin.
   c. There are reports of cross-reactivity to fenamates in aspirin-sensitive patients.

F. Tolmetin

1. **Pharmacokinetics.** Tolmetin is rapidly and completely absorbed from the gastrointestinal tract. Peak plasma levels are achieved within 20–60 minutes after dosing, and the plasma half-life is about 5 hours. Tolmetin is extensively bound to plasma proteins and excreted virtually completely in the urine.

2. **Pharmacologic effects**
   a. Tolmetin is an NSAID that is more potent than aspirin but less potent than indomethacin.
   b. It is thought to preferentially inhibit CNS cyclooxygenase.
   c. Tolmetin also produces analgesic and antipyretic effects.

3. **Therapeutic uses.** The major therapeutic indication for tolmetin is for the treatment of **juvenile rheumatoid arthritis, adult rheumatoid arthritis,** and **osteoarthritis**.

4. **Adverse effects** are those common to most of the other NSAIDs, including:
   a. Gastrointestinal discomfort
   b. CNS symptoms
   c. Cross-reactivity in aspirin-sensitive patients
   d. Anaphylactoid reactions in some patients who are not aspirin-sensitive.

G. Propionic acid derivatives

1. **General considerations**
   a. Propionic acid derivatives include:
      (1) Ibuprofen
      (2) Naproxen
      (3) Fenoprofen
      (4) Ketoprofen
      (5) Flurbiprofen
      (6) Oxaprozin
   b. These agents offer significant advantages over aspirin and indomethacin because they are better tolerated at anti-inflammatory doses.
   c. All of these compounds can induce gastrointestinal side effects or alter platelet function; some may alter leukocyte function and motility.
   d. Drug interactions
      (1) Potential adverse drug interactions may result from the high degree of plasma albumin binding and the impact that this may have on **oral anticoagulants**.
      (2) Propionic acid derivatives may reduce the diuretic and natriuretic effects of **furosemide,** as well as the antihypertensive effects of **thiazides, β-adrenergic antagonists,** and **ACE inhibitors**.

2. **Ibuprofen** (Figure 9-4)
   a. Pharmacokinetics. Oral absorption is rapid, with peak plasma levels occurring within 1–2 hours and a half-life of about 2 hours. Excretion is rapid and complete, with more than 90% appearing in the urine, mostly as metabolites or conjugates.

$$(CH_3)_2CHCH_2- \bigcirc -\underset{\underset{CH_3}{|}}{CH}COOH$$

FIGURE 9-4. Ibuprofen.

b. **Pharmacologic effects.** Ibuprofen is equal to aspirin in its anti-inflammatory effect, but it is a more effective analgesic than aspirin or acetaminophen.

c. **Therapeutic uses.** As an NSAID, ibuprofen is used for the treatment of **arthritis** and **osteoarthritis**.

d. **Adverse effects**
   (1) Gastrointestinal effects occur in approximately 5%–15% of patients, but the incidence of these events is less than with aspirin or indomethacin. Nevertheless, ibuprofen should be used cautiously in patients with known peptic ulceration or gastric intolerance to other aspirin-like drugs.
   (2) Ibuprofen should not be used during pregnancy or nursing.
   (3) Ibuprofen is a potent inhibitor of cyclooxygenase and prolongs bleeding time.

3. **Naproxen** (Figure 9-5)
   a. **Pharmacokinetics**
      (1) **Absorption.** Peak concentrations occur within 2–4 hours, but naproxen's half-life is approximately 14 hours, permitting twice-a-day dosing.
      (2) **Distribution.** Naproxen is highly bound to plasma proteins. It does cross the placenta and appears in the milk of lactating women at about 1% of the maternal plasma level.
      (3) **Excretion** is primarily in the urine.
   b. **Therapeutic uses.** As an NSAID, naproxen is used for the treatment of **rheumatoid arthritis** and **osteoarthritis**.
   c. **Adverse effects**
      (1) Whereas the incidence of gastrointestinal and CNS effects approximates those of indomethacin, naproxen is better-tolerated.
      (2) Less common are pruritus and dermatologic problems.
      (3) Isolated cases of jaundice, renal dysfunction, angioneurotic edema, thrombocytopenia, and agranulocytosis have been reported.

4. **Fenoprofen**
   a. **Pharmacokinetics.** Oral absorption is rapid, although not as complete (85%) as for ibuprofen; peak plasma levels occur at approximately 2 hours, with a half-life of approximately 3 hours. Similarly, there is a high degree of plasma protein binding and virtually complete elimination via the urine.
   b. **Adverse effects**
      (1) Gastrointestinal effects account for the majority (15%) of reports, but these are generally milder than with equal doses of aspirin, and discontinuation is rarely required.
      (2) CNS effects include tinnitus, vertigo, lassitude, confusion, and anorexia.

5. **Ketoprofen**
   a. **Pharmacokinetics.** Ketoprofen exhibits a profile similar to that of ibuprofen, with a slightly longer half-life in elderly patients.
   b. **Therapeutic uses.** Like ibuprofen, ketoprofen is used to treat **arthritis** and **osteoarthritis**. It is also approved for ophthalmic use to relieve itching associated with **seasonal allergic conjunctivitis**.

FIGURE 9-5. Naproxen.

c. Adverse effects

(1) Gastrointestinal effects (30%) are generally less severe than those seen with aspirin and may be reduced further by taking the drug with food, milk, or antacids.

(2) Renal function should be monitored in patients older than 60 years of age or with impaired renal function because ketoprofen can cause fluid retention and transient increases in plasma creatinine levels.

(3) Patients treated concurrently with ketoprofen and methotrexate can develop life-threatening methotrexate hepatotoxicity.

6. Flurbiprofen

a. Pharmacokinetics. Flurbiprofen has a profile similar to that of ibuprofen, but its plasma half-life is approximately 6 hours.

b. Therapeutic uses

(1) Flurbiprofen tablets are used to treat the signs and symptoms of **rheumatoid arthritis** and **osteoarthritis**.

(2) Flurbiprofen is available in an ophthalmic dosage form for the treatment of **postoperative miosis**.

    (a) Trauma of intraocular surgery releases PGs, which cause progressive miosis.

    (b) Flurbiprofen decreases miosis without affecting intraocular pressure.

c. Adverse effects

(1) The profile is similar to that of other propionic acid derivatives with regard to the incidence of gastrointestinal and CNS effects.

(2) Flurbiprofen may exacerbate herpes simplex keratitis and delay wound healing. A foreign body sensation is the most common adverse effect.

7. Oxaprozin

a. Pharmacokinetics. Oxaprozin is orally absorbed and reaches peak serum concentrations in 3–5 hours. It is metabolized in the liver and excreted in bile and urine. The elimination half-life is 50–60 hours and increases with the patient's age.

b. Therapeutic uses. Oxaprozin is comparable in effectiveness to ibuprofen and other NSAIDs for treatment of **rheumatoid arthritis** or **osteoarthritis**. Its long half-life permits once-a-day dosing.

c. Adverse effects

(1) The incidence of gastrointestinal side effects may be slightly higher than for ibuprofen.

(2) Renal toxicity, hepatic toxicity, and prolonged bleeding may occur.

H. | Piroxicam

1. Chemistry. Piroxicam is one of the oxicam derivatives, a class of enolic acids.

2. Pharmacokinetics. Oral absorption is virtually complete, with peak plasma levels occurring 3–5 hours after dosing.

a. The plasma half-life is estimated to be approximately 50 hours, which allows once-daily dosing.

b. Steady-state plasma levels are achieved within 7–12 days, and maximal therapeutic responses occur within 2 weeks.

3. Pharmacologic effects

a. As an **anti-inflammatory agent,** piroxicam is equipotent to indomethacin, aspirin, and naproxen. Piroxicam may inhibit activation of neutrophils, suggesting an additional mode of anti-inflammatory action.

b. As with other cyclooxygenase inhibitors, piroxicam is both **analgesic** and **antipyretic**.

4. Therapeutic uses. Piroxicam is approved for use in the treatment of **rheumatoid arthritis** and **osteoarthritis,** but it has also been used in ankylosing spondylitis, musculoskeletal disorders, dysmenorrhea, postoperative pain, and gout.

5. Adverse effects
   a. Gastrointestinal side effects are most common. The longer half-life of piroxicam may cause a higher incidence of gastrointestinal bleeding than other NSAIDs.
   b. Piroxicam may have cross-reactivity in patients who are aspirin-sensitive.

I. Nabumetone

1. **Chemistry.** Nabumetone is a naphthoquinone.

2. **Pharmacokinetics**
   a. Nabumetone is absorbed in the duodenum as **nabumetone,** a weak cyclooxygenase inhibitor, and converted in the liver to **6-MNA,** a strong cyclooxygenase inhibitor.
   b. Peak serum concentrations of 6-MNA occur in 5 hours, with a terminal half-life of 24 hours.

3. **Therapeutic uses.** Nabumetone is effective for the treatment of **rheumatoid arthritis** and **osteoarthritis**.

4. **Adverse effects**
   a. As an inactive prodrug, nabumetone may cause less local gastric irritation.
   b. Gastrointestinal, CNS, and photosensitive adverse reactions occur.

J. Etodolac

1. **Chemistry.** Etodolac is a pyranone acid derivative.

2. **Pharmacokinetics**
   a. Absorption. Etodolac is well absorbed orally; it reaches a peak serum concentration in 1–2 hours.
   b. Distribution. More than 99% of etodolac is bound to plasma proteins.
   c. Metabolism and excretion. Etodolac is metabolized in the liver and excreted in the urine. Its elimination half-life is 6–7 hours.

3. **Therapeutic uses.** Etodolac is used in the treatment of **osteoarthritis** and as an analgesic.

4. **Adverse effects** include abdominal pain and dyspepsia. Gastrointestinal ulceration occurs in less than 0.3% of patients.

K. Phenylbutazone

1. **Chemistry.** Phenylbutazone, one of a group of drugs derived from pyrazolon, is a congener of antipyrene.

2. **Pharmacokinetics.** Phenylbutazone is rapidly and completely absorbed, with peak plasma levels occurring within 2 hours. The half-life is notably long, 50–65 hours. Significant concentrations may persist in synovial fluid for up to 3 weeks after treatment.

3. **Pharmacologic effects**
   a. Phenylbutazone is an effective anti-inflammatory agent, but toxicity prohibits its long-term use.
   b. Phenylbutazone possesses anti-inflammatory and analgesic activity that is qualitatively similar to that of aspirin. Its analgesic effect against nonrheumatic pain, however, is less than that of aspirin.

4. **Therapeutic uses.** Because phenylbutazone is poorly tolerated by many patients, it is not used as an antipyretic or general analgesic agent.
   a. Phenylbutazone is chiefly used in the short-term therapy of **acute gout** and in **acute** exacerbations of **rheumatoid arthritis,** but only after other agents have failed.
   b. Brief courses of the drug may be beneficial in the treatment of **osteoarthritis** and **ankylosing spondylitis**.

5. **Administration.** Phenylbutazone is administered orally. It should be taken with meals to lessen gastric irritation.

6. Adverse effects
   a. Significant salt and water retention occur through a direct effect on renal tubules; this can cause cardiac decompensation and acute pulmonary edema.
   b. Phenylbutazone can cause agranulocytosis or aplastic anemia. Phenylbutazone has a direct effect in reducing platelet function.
   c. As many as 10%–50% of patients experience nausea, vomiting, or skin rashes.
   d. Peptic ulceration has been reported.

7. Drug interactions
   a. Phenylbutazone may displace:
      (1) Oral anticoagulant drugs
      (2) Oral hypoglycemic drugs
      (3) Sulfonamides
      (4) Protein-bound thyroid hormone, thus complicating interpretations of thyroid function tests
   b. Induction of hepatic enzymes, or mixed function oxidases (MFOs), can disturb the metabolism of other active moieties.
   c. The effects of insulin may be potentiated by phenylbutazone.

L. Diclofenac

1. Chemistry. Diclofenac is the first of a series of phenylacetic acid derivatives developed as anti-inflammatory agents.

2. Pharmacokinetics
   a. Oral absorption is rapid and complete, with peak plasma levels achieved within 2 hours.
   b. There is a substantial first-pass effect, reducing systemic levels by as much as 50%.
   c. Diclofenac is highly protein-bound in plasma, and its half-life is 1–2 hours.
   d. Diclofenac accumulates in synovial fluid, which may account for its long-lived therapeutic effect, despite its short plasma half-life.

3. Pharmacologic effects
   a. Diclofenac is a potent anti-inflammatory, antipyretic, and analgesic agent; it is a more potent inhibitor of cyclooxygenase than indomethacin or naproxen.
   b. Additionally, diclofenac appears to alter the release or uptake of fatty acids, reducing intracellular levels of arachidonate in leukocytes.

4. Therapeutic uses. Diclofenac is approved for use in the treatment of **rheumatoid arthritis, osteoarthritis,** and **ankylosing spondylitis**. It may also be useful for short-term treatment of acute **musculoskeletal injury, tendinitis, bursitis, postoperative pain,** and **dysmenorrhea**.

5. Adverse effects. Approximately 30% of diclofenac patients report an adverse event, with about 2% discontinuing therapy.
   a. Gastrointestinal symptoms (20%) are the most common; bleeding, ulceration, and perforation have been reported.
   b. Elevated hepatic transaminase levels occur in about 15% of diclofenac patients. Hepatic transaminases should be monitored for the first 8 weeks of therapy. Hepatitis and jaundice have been reported.
   c. Diclofenac is not recommended for children, nursing mothers, or women who are pregnant.

M. Ketorolac

1. Chemistry. Ketorolac is a member of the pyrrolo-pyrrole group of NSAIDs.

2. Pharmacokinetics
   a. Absorption. Ketorolac is completely absorbed following intramuscular injection and reaches peak plasma concentrations in 1 hour. It is highly protein-bound and has a terminal half-life of 4–6 hours.
   b. Excretion. Ketorolac is excreted in the urine.

3. **Therapeutic uses.** Ketorolac is as effective as morphine or meperidine for the **short-term relief of moderate to severe pain**. Unlike narcotic analgesics, ketorolac does not produce respiratory depression.

4. **Adverse effects** are similar to those associated with the short-term use of oral NSAIDs (e.g., **drowsiness, dyspepsia, gastrointestinal pain,** and **nausea**). Serious gastrointestinal bleeding has not been reported.

III. DISEASE-MODIFYING ANTIRHEUMATIC DRUGS (DMARDs) encompass a wide range of compounds used in conjunction with NSAIDs to modify the immunologic response.

A. General considerations

1. Although NSAIDs may provide symptomatic relief for joint pain and morning stiffness, occult joint damage may still be occurring.
   a. DMARDs interfere with the pathogenesis of rheumatoid arthritis (Figure 9-6).
   b. Radiologic assessments of joint involvement and erosions are a valuable corroboration of the clinical efficacy of any drug regimen.

FIGURE 9-6. Overview of the pathogenesis of rheumatoid arthritis and the possible sites of action of the second-line agents. *AM* = antimalarials; *AZ* = azathioprine; *CP* = cyclophosphamide; *CS* = cyclosporine; *G* = gold; *M* = methotrexate; *P* = penicillamine; *S* = sulfasalazine. [Redrawn and modified with permission from Cash JM, Klippel JH: Second-line drug therapy for rheumatoid arthritis. *N Engl J Med* 330(19):1370, 1994.]

2. Because degenerative lesions do not regress once formed, there is an increasing tendency to institute DMARD therapy early in progressive cases; however, DMARDs are generally not the first drugs used to treat patients with arthritis.

3. Combination therapy with second-line agents has generally failed to be beneficial.

B. Gold

1. **Chemistry.** Most gold preparations used are aurous salts in which the gold is attached to sulfur.

2. **Pharmacokinetics**
   a. **Aurothioglucose** and **gold sodium thiomalate** are given by intramuscular injection.
      (1) Peak plasma levels occur within 2–6 hours, and virtually all (95%) is protein bound.
      (2) The plasma half-life is about 7 days for a 50-mg dose.
   b. **Auranofin** is given orally with about 25% absorption. Steady-state concentrations are achieved within 8–12 weeks of treatment.
      (1) A 6-month regimen of 6 mg/d yields about 20% gold accumulation as compared with injectable gold compounds.
      (2) With auranofin, the half-life of gold in the body is about 80 days.
   c. With long-term chrysotherapy, gold deposits build up. Gold can be detected in the urine up to 1 year after cessation of chrysotherapy.

3. **Pharmacologic effects**
   a. Gold preparations (i.e., aurothioglucose, gold sodium thiomalate, auranofin) have minimal anti-inflammatory activity.
   b. The primary mechanisms of action may be in the **inhibition of mononuclear phagocyte maturation and function**.
      (1) Gold is sequestered in mononuclear phagocytes within the inflamed synovium.
      (2) Gold thiomalate reduces migration and phagocytic activity of macrophages in inflammatory exudates, as well as lysosomal enzyme activity.
      (3) Gold may suppress cellular immunity.

4. **Therapeutic uses.** Even though parenteral gold has been accepted as the most effective second-line drug, its use has declined and its continued role challenged.
   a. Gold therapy is of little use in advanced arthritis or in mild disease.
   b. Chrysotherapy is sometimes beneficial in **juvenile rheumatoid arthritis, palindromic rheumatism, psoriatic arthritis,** and other connective tissue disorders.

5. **Preparations and administration**
   a. **Aurothioglucose** is water-soluble (50% gold), but it is given by intramuscular injection as a sterile suspension in fixed oil; each dose contains 50 mg/mL.
   b. **Gold sodium thiomalate.** Water-soluble gold sodium thiomalate (50% gold) is also given by intramuscular injection.
   c. **Auranofin** (29% gold) is taken orally for active rheumatoid arthritis.
      (1) Initial clinical responses may not be detected until 10–12 weeks of therapy.
      (2) Therapy should be discontinued if, after 3 additional months, response is still inadequate.
      (3) Auranofin may be somewhat less effective than injectable gold for rheumatoid arthritis, but it is less toxic and better tolerated.

6. **Adverse effects** occur in 25%–50% of patients on chrysotherapy. Cutaneous reactions, ranging from vasodilation and "nitroid" reactions to exfoliative dermatitis and lesions of the mucous membrane, are often observed with gold thiomalate but rarely with aurothioglucose.

C. Methotrexate produces an antirheumatic effect within 6 weeks of treatment.

1. **Pharmacokinetics.** Aspirin and other NSAIDs increase methotrexate's toxicity by slowing its rate of excretion.

2. Adverse effects
   a. Methotrexate is immunosuppressive, and infections (e.g., herpes zoster, *Pneumocystis carinii*) can occur.
   b. Lymphomas associated with Epstein-Barr virus infection have occurred but are reversed by discontinuation of therapy.
   c. At recommended doses, severe toxicity is rare; however, the drug is teratogenic.
   d. Methotrexate is **contraindicated** in patients with renal insufficiency or hemodynamic instability.

D. **Azathioprine** and **cyclophosphamide** are immunosuppressive drugs used to treat refractory rheumatoid arthritis. Some patients cannot tolerate these agents.

E. **Cyclosporine** is a fungus-derived cyclic peptide used only for patients with severe, progressive disease.

   1. Pharmacokinetics. Oral bioavailability of cyclosporine ranges from 20%–50% and its half-life is about 6 hours. It is metabolized in the liver and most is then excreted in the bile.

   2. Mechanism of action
      a. Cyclosporine is a highly selective **inhibitor of helper T cells**. It inhibits the production of interleukin-2 (IL-2) by helper T cells and reduces the production and release of other lymphokines in response to an antigenic stimulus.
      b. Cyclosporine also **binds to** lymphoid proteins called **cyclophilins** and **to isomerase enzymes,** which aid in the folding of certain proteins.

   3. Therapeutic uses. Cyclosporine is used in combination with prednisone to **sustain cardiac, renal, and hepatic transplants**. One-year survival is approximately 75%.

   4. Adverse effects. The major adverse effect is nephrotoxicity, a dose-related phenomenon that occurs in 25%–75% of patients treated with the drug. Both the glomerular filtration rate and renal plasma flow are reduced, but these effects are usually reversible. Neurologic toxicity, hypertension, and increased incidence of infections are also seen.

F. **Glucocorticoids**

   1. Therapeutic uses. Patients with severe rheumatoid arthritis may benefit from 5–10 mg/d of oral **prednisone;** patients with vasculitis may require higher doses. The adverse effects of long-term systemic corticosteroids usually preclude their use for all but the most severe forms of rheumatoid arthritis.

   2. Administration. An acutely inflamed rheumatoid joint may be helped by an intra-articular injection.

G. **Penicillamine**

   1. Therapeutic uses. Penicillamine in high doses can be effective in patients with refractory rheumatoid arthritis and may delay progression of erosions.

   2. Adverse effects. Penicillamine is highly toxic and teratogenic, and the most common adverse effects are similar to those of parenteral gold.

H. **Hydroxychloroquine,** an antimalarial agent, is frequently effective for rheumatoid arthritis and is usually well-tolerated.

I. **Sulfasalazine** appears to be as effective as penicillamine but it is less toxic. Gastrointestinal disturbances and rashes are common. Sulfasalazine may prevent progression of joint damage.

J. **Capsaicin,** an alkaloid found in hot peppers, is used to topically relieve arthritic pain.

IV. DRUGS USED IN THE TREATMENT OF GOUT

A. General considerations

1. **Mechanism of gouty inflammation**
   a. When the plasma is supersaturated with urate, needle-shaped crystals of monosodium urate precipitate in joint tissue.
   b. An acute inflammatory reaction occurs, resulting in the ingestion of monosodium urate crystals by polymorphonuclear leukocytes.
   c. Lysosomal enzymes are released by the granulocytes, producing a decrease in the local pH in the joint tissue.
   d. With a decreased pH, further urate precipitation occurs in joints and cartilage.

2. **Precipitating factors. Acute gouty arthritic episodes** can be precipitated by excessive alcohol consumption, by kidney disease, and possibly by high-purine diets or external stresses. If the gout is a secondary phenomenon unrelated to a genetic defect, the underlying cause of the hyperuricemia must be determined.

3. **Hyperuricemia** is not always accompanied or followed by gout; but when gout occurs, it is preceded by hyperuricemia.
   a. **Normal handling of uric acid.** Twenty-five percent of the body's uric acid is degraded in the gastrointestinal tract by bacterial enzymes. Seventy-five percent is renally excreted. Ninety-eight percent of the filtered uric acid is reabsorbed in the proximal tubule and then secreted in the distal portion of the proximal tubule.
   b. **Causes of hyperuricemia**
      (1) Excessive uric acid synthesis associated with myeloproliferative disorders and malignancies, especially after antineoplastic or radiation therapy, can cause hyperuricemia. Conditions that lead to high rates of cell formation and destruction increase serum levels of purines, because purines are derived from nucleic acids.
      (2) A primary defect in the rate of purine synthesis can cause hyperuricemia.
      (3) Decreased renal excretion of uric acid can be caused by certain drugs (e.g., thiazides) or by a genetic deficiency.
      (4) Sex-linked uricaciduria (e.g., in Lesch-Nyhan syndrome) can result from a lack of the enzyme hypoxanthine–guanine phosphoribosyltransferase.

B. Probenecid

1. **Mechanism of action and pharmacologic effects**
   a. At therapeutic doses, probenecid lowers serum levels of uric acid by inhibiting the proximal tubular reabsorption of uric acid.
      (1) In low doses, probenecid blocks the tubular secretion of uric acid, while at therapeutic doses probenecid is uricosuric.
      (2) When approximately 1 g of probenecid is administered daily, urinary excretion of uric acid increases by 50%, resulting in a corresponding decrease in serum urate.
      (3) The metabolic products of probenecid are also uricosuric.
   b. As a general inhibitor of the tubular secretion of organic acids, probenecid also increases serum levels of other organic acids, such as penicillin.
   c. Probenecid has no analgesic activity.

2. **Pharmacokinetics.** Probenecid is rapidly absorbed from the gastrointestinal tract.

3. **Therapeutic uses**
   a. By virtue of its uricosuric effects, probenecid is useful for the treatment of **chronic gout**.
   b. By virtue of its effects on organic acid excretion, probenecid is also used to prolong the effects of penicillin [see Chapter 12 II B 2 d (1) (b) (ii)].

   4. Administration. Probenecid is administered orally.
      a. The action of probenecid is blocked by the administration of aspirin.
      b. Because of its biphasic action [see IV B 1 a (1)], therapy with probenecid should not be initiated during an acute attack of gout.

   5. Adverse effects. Probenecid is well tolerated, the most common adverse effects being gastrointestinal disturbances and hypersensitivity reactions, such as skin rash and drug fever.

C. **Sulfinpyrazone**

   1. Chemistry. Sulfinpyrazone is a sulfoxide derivative of phenylbutazone.

   2. Mechanism of action and pharmacologic effects
      a. Sulfinpyrazone inhibits the proximal tubular reabsorption of uric acid. A hydroxy metabolite is also a potent uricosuric substance.
      b. Sulfinpyrazone also inhibits PG synthesis and interferes with a number of platelet functions, including adherence to subendothelial cells.

   3. Pharmacokinetics. After oral administration, sulfinpyrazone is well absorbed from the gastrointestinal tract and most is excreted unchanged in the urine.

   4. Therapeutic uses
      a. Sulfinpyrazone is used for the treatment of **chronic gout**.
      b. Because of its effects on platelets, it is being examined as an antithrombotic agent.

   5. Administration. Sulfinpyrazone is given orally. Administration with meals is recommended. As with probenecid, sulfinpyrazone therapy should not be initiated during an acute gouty attack.

   6. Adverse effects are similar to those seen with probenecid.

D. **Colchicine**

   1. Chemistry. Colchicine is an alkaloid derivative.

   2. Mechanism of action
      a. Colchicine inhibits the migration of polymorphonuclear leukocytes to the inflammatory area. It is proposed that colchicine produces ultrastructural alterations in leukocytes by attaching to the microtubular protein (tubulin) that is involved in cell motility and, thus, prevents the migration of granulocytes and inhibits phagocytic activity.
      b. Colchicine also blocks cell division by binding to mitotic spindles (mitotic blockade).

   3. Pharmacokinetics
      a. Colchicine is rapidly absorbed from the gastrointestinal tract.
      b. Large amounts of the drug and its metabolites reenter the intestinal tract in the bile and intestinal secretions.
      c. This high local concentration of drug, together with the rapid turnover of intestinal epithelial cells, which makes the cells particularly susceptible to mitotic blockade by colchicine, leads to altered function of the intestinal mucosa and produces one of the drug's major untoward effects, diarrhea.

   4. Therapeutic uses. Colchicine is effective in the treatment of **acute attacks of gout** and is also effective if given **prophylactically to prevent such attacks**.

   5. Administration. In an acute attack of gout, colchicine is usually administered orally in intermittent doses until pain disappears or gastrointestinal symptoms occur.
      a. The patient usually experiences a marked improvement in joint symptoms within 12 hours.
      b. A total of no more than 10 mg should be administered in one such course of therapy.
      c. Colchicine is excreted unchanged by the liver and kidney; therefore, the dosage may have to be reduced if renal or liver disease is present.

6. Adverse effects

a. Nausea, vomiting, and abdominal pain with diarrhea are warning signs that more serious toxicity could result and may indicate a need to discontinue colchicine therapy.

b. The most serious untoward effects that occur with chronic administration are agranulocytosis, aplastic anemia, myopathy, and alopecia.

c. A fatal dose of colchicine can be as little as 8 mg in 24 hours.

E. **Allopurinol**

1. Chemistry. Allopurinol is an isomer of hypoxanthine, a purine.

2. Mechanism of action

a. Allopurinol, together with its primary metabolite alloxanthine, prevents the terminal steps in uric acid synthesis by inhibiting the enzyme xanthine oxidase, which converts xanthine or hypoxanthine to uric acid. Hyperuricemia is, thus, reversed by the blockade of uric acid production.

b. Allopurinol acts as a competitive inhibitor, while alloxanthine acts noncompetitively.

c. The inhibition of xanthine oxidase causes serum levels of the catabolic intermediates xanthine and hypoxanthine to increase. Renal clearance of these substances, however, is rapid, and their increased plasma concentrations do not exceed their solubility. Thus, crystallization within joint tissue does not occur as it would with comparable levels of uric acid.

3. Administration. Allopurinol is administered orally. Starting with a low dose may lessen the probability of precipitating recurrent acute gouty attacks.

4. Adverse effects. Allopurinol is well tolerated.

a. The most common untoward effects are **hypersensitivity reactions,** including cutaneous reactions.

b. Acute attacks of gout occur more frequently during initial therapy with allopurinol.

(1) This may be due in part to the active dissolution of microcrystalline deposits of sodium urate (tophi) within subcutaneous tissue, resulting in transient periods of hyperuricemia and crystal deposition in joint tissue.

(2) To reduce this complication, simultaneous prophylactic therapy with colchicine is indicated.

F. **Nonsteroidal anti-inflammatory agents used in the treatment of gout**

1. Indomethacin may provide symptomatic relief in acute attacks. The dosage of indomethacin must be reduced for patients who are also taking probenecid, since the latter increases the plasma levels of indomethacin (see II C).

2. Phenylbutazone is an alternative drug to indomethacin in the treatment of acute gouty arthritis (see II K).

3. Aspirin and other salicylates, although they may provide symptomatic relief, actually antagonize the action of the uricosurics probenecid and sulfinpyrazone. Therefore, the salicylates are contraindicated when probenecid or sulfinpyrazone is being administered.

DIRECTIONS: Each of the numbered items or incomplete statements in this section is followed by answers or by completions of the statement. Select the ONE lettered answer or completion that is BEST in each case.

1. Which one of the following is an action of colchicine?

(A) It produces uricosuria
(B) It produces constipation
(C) It produces polycythemia
(D) It stimulates cell division
(E) It inhibits migration of granulocytes

2. Aspirin could be used prophylactically for which one of the following conditions?

(A) Noncardiogenic pulmonary edema
(B) Thromboembolism
(C) Metabolic acidosis
(D) Peptic ulcers
(E) Hypertension

3. The major therapeutic use for gold is in the treatment of

(A) advanced rheumatoid arthritis
(B) acute gout
(C) chronic ankylosing spondylitis
(D) early progressive rheumatoid arthritis
(E) chronic gout

4. A hemophiliac patient has rheumatoid arthritis. Which drug might be prescribed to relieve the pain?

(A) Acetaminophen
(B) Acetylsalicylic acid
(C) Phenylbutazone
(D) Ibuprofen
(E) Naproxen

5. Which of the following drugs used in the treatment of gout has as its primary effect the reduction of uric acid synthesis?

(A) Allopurinol
(B) Sulfinpyrazone
(C) Colchicine
(D) Aspirin
(E) Indomethacin

DIRECTIONS: Each of the numbered items or incomplete statements in this section is negatively phrased, as indicated by a capitalized word such as NOT, LEAST, or EXCEPT. Select the ONE lettered answer or completion that is BEST in each case.

6. True statements concerning characteristics of anti-inflammatory drugs include all of the following EXCEPT

(A) aspirin is uricosuric in high doses
(B) sulindac has a long half-life
(C) indomethacin causes frontal headaches
(D) ibuprofen has more potent anti-inflammatory effects than aspirin
(E) brief courses of phenylbutazone may have value in the treatment of ankylosing spondylitis

7. Characteristics of probenecid include all of the following EXCEPT

(A) it promotes the renal tubular secretion of penicillin
(B) it is useful in the treatment of gout
(C) at appropriate doses, it promotes the excretion of uric acid
(D) it has a mechanism of action similar to that of sulfinpyrazone
(E) the metabolic products of probenecid are uricosuric

8. A 58-year-old patient with long-standing rheumatoid arthritis has been taking twelve aspirin tablets daily for 2 years. Though aspirin has produced clear therapeutic benefit, she is now complaining of epigastric distress. All of the following statements are true EXCEPT

(A) the epigastric distress is likely to be dose- and time-related
(B) PGI$_2$ levels are likely to be increased
(C) the pain is probably the result of peptic ulcers or erosive gastritis
(D) concurrent administration of misoprostol might have prevented this complication

9. Ibuprofen can be bought over-the-counter for use as an analgesic. All of the following statements concerning this drug are true EXCEPT that

(A) it is a more effective analgesic than aspirin
(B) it is a more effective anti-inflammatory agent than aspirin
(C) it is used for the treatment of rheumatoid arthritis
(D) it is used for the treatment of osteoarthritis
(E) it can cause gastrointestinal complaints

10. All of the following are undesirable effects of the salicylates EXCEPT

(A) exfoliation of gastric mucosal cells
(B) inhibition of peripheral PGE$_2$ and PGF$_{2\alpha}$ synthesis
(C) stimulation of the chemoreceptor trigger zone (CTZ)
(D) salicylism
(E) decreased gastric mucus secretion

DIRECTIONS: Each set of matching questions in this section consists of a list of four to twenty-six lettered options (some of which may be in figures) followed by several numbered items. For each numbered item, select the ONE lettered option that is most closely associated with it. To avoid spending too much time on matching sets with large numbers of options, it is generally advisable to begin each set by reading the list of options. Then, for each item in the set, try to generate the correct answer and locate it in the option list, rather than evaluating each option individually. Each lettered option may be selected once, more than once, or not at all.

Questions 11–14

Match each description with the appropriate disease-modifying antirheumatic drug (DMARD).

(A) Methotrexate
(B) Aurothioglucose
(C) Glucocorticoids
(D) Hydroxychloroquine
(E) Penicillamine

11. An antimalarial agent frequently used for rheumatoid arthritis

12. Has emerged as the most frequently used second-line drug in the treatment of rheumatoid arthritis

13. *Pneumocystis carinii* infections, herpes zoster infections, and lymphomas associated with Epstein-Barr virus infection are complications of therapy with this drug

14. An injectable agent of little use in advanced arthritis

Questions 15–19

For each of the characteristics listed below, choose the drug that is most likely to show that characteristic.

(A) Aspirin
(B) Acetaminophen
(C) Phenylbutazone
(D) Probenecid
(E) Ibuprofen

15. Produces significant fluid retention

16. Possesses no analgesic activity

17. A uricosuric whose action is antagonized by salicylates

18. Possesses no anti-inflammatory activity but is a central prostaglandin (PG) inhibitor

19. Increases depth of respiration

Questions 20–22

Match each description with the appropriate nonsteroidal anti-inflammatory drug (NSAID).

(A) Ketoprofen
(B) Oxaprozin
(C) Nabumetone
(D) Phenylbutazone
(E) Indomethacin

20. Used to treat patent ductus arteriosus in neonates

21. Approved for ophthalmic use to relieve itching associated with seasonal allergic conjunctivitis

22. The metabolite, 6-MNA, is a much stronger cyclooxygenase inhibitor than the parent compound

1. The answer is E *[IV D 2 a]*. Colchicine is effective for the treatment and prophylaxis of acute gout. It inhibits the migration of polymorphonuclear leukocytes by attaching to tubulin, a microtubular protein involved in cell motility. Colchicine blocks cell division by binding to mitotic spindles. It is not uricosuric. Adverse effects include abdominal pain and diarrhea. Chronic administration can cause agranulocytosis and aplastic anemia.

2. The answer is B *[II A 3 e (1)]*. The prophylactic use of aspirin to reduce the risk of thromboembolic events has widened. Long-term salicylate therapy in older patients can cause noncardiogenic pulmonary edema. Toxic doses of aspirin depress the medulla and ultimately cause the accumulation of organic acids, resulting in a metabolic acidosis. Salicylates depress prostacyclin, which inhibits gastric acid secretion, thereby reducing cytoprotection. Aspirin has no use in the treatment of hypertension.

3. The answer is D *[III B 4]*. The major therapeutic use of gold is in the treatment of early, progressive rheumatoid arthritis, particularly when it is unresponsive to salicylates and other types of nonsteroidal anti-inflammatory therapy. Gold therapy is of little use in advanced rheumatoid arthritis. Gold is not used in the treatment of acute or chronic gout or ankylosing spondylitis. Therapeutic drugs for gout include probenecid, sulfinpyrazone, colchicine, allopurinol, indomethacin, and phenylbutazone. Drugs used for the treatment of ankylosing spondylitis include sulindac, phenylbutazone, and indomethacin.

4. The answer is A *[II B 4 a]*. All of the agents listed in the question except acetaminophen are capable of reducing platelet aggregation and, thus, prolonging bleeding times. Therefore, acetaminophen might be useful for relieving the pain of arthritis in a hemophiliac patient, who is already at risk for deficient hemostasis.

5. The answer is A *[IV E 2 a]*. The only agent listed in the question that interferes with the synthesis of uric acid is allopurinol. It does this by inhibiting xanthine oxidase, which converts xanthine and hypoxanthine to uric acid. Sulfinpyrazone is a uricosuric agent, while colchicine acts by preventing the migration of granulocytes. Indomethacin is a nonsteroidal

anti-inflammatory agent; it is useful for symptomatic relief in acute attacks of gout. Aspirin is useful for symptomatic relief in acute attacks of gout; at high dosages it can be uricosuric.

6. The answer is D *[II G 2 b]*. High doses of aspirin are uricosuric, and sulindac has a long half-life. Central nervous system (CNS) complaints, including frontal headache, frequently occur with indomethacin. Ibuprofen is not a more potent anti-inflammatory agent than aspirin; it is equipotent. Phenylbutazone is quite toxic, and its use is reserved for the short-term treatment of gout and ankylosing spondylitis.

7. The answer is A *[IV B–C]*. Probenecid prolongs penicillin blood levels by inhibiting the secretion of penicillin by the proximal tubule. Probenecid is a uricosuric agent that is useful in the treatment of gout because it blocks the reabsorption of uric acid in the kidney. Sulfinpyrazone has a similar mechanism of action, namely, inhibiting the renal tubular reabsorption of uric acid. The metabolic products of probenecid are uricosuric.

8. The answer is B *[II A 3 f (2)]*. Because gastric cytoprotection is reduced by aspirin, peptic ulcers or erosive gastritis is a likely source of this patient's epigastric pain. PGI_2 (prostacyclin) has a cytoprotective effect on gastric mucosal cells and it inhibits gastric acid secretion. Salicylates decrease PGI_2 levels. Misoprostol (a synthetic PGE_1 analog) prevents nonsteroidal anti-inflammatory drug (NSAID)-induced gastric ulcers, but not duodenal ulcers. The epigastric distress is likely related to the dose and length of use of the aspirin.

9. The answer is B *[II G 2]*. Ibuprofen is equivalent to aspirin in its anti-inflammatory effect, although it is a more effective analgesic than aspirin. As a nonsteroidal anti-inflammatory drug (NSAID), ibuprofen is effective for the treatment of rheumatoid arthritis and osteoarthritis. Ibuprofen can cause adverse gastrointestinal and central nervous system (CNS) effects, but it appears to be better tolerated than aspirin gastrointestinally. It is also safer than aspirin when taken in overdose amounts.

10. The answer is B *[I A 1 a; II A 3 f]*. Salicylates (e.g., aspirin) inhibit prostaglandin (PG) synthesis and, thus, have excellent anti-inflammatory properties. For example, the enzyme cyclooxygenase is irreversibly inactivated by aspirin, and this blocks the synthesis of PGE_2 and $PGF_{2\alpha}$. Both of these PGs are thought to be involved in inflammation-associated vasodilation, pain, and edema. The salicylates can cause epigastric distress and stimulate the chemoreceptor trigger zone (CTZ). Dose-related gastric ulceration and hemorrhage can occur, caused in part by exfoliation of gastric mucosal cells. Because the formation of PGI_2 (prostacyclin), which is known to inhibit gastric acid secretion, is suppressed, protective gastric mucus secretion is suppressed and gastric secretion increases. Salicylism is a mild salicylate intoxication and usually occurs with repeated ingestion of moderately large doses of salicylates. Salicylism is characterized by headache, dizziness, tinnitus, mental confusion, hyperventilation, and nausea.

11–14. The answers are: 11-D *[III H]*, **12-A** *[III C]*, **13-A** *[III C 2 a–b]*, **14-B** *[III B 2 a, 4]*. Hydroxychloroquine, an antimalarial agent, is frequently used to treat rheumatoid arthritis. It is usually well tolerated.

Methotrexate produces an antirheumatic effect within 6 weeks of initiation of treatment. It is the most frequently used second-line agent; however, it is immunosuppressive, and use of methotrexate can lead to infections with *Pneumocystis carinii* and herpes zoster virus. Lymphomas associated with Epstein-Barr virus infection have occurred but are reversed with discontinuation of therapy.

Aurothioglucose, a gold preparation, is administered by intramuscular injection. It used to be considered one of the more effective second-line drugs, but its use has declined.

15–19. The answers are: 15-C *[II K 6 a]*, **16-D** *[IV B 1 c]*, **17-D** *[IV B 4 a]*, **18-B** *[II B 3 a]*, **19-A** *[II A 3 d]*. Phenylbutazone, by a direct effect on renal tubules, causes salt and water retention.

Probenecid is the only agent listed that has no analgesic activity. Probenecid at therapeutic doses is uricosuric; it acts by inhibiting proximal tubular reabsorption of uric acid. Its action is antagonized by the salicylates.

Acetaminophen is a central prostaglandin (PG) inhibitor, but it exerts no anti-inflammatory activity.

Aspirin in full therapeutic doses causes an increase in alveolar ventilation characterized by an increase in the depth of respiration. Higher doses lead to hyperventilation and respiratory alkalosis. Toxic doses result in respiratory and metabolic acidosis.

20–22. The answers are: 20-E *[II C 4 b]*, **21-A** *[II G 5 b]*, **22-C** *[II I 2]*. Although the primary use of indomethacin is in the treatment of arthritic disorders, including acute gout, it has been used to treat patent ductus arteriosus in neonates and Bartter's syndrome (i.e., juxtaglomerular cell hyperplasia).

Ketoprofen is similar to ibuprofen, but it has a slightly longer half-life in elderly patients. It can be used ophthalmically to relieve itching associated with seasonal allergic conjunctivitis.

Nabumetone, a weak cyclooxygenase inhibitor, is absorbed in the duodenum. It is then converted in the liver to 6-MNA, a strong cyclooxygenase inhibitor. Because nabumetone is a relatively inactive prodrug, it may cause less gastric irritation.

Chapter 10

Hormones, Antagonists, and Other Agents Affecting Endocrine Function

---

I. ENDOCRINE FUNCTION

A. Hypothalamic–pituitary relationship

1. **Releasing hormones.** Pituitary (**adenohypophyseal**) function is mediated by neurohumoral substances, or releasing hormones, from the hypothalamus, which are transported via a rich capillary network in the region of the median eminence. These releasing hormones affect both the synthesis and release of pituitary hormones. Five hypothalamic releasing hormones have been well characterized.
   a. **Gonadotropin-releasing hormone (GnRH)**
   b. **Growth hormone-releasing hormone (GHRH)**
   c. **Melanocyte-releasing hormone (MSH)**
   d. **Thyrotropin-releasing hormone (TRH)**
   e. **Corticotropin-releasing hormone (CRH)**

2. **Vasopressin** and **oxytocin,** bound to a large carrier protein, neurophysin, are also produced by the hypothalamus. The active hormone is released from the posterior pituitary.

3. Some hypothalamic hormones are **inhibitory,** such as **somatostatin** and **dopamine,** which suppress prolactin release.

B. Pituitary hormones

1. Pituitary hormones comprise three major groups:
   a. **Somatomammotropins**
      (1) Growth hormone
      (2) Prolactin
      (3) Placental lactogen
   b. **Glycoproteins**
      (1) Luteinizing hormone (LH)
      (2) Follicle-stimulating hormone (FSH)
      (3) Human chorionic gonadotropin (hCG)
      (4) Thyroid-stimulating hormone (TSH)
   c. **Corticotropin and related peptides**
      (1) Adrenocorticotropic hormone (corticotropin, ACTH)
      (2) α-Melanocyte-stimulating hormone (α-MSH)
      (3) β-Melanocyte-stimulating hormone (β-MSH)
      (4) β-Lipoprotein (β-LPH)
      (5) γ-Lipoprotein (γ-LPH)

2. **Mechanism of action**
   a. Many hormones affect signal transduction through one of three major mechanisms.
      (1) **Cyclic adenosine monophosphate** (cAMP), or the **second messenger,** is increased via adenyl cyclase; cAMP activates protein kinases. Calcium (Ca^{2+}) levels are also affected. It appears that guanine nucleotide proteins (G proteins) may activate membrane-bound phospholipase C and account for the increased membrane fluidity, Ca^{2+} flux, and "flip-flop" of lipids in the membrane bilayer.

(2) Insulin and certain growth factors may act as membrane-bound receptors, which are also protein kinases.

(3) Steroid hormones bind to a membrane-bound receptor and become internalized via endocytosis. These hormone–receptor complexes access cytosolic or nuclear receptor proteins to act on DNA.

b. Feedback inhibition of hormone synthesis and release can be manipulated for therapeutic goals or used diagnostically to determine the level of endocrine dysfunction.

II. ENDOCRINE DYSFUNCTION

A. Pituitary anterior lobe disorders

1. Hypopituitarism in the adult (Sheehan's syndrome)

2. Pituitary dwarfism (in children)

3. Selective pituitary hormone deficiencies

4. Hypersecretion of pituitary hormones
   a. Acromegaly and gigantism (growth hormones)
   b. Cushing's syndrome (ACTH)
   c. Galactorrhea (prolactin)

B. Pituitary posterior lobe disorders. Diabetes insipidus results from insufficient production of vasopressin [antidiuretic hormone (ADH)].

C. Thyroid dysfunction

1. **Hypothyroidism**
   a. Cretinism and juvenile in children
   b. Myxedema in adults

2. **Hyperthyroidism**
   a. Thyrotoxicosis, Graves' disease, Plummer's disease
   b. Thyroid storm or crisis

3. **Goiter**

4. **Thyroiditis**
   a. Hashimoto's disease (autoimmune)
   b. Subacute granulomatous thyroiditis
   c. Riedel's (fibrous) thyroiditis

5. **Thyroid neoplasms**

D. Adrenal dysfunction

1. **Hyposecretion**
   a. Addison's disease (primary insufficiency)
   b. Secondary adrenal insufficiency

2. **Hypersecretion**
   a. Cushing's syndrome
   b. Congenital adrenal hyperplasia
   c. Adrenal virilism (adrenogenital syndrome)
   d. Hyperaldosteronism

3. **Pheochromocytoma**

4. **Nonfunctional adrenal masses**

E. | **Parathyroid dysfunction**

1. Hypoparathyroidism (postoperative tetany)

2. Hyperparathyroidism

F. | **Gonadal dysfunction**

1. Male hypogonadism

2. Testicular feminization syndrome

3. Precocious puberty

G. | **Carbohydrate metabolism disorders**

1. Diabetes mellitus

2. Hypoglycemia

3. Genetic disorders
   a. Galactosemia
   b. Fructose intolerance
   c. Glycogen storage disorders

III. HORMONES AND AGENTS AFFECTING ENDOCRINE FUNCTION

A. | **Growth hormone** is a somatomammotropin, as are prolactin and placental lactogen. They are structurally similar and probably evolved from a common ancestral gene.

1. **Activity, regulation, and mechanism of action**
   a. Growth hormone synthesis and release is controlled by both GHRH and somatostatin.
   b. Growth hormone is secreted by pituitary somatotrophic cells, which comprise up to 50% of all pituicytes; growth hormone is the most abundant and may comprise 10%–15% of the gland's dry weight.
   c. Growth hormone secretion is pulsatile, with about 0.5 mg/d released in 6–8 distinct but irregular bursts.
   d. Secretion may be elicited by hypoglycemia, exercise, stress, emotional excitement, a protein-rich meal, and after the onset of deep sleep.
   e. **Physiologic actions** include:
      (1) Statural growth as well as balanced systemic growth
      (2) Retention of protoplasmic nitrogen, increased amino acid transport, and decreased plasma urea levels
      (3) A diabetogenic effect on carbohydrate and lipid metabolism, which shifts the source of fuel from carbohydrates to lipids
   f. The **mechanism of action** for growth hormone is unknown but does not appear to involve changes in cyclic nucleotide levels, intracellular Ca^{2+}, or other familiar mechanisms of signal transduction.
      (1) Growth hormone may act by stimulating synthesis or release of **somatomedins,** which are identical to polypeptides known as **insulin-like growth factors (IGF) 1 and 2**.
      (2) IGF-1 appears to mediate growth hormone activity, enhancing sulfate incorporation into proteoglycans, increasing protein synthesis and RNA.
      (3) Low levels of IGF-1 are associated with **dwarfism.**
      (4) Like insulin, the IGF-1 receptor has protein kinase activity, which mediates hormonal signal transduction.

2. Growth hormone deficiency
   a. Etiology. Growth hormone deficiency may be a result of:
      (1) Adult hypopituitarism (Sheehan's syndrome), which, in conjunction with low cortisol levels, may lead to hypoglycemia.
      (2) Juvenile hypopituitarism, the result of either craniopharyngioma or an idiopathic etiology, causes **pituitary dwarfism**.
   b. Treatment. Recombinant DNA (rDNA)–derived growth hormone is used to treat disorders caused by growth hormone deficiency in children, including pituitary dwarfism.
      (1) Preparations. There are two synthetic versions of growth hormone.
         (a) Somatropin (191 amino acids) is the same as endogenous growth hormone. Recently, the Food and Drug Administration (FDA) approved **Humatrope** as a new brand of somatropin.
            (i) Humatrope has been approved for the treatment of growth failure in children with chronic renal failure.
            (ii) Unapproved uses include growth promotion in children with Turner's syndrome and acceleration of wound healing in children with large, cutaneous burns.
         (b) Somatrem (Protropin) has an extra methionine amino acid on the *N*-terminus.
      (2) Adverse effects. Usually, there are no serious adverse effects from growth hormone administration. However, the long-term safety of the growth hormone preparations is unknown.
         (a) Intracranial hypertension with papilledema has been reported.
         (b) Mild hyperglycemia and **glucosuria** may occur.
      (3) Contraindications. Growth hormone preparations are contradicted in patients with:
         (a) Closed epiphyses
         (b) Active tumors or neoplasia
         (c) Active or unhealed intracranial lesions

3. Hypersecretion of growth hormone can result in **acromegaly** and **gigantism**.
   a. Etiology. More than 90% of the cases of acromegaly are caused by growth hormone–secreting adenomas, or somatotropinomas.
   b. Treatment
      (1) The use of **bromocriptine,** a dopaminergic agonist, in acromegaly is paradoxical because dopamine stimulates growth hormone secretion in normal individuals.
      (2) Analogues of somatostatin, such as **octreotide,** offer therapeutic promise with minimal side effects.

B. | **Prolactin**

1. Activity, regulation, and mechanism of action
   a. Prolactin is synthesized and stored in pituitary lactotrophs, but **secretion is primarily under negative control by the hypothalamus.**
      (1) Dopamine is putatively considered the **prolactin release–inhibiting hormone (PRIH).**
      (2) Opioid peptides and **TRH** also affect prolactin secretion.
   b. Prolactin release mirrors that of growth hormone with regard to stimuli such as sleep, exercise, circadian rhythms, and estrogen levels.
   c. The **primary physiologic action** of prolactin is **lactation**. Prolactin, in a complex interaction with hormones of the adrenal cortex, thyroid, and ovaries, prepares the breast for secretion postpartum. Insulin, growth hormone, and oxytocin are also involved.
      (1) During pregnancy, high estrogen and progestin levels inhibit prolactin activity, but after birth, these hormone levels drop, leaving the actions of prolactin unopposed.
      (2) Breast-feeding elevates prolactin levels, which mediates an antigonadotropic effect, causing a lack of ovulation. This natural contraception diminishes over several months as the prolactin release to the sucking response wanes.

(3) Prolactin induces rapid increases in RNA synthesis for milk production proteins and lactose synthesis.

2. Prolactin-secreting disorders
   a. Etiology. Hyperprolactinemia may be caused by:
      (1) Dopaminergic antagonist drug therapy
      (2) Infiltrative disorders of the hypothalamus or pituitary
      (3) Hypothyroidism
      (4) Use of oral contraceptives
      (5) Prolactin-secreting tumors
   b. Significance. Prolactin may contribute to the development of mammary tumors.
      (1) In animal models, drugs that enhance prolactin secretion (e.g., reserpine, haloperidol, phenothiazines) facilitate tumor growth.
      (2) In patients with breast tumors, prolactin levels are normal; however, prolactin may play a permissive role.
   c. Treatment of galactorrhea, amenorrhea, and **infertility** resulting from hyperprolactinemia
      (1) Levodopa (L-dopa), a precursor to dopamine synthesis, has been used with initial and variable success, but some patients become refractory.
      (2) Bromocriptine, an ergot derivative and dopaminergic agonist, is often used to treat pituitary adenomas. Bromocriptine is no longer indicated for the prevention of physiologic lactation because it increases the risk of stroke and seizure in the postpartum period.
         (a) Galactorrhea and amenorrhea usually abate within weeks, and pregnancy is possible. (Bromocriptine restores ovulatory menses in approximately 80% of women with hyperprolactinemia.)
         (b) Bromocriptine should be discontinued during pregnancy.
         (c) Tumor regression has been noted, but the mechanism is unknown.
         (d) Cessation of bromocriptine therapy generally allows a recurrence of symptoms (and tumors).
      (3) Cabergoline is a new, selective, potent, and long-acting dopamine agonist that appears more effective and better tolerated than bromocriptine in women with hyperprolactinemic amenorrhea.

C. Human placental lactogen

1. Activity
   a. Placental lactogen has both growth-promoting and lactogenic activity.
   b. Its amino acid sequence is 83% identical to growth hormone and 30% identical to prolactin.

2. Function
   a. The function of human placental lactogen is not clearly defined but it is synthesized by the syncytiotrophoblasts of the placenta for release into the maternal circulation.
   b. Placental lactogen stimulates growth and development of the mammary gland.
   c. Placental lactogen is also luteotropic and may stimulate steroid production by the corpus luteum.

D. Gonadotropic hormones, FSH, LH, hCG, and inhibin, are also collectively known as glycoprotein hormones.

1. Activity, regulation, and mechanism of action
   a. FSH and LH
      (1) Production and secretion. FSH and LH are produced and secreted by the gonadotropic cells of the pituitary. As with other hormones under hypothalamic control, their release is modulated by plasma steroid concentrations or by the combined effect of their action (feedback inhibition).
         (a) At puberty, gonadotropin secretion doubles, reflecting increases in the frequency and amplitude of GnRH pulses.

        (b) In men, FSH and LH plasma levels are fairly stable; in women, plasma levels vary with the stage of the menstrual cycle.

     (2) Hormonal control of ovulation and the menstrual cycle is complex due to several levels of interaction and feedback inhibition.

        (a) The **preovulatory,** or **follicular, phase** is characterized by rising LH and FSH levels, which mediate ovulation and follicular growth, respectively. Ovarian estrogen production increases.

        (b) Ovulation is associated with LH and FSH spikes, often three- to six-fold higher than during menstruation. Estrogen production peaks also.

        (c) The **postovulatory,** or **luteal, phase** is characterized by proliferation of the vaginal and uterine mucosae. Menstruation is then initiated by the cessation of progesterone production.

           (i) As the **corpus luteum** involutes, estrogen and progesterone levels decline, causing endometrial and uterine degeneration, and menstruation begins.

           (ii) The degeneration of the corpus luteum may be mediated by a luteolytic substance, **prostaglandin $F_{2\alpha}$ ($PGF_{2\alpha}$),** or it may be programmed to degenerate at a fixed interval without external signals.

  b. hCG is secreted by the syncytiotrophoblasts of the fetal placenta as early as 1 week after ovulation.

    (1) hCG **maintains luteal function** and suppresses LH release.

    (2) hCG can be detected in the urine; levels peak at about 6 weeks after conception and stabilize at a lower level during pregnancy.

2. Oral contraceptives

  a. Types of formulations

    (1) Combination preparations are the most common oral contraceptives used.

      (a) Combination preparations contain both an **estrogen** and a **progestin.**

        (i) The estrogen used is either **ethinyl estradiol** or **mestranol.**

        (ii) The progestin used is **norethindrone acetate,** or **norgestrel,** or **ethylnodiol diacetate. Desogestrel, norgestimate,** and **gestodene** are new progestins that are considered less androgenic than other progestins. When used with estrogen as oral contraceptives, these progestins appear to be as effective as other progestins but have fewer androgenic-related adverse effects.

      (b) The **primary mechanism of action** appears to be suppression of the midcycle surge of LH and FSH, thereby suppressing ovulation and ovarian follicle growth.

      (c) Benefits. Recent evidence suggests that health benefits of combination preparations outweigh the risks: use results in a lower incidence of endometrial and ovarian cancer, and thromboembolic events are rare (particularly with lower doses of estrogen, which presumably increases clotting factor levels and platelet aggregation). Table 10-1 summarizes the beneficial effects of progestin.

    (2) Sequential preparations (estrogen for 14–16 days followed by 5–6 days of combined estrogen and progestin) were removed from the market due to reports of increased incidence of endometrial tumors.

    (3) Biphasic or **triphasic preparations,** which replaced sequential preparations, have a fixed estrogen level, but the progestin level varies to reflect changes in the menstrual cycle. This approach may minimize "breakthrough" or irregular bleeding.

TABLE 10-1. Effects of Progestins

↑ Low-density lipoprotein (LDL)
↓ High-density lipoprotein (HDL)
↓ Risk of endometrial cancer
↓ Endometrial hyperplasia

(4) Single-entity preparations

(a) The **"minipill"** contains progestin alone and may act by thickening the consistency of cervical mucus, which is a barrier to sperm. It has a higher failure rate than other oral contraceptives and may cause irregular bleeding.

(b) The **"morning after" pill,** or postcoital preparation, contains diethylstilbestrol (DES). DES must be started within 72 hours and continued (25 mg twice daily) for 5 days despite any nausea and vomiting. If DES is not effective, abortion may be considered due to the increased risk of vaginal carcinoma in children exposed in utero to estrogen and DES.

b. Adverse effects

(1) The development of certain types of **cancer** has been studied with oral contraceptives, but actual culpability is clouded by the long latency period and multiple risk factors.

(a) Estrogens are tumorigenic, causing tumors of the breast, uterus, testis, bone, and other tissues.

(b) There is an increased incidence of vaginal and cervical cancer in women who were exposed in utero to DES.

(c) Studies examining breast cancer rates among birth control users are conflicting and complicated. The risk of breast cancer might be slightly increased in women younger than 35 years of age. Oral contraceptives are contraindicated in patients with known or suspected neoplasms. Close monitoring of patients with fibrocystic disease, history of breast cancer, or breast nodules is advised.

(2) Nausea, vomiting, breast tenderness, weight gain, dizziness, and **headaches** are all associated with oral contraceptive use.

(3) Depression, irritability, ocular disturbances, and an **increased incidence of gallbladder disease** have been noted.

(4) Oral contraceptives **may cause birth defects if taken during the first trimester** of pregnancy.

3. Levonorgestrel implants (Norplant)

a. Mechanism of action. Contraception is achieved by subdermal implantation of six flexible silastic tubes containing a progestin, levonorgestrel. Levonorgestrel inhibits ovulation and causes thickening of cervical mucus.

(1) The amount of hormone initially released is about 85 ng/d but drops to about 50 ng/d at 9 months. At 18 months, the level is about 35 ng/d, which eventually declines to approximately 30 ng/d.

(2) Effective contraception may be achieved within 1 day (when implantation takes place during the first 7 days of menstruation) and lasts up to 5 years.

b. Adverse effects

(1) Bleeding irregularities diminish over time.

(2) Delayed follicular atresia and **ectopic pregnancy** are rare complications.

(3) Thromboembolic disorders may require removal of the steroid implants. Removal should also be considered in cases of prolonged immobilization or illness.

(4) Cardiovascular side effects are increased in women who smoke.

c. Contraindications include:

(1) Active **thrombophlebitis** or **thromboembolic disease**

(2) Undiagnosed **abnormal genital bleeding**

(3) Known or suspected **pregnancy**

(4) Hepatic disease; benign or malignant **liver tumors**

(5) Known or suspected **breast cancer**

4. Noncontraceptive uses (estrogens and progestins)

a. Prevention of cardiovascular disease in postmenopausal women. In postmenopausal women, estrogen therapy can reduce morbidity and mortality from myocardial infarction. However, it should be noted that estrogens increase the risk of heart attacks in men and, possibly, premenopausal women.

TABLE 10-2. Role of Estrogen in Decreasing Risk of Coronary Artery Disease in Postmenopausal Women

↑ High-density lipoprotein (HDL)
↑ Low-density lipoprotein (LDL) receptors ↓ LDL cholesterol
↓ Thromboxane effects on blood vessels
↑ Prostacyclin production
↓ Cholesterol deposition in vessels

    (1) Mechanism of action (Table 10-2). Estrogen decreases low-density lipoprotein (LDL) levels and increases high-density lipoprotein (HDL) levels. Atherosclerosis is correlated with elevated LDL levels and low HDL levels.

    (2) Adverse effects. Postmenopausal women taking only estrogen may have a 5- to 15-fold increased risk of developing endometrial cancer. Epidemiologic studies show a lower incidence when estrogen levels are reduced or accompanied by progestin.

b. Postmenopausal osteoporosis results from the loss of both hydroxyapatite (calcium phosphate complexes) and protein matrix (colloid), resulting in compromised skeletal integrity.

    (1) Estrogen therapy reduces the incidence of hip fracture by 50%.

        (a) Several months of estrogen therapy may be necessary to effect a positive Ca^{2+} balance. Doses of 15–25 ng/d are required to maintain or increase bone density.

        (b) The positive effects may be rapidly lost when estrogen therapy is discontinued.

        (c) The risk-to-benefit ratio is highest for women who have undergone hysterectomy or oophorectomy because the risk of endometrial carcinoma (from estrogens) is no longer an issue.

    (2) Other agents for postmenopausal osteoporosis treatment include:

        (a) Calcium citrate malate can increase bone mineral density and peak bone mass. Calcium supplementation has little effect in the first years after menopause but may increase bone mass in older postmenopausal women.

        (b) Salmon calcitonin is a peptide hormone that inhibits bone resorption; it is approved for treatment of osteoporosis. Human calcitonin is also available but is not yet approved for this indication.

            (i) Although calcitonin relieves bone pain resulting from vertebral collapse, unlike estrogen, it does not decrease cortical bone loss in the extremities.

            (ii) Allergic reactions and development of neutralizing antibodies to salmon calcitonin occur.

        (c) Bisphosphonates adsorb to apatite crystals, inhibiting osteoclast activity and decreasing bone resorption.

            (i) Etidronate (orally administered), used for the treatment of Paget's disease, has been used to treat osteoporosis; it inhibits mineralization of osteoid.

            (ii) Pamidronate may also increase bone mass but is only approved for the treatment of hypercalcemia resulting from malignancy.

        (d) Vitamin D may be effective in treating established osteoporosis by increasing calcium absorption from the gut.

c. Estrogen replacement therapy

    (1) Menopausal symptoms. Estrogen is used during and after menopause to relieve **vasomotor symptoms, hot flashes,** and **atrophic vaginitis.** Low-dose progestational agents (e.g., **megestrol**) can decrease the frequency of hot flashes in women (and men) and may be used when estrogen replacement therapy is contraindicated.

    (2) Dysmenorrhea can be treated with estrogens or a nonsteroidal anti-inflammatory drug (NSAID).

    (3) Failure of ovarian development (dysgenesis) may result in dwarfism due to hypopituitarism. Estrogen therapy at puberty in combination with an androgen for growth spurt can satisfactorily emulate endogenous release.

d. Antineoplastic uses of certain hormones have evolved, allowing manipulation of cancer development.

  (1) Progestins are used in the treatment of endometrial, breast, and prostate carcinomas and in hypernephromas.

  (2) Antiandrogens and **DES** are used in the treatment of prostatic cancer.

  (3) Antiandrogens and **GnRH agonists** have been used in the treatment of prostate cancer. **Leuprolide,** a peptide analogue, inhibits LH and FSH release by chronically stimulating, desensitizing, and down-regulating pituitary GnRH receptors.

   (a) Leuprolide produces responses equal to DES with less toxicity.

   (b) A leuprolide-induced transient flare-up of the disease can be prevented by concurrent use of flutamide, an antiandrogen.

   (c) Leuprolide is given as an injectable depot or by single administration.

  (4) Antiestrogens, such as **tamoxifen,** and **androgens** are used in the treatment of breast cancer.

   (a) Tamoxifen, after oral dosing, reaches peak blood levels within 4–7 hours; it has a biphasic half-life of 7–14 hours and 4–7 days. Steady-state levels are achieved within 4 weeks.

   (b) Tamoxifen is primarily indicated for:

      (i) Initial endocrine control of breast cancer

      (ii) Palliative treatment of advanced breast cancer in postmenopausal women. Premenopausal women do not respond as well as women who have been postmenopausal for years.

   (c) Tamoxifen has a relatively safe toxicity profile but **adverse effects** include:

      (i) Hot flashes, nausea, and vomiting

      (ii) Menstrual irregularities, vaginal bleeding, and discharge

      (iii) Pruritus vulvae and dermatitis

      (iv) Pain or inflammation at the tumor site, which is associated with a good response

5. Fertility drugs

 a. Clomiphene is a nonsteroidal partial antagonist that induces ovulation presumably by blocking hypothalamic estrogen receptors. The disrupted feedback inhibition results in **enhanced gonadotropin secretion. In men, gametogenesis** and **steroidogenesis** are also increased.

  (1) Effectiveness. After clomiphene treatment, 80% of women ovulate, 30%–40% become pregnant, and 10% of these pregnancies are multiple births. Clomiphene has little or no effect in postmenopausal women.

  (2) Adverse effects

   (a) In premenopausal women, ovulation may be accompanied by the formation of **ovarian cysts** and **ovarian hypertrophy**.

   (b) Prolonged use of clomiphene may increase the risk of **ovarian tumors**.

 b. Gonadotropins

  (1) Mechanism of action. Human menopausal gonadotropin (**Pergonal**) contains equal amounts of FSH and LH, whereas urofollitropin (**Metrodin**) contains only FSH. These agents **stimulate ovarian follicle development** but **require a sequential dose of hCG to induce ovulation**. They are administered parenterally.

  (2) Effectiveness. Multiple births have been reported in 17%–20% of all treated pregnancies.

  (3) Indications. This treatment is reserved for:

   (a) Women with low basal gonadotropin levels and low endogenous estrogen

   (b) Women who do not respond to clomiphene or cannot tolerate it

   (c) Men, to augment spermatogenesis (with hCG)

  (4) Contraindications. These agents are contraindicated in:

   (a) Women with primary ovarian failure

   (b) Patients with uncontrolled thyroid or adrenal dysfunction

   (c) Patients with intracranial lesions, such as a pituitary tumor

   (d) Pregnancy

      (e) Women with abnormal bleeding

      (f) Women with ovarian cysts or enlargement not due to polycystic ovary syndrome

    (5) One important **adverse effect** is the development of **ovarian hyperstimulation syndrome (OHSS),** which is characterized by increased vascular permeability.

6. Progestins (noncontraceptive uses) and antiprogestins

    a. Progestins may be indicated for:

      (1) Dysfunctional uterine bleeding

      (2) Dysmenorrhea

      (3) Premenstrual syndrome

      (4) Endometriosis

      (5) Suppression of postpartum lactation

      (6) Carcinoma

      (7) Hypoventilation

    b. Antiprogestins. Mifepristone (RU-486) is used as a contraceptive and abortifacient.

      (1) Mechanism of action. Mifepristone is a competitive antagonist at both progesterone and glucocorticoid receptors. Its actions include:

        (a) Inhibition of ovulation during the follicular phase by blocking hypothalamic–pituitary progesterone receptors, which suppresses midcycle gonadotropin release

        (b) During the luteal phase, inhibition of progesterone action on the uterus, which induces prostaglandin release from the endometrium

        (c) Termination of pregnancy by facilitating luteolysis, menstruation, uterine motility, softening of the cervix, and detachment of the embryo

      (2) Mifepristone is also being studied for use in:

        (a) Induction of labor after intrauterine death

        (b) Cervical ripening in anticipation of a second-trimester abortion

        (c) Adjunctive treatment of progesterone-sensitive tumors

7. Androgens and antiandrogens

    a. Androgens. The actions of the androgenic hormones manifest in early embryonic growth (sex differentiation), early neonatal life (anabolic growth), puberty, and adult sexual life.

      (1) Synthesis and secretion. Testosterone is synthesized in the testis, ovary, and adrenal cortex. In target tissues, like the seminiferous tubules or Sertoli cells, testosterone is reduced to **dihydrotestosterone**.

        (a) The gonadotropic LH appears to mediate its effect through cAMP on the Leydig cells to convert cholesterol to androgens. Growth hormone and estrogen may have synergistic and antagonistic actions, respectively, on LH-mediated effects.

        (b) FSH also affects LH-mediated actions on the Leydig cells, but the major effect of FSH is on the Sertoli cells of the seminiferous tubules and, thus, spermatogenesis.

        (c) Feedback inhibition of gonadotropin release may encompass not only plasma cerebrospinal fluid (CSF) levels of hormones but also estrogens formed locally in the brain and **inhibin,** a peptide produced in the Sertoli cells and ovary.

      (2) Androgen replacement therapy

        (a) Therapeutic uses include:

          (i) Induction of puberty and maintenance of sex characteristics in adults with testicular failure, accidental castration, or hypogonadism

          (ii) Stimulation of erythropoietin secretion in some types of refractory anemia

          (iii) Induction of anabolic effects (weight gain) in undernourished patients or in the terminally ill. (This application is a controversial and dangerous form of abuse among professional athletes.)

          (iv) Replacement therapy in women with hypopituitarism; androgens are given in conjunction with other hormones (i.e., thyroid, growth, adrenal corticosteroid, estrogen hormones)

   (v) Breast cancer therapy because of its antiestrogenic effect

   (vi) Treatment of short stature not due to pituitary insufficiency; androgen treatment in children younger than 9 years old may have negative consequences

   (vii) Treatment of hereditary angioneurotic edema, a condition in which complement activation is unopposed, leading to increased vascular permeability and angioedema; the benefit of androgens is likely manifested on liver function rather than on androgenic action

  (b) Preparations are available for oral, injectable, or transdermal (scrotal skin) administration.

   (i) The greatest androgenic potency is with agents that are 17-β esters of testosterone and given by injection.

    Substitution at the 17-β position affects lipid solubility and duration of action.

    In order of decreasing duration, the 17-β esters are testosterone ethanate > cypionate > propionate > acetate.

   (ii) The 17-α alkylated derivatives (e.g., methyltestosterone, Fluoxymesterone, oxandrolone, norethindrone) are orally active and less androgenic.

  (c) Adverse effects are divided into three major areas (Table 10-3).

 b. Antiandrogens

  (1) Androgen receptor antagonists, like **cyproterone** and **flutamide,** are potentially useful in treating prostate cancer, acne, male-pattern baldness, virilizing syndromes, and precocious puberty, and inhibiting the sex drive in men who are sex offenders.

  (2) Finasteride

   (a) Mechanism of action. Finasteride, a 4-azasteroid, is a specific inhibitor of steroid 5α-reductase, which catalyzes the conversion of testosterone to dihydrotestosterone.

TABLE 10-3. Adverse Effects of Androgen Replacement Therapy

	Virilizing Effects	Feminizing Effects*	Toxic Effects†
Women	Acne		Edema
	Facial hair		Jaundice and cholestatic hepatitis‡
	Deepening of voice		
	Menstrual irregularities		Peliosis hepatitis
	Male-pattern baldness		Hepatic carcinoma
	Altered musculature		Skewing of diagnostic tests
	Hypertrophy of the clitoris		
	Masculinization of female embryos following in utero exposure		
Children	Premature closure of the epiphyseal plates		
	Altered bone development		
Men	Inhibition of gonadotropin release	Gynecomastia	
	Reduced spermatogenesis lasting months after discontinuation		

*Exacerbated in children and men with poor liver function.
†All patients.
‡Especially with the 17-α alkyl substituted androgens.

      (i) Dihydrotestosterone is responsible for the development of prostatic hypertrophy.

      (ii) Finasteride does not interfere with testosterone-dependent functions, such as potency and libido.

    (b) Pharmacokinetics

      (i) Absorption. 60% of the dose is absorbed from the gastrointestinal tract.

      (ii) Fate. Finasteride is metabolized in the liver.

      (iii) Excretion. Finasteride is excreted in the urine and feces.

    (c) Therapeutic uses and administration

      (i) For the treatment of **benign prostatic hyperplasia,** 5 mg of finasteride are administered once daily, for up to 6–12 months to determine patient response.

        In responsive patients, the drug should be continued indefinitely or the prostate will return to its former size.

      (ii) Early clinical investigation suggests that finasteride might be useful for the treatment of **prostate cancer**. Men with 5α-reductase deficiency do not develop this disease.

    (d) Adverse effects. Finasteride may cause abnormal fetal development. Pregnant women should avoid contact with crushed tablets or the semen of men being treated with finasteride.

  c. Male contraceptives

    (1) Gossypol, a phenolic derivative of the cotton plant, is a potent azoospermic agent and impairs sperm motility, both of which are reversible effects. Adverse effects include those seen in cottonseed poisoning:

      (a) Hypokalemia and weakness

      (b) Diarrhea, edema, dyspnea, and neuritis

      (c) Paralysis at high doses

    (2) Gonadal steroids, such as **estrogen** and **progesterone,** are azoospermic and depress libido and potency; gynecomastia can occur.

    (3) An experimental regimen combining an **androgen** and a **progestin** has produced variable results. Azoospermia develops over months; recovery after discontinuation also takes months.

    (4) Potent **agonists and antagonists of GnRH,** given **with testosterone,** produce variable azoospermia.

E. Thyroid hormones

1. Synthesis

  a. Thyroglobulin, a large protein of 600,000 molecular weight, is synthesized in the thyroid gland.

    (1) The tyrosines on the molecule are iodinated and coupled by a peroxidase. The iodinated thyroglobulin is secreted into the lumen of the gland.

    (2) The hypothalamus releases **TRH,** which stimulates the pituitary gland to release **thyrotropin**. In the thyroid gland, thyrotropin stimulates the uptake of thyroglobulin from the lumen back into the cell where it is broken down to yield the thyroid hormones.

  b. There are two forms of thyroid hormone (Figure 10-1): **thyroxine (T_4),** which is relatively inactive, and **triiodothyronine (T_3),** which is converted from T_4 by the enzyme thyronine 5′-deiodinase. T_3 is the active hormone.

2. Physiologic effects

  a. Thyroid hormones regulate growth and development, principally through the interaction of T_3 with nuclear receptors that bind to the regulatory regions of genes and modify their expression.

  b. They exert a calorigenic effect by increasing the basal metabolic rate.

  c. Thyroid hormones accelerate carbohydrate utilization and enhance lipolytic reactions, one consequence of which is a decrease in plasma cholesterol.

  d. They inhibit pituitary secretion of thyrotropin by negative feedback.

FIGURE 10-1. Structures of thyroxine (A) and triiodothyronine (B).

    e. They are cardiovascular stimulants.
    f. T_3 is an essential factor in the normal secretion of growth hormone in humans.

3. Therapeutic uses
    a. Thyroid hormone therapy is used for the treatment of **hypothyroidism (myxedema),** including **myxedema coma**.
    b. If thyroid hormone therapy is begun early after birth in hypothyroid infants, the consequences of **cretinism** are prevented.
    c. Thyroid hormone is used in patients with **simple goiter** and in patients with **nodular goiter** who are deficient in the secretion of thyroid hormone. In the case of nodular goiter, carcinoma should be ruled out.

4. Preparations and administration
    a. Thyroid tablets are made from extracts of the thyroid gland.
    b. Thyroglobulin is a purified extract of pig thyroid.
    c. Levothyroxine sodium is the sodium salt of L-thyroxine.
    d. Liothyronine sodium is the sodium salt of L-triiodothyronine.
    e. Equivalent clinical responses are obtained from the daily administration of about 60 mg of thyroid, 60 mg of thyroglobulin, 100 µg of levothyroxine, or 25 µg of liothyronine.

5. Adverse effects
    a. Cardiac effects are the most important and call for care in initiating therapy. **Palpitations** caused by thyroid hormones can be treated with β-adrenergic blocking agents.
    b. Levothyroxine can cause **thyrotoxicosis**. During long-term administration, serum T_4 levels may rise without a change in dose.

6. Thyroid hormone inhibitors
    a. Types and mechanisms of action are summarized in (Table 10-4).
    b. Antithyroid agents
        (1) Pharmacokinetics
            (a) The prototype agent, **propylthiouracil,** is rapidly absorbed and has a short half-life (2 hours). It has a shorter duration of action than methimazole (half-life, 3–5 hours). Methimazole (but not propylthiouracil) is effective when administered once daily.

TABLE 10-4. Actions of Thyroid Hormone Inhibitors

Class	Mechanism of Action
Antithyroid agents	
Propylthiouracil	Inhibits peroxidase, thus inhibiting the organification of iodine
	Inhibits the peripheral conversion of T_4 to T_3
Methimazole*	Inhibits peroxidase, thus inhibiting the organification of iodine
Iodide	Unknown
Iodine-containing compounds	
Lugol's solution	Inhibits the release of T_3 and T_4
β-Adrenergic antagonists	
Propranolol	Reduces activity of thyroid hormone on target tissues
Radioactive iodine	Rapidly concentrates in the colloid of thyroid follicles, damaging the gland through cytotoxic effects
Ionic inhibitors	Competitively inhibit iodine uptake; seldom used

T_3 = triiodothyronine; T_4 = thyroxine.
*Methimazole is the active metabolite of propylthiouracil.

(b) Antithyroid agents cross the placenta and are found in breast milk, methimazole to a greater extent than propylthiouracil. Both drugs concentrate in the thyroid and are excreted renally.

(2) Therapeutic uses. Antithyroid agents are most frequently used to treat children, young adults, and pregnant women with hyperthyroidism resulting from Graves' disease. They may be used:

(a) Alone

(b) With radioiodine while awaiting the beneficial effects of radiation to occur

(c) Before surgical treatment of hyperthyroidism

(3) Adverse effects

(a) The most serious adverse effect is **idiosyncratic agranulocytosis**. Because this risk is lower with methimazole, methimazole is preferred over propylthiouracil.

(b) The most common adverse effect is **transient leukopenia**.

(c) Other complaints include **maculopapular rash, fever,** and **joint pain**.

c. Iodide

(1) Therapeutic uses in hyperthyroidism

(a) Iodide is used preoperatively to control hyperthyroidism in Graves' disease because it reduces the size of the gland and makes the gland firmer by inhibiting the release of thyroid hormone for a few days or weeks.

(b) It is best to control the hyperthyroidism first with an antithyroid agent, such as propylthiouracil. Iodide is then begun 10 days before the operative procedure.

(2) Preparations and administration

(a) Lugol's solution contains 5% iodine, which is reduced to iodide in the intestine, and 10% potassium iodide.

(b) Potassium iodide is available for oral use in both solution and solid forms.

(3) Adverse effects

(a) Preparations containing iodine or iodide can produce an acute hypersensitivity reaction, resulting in angioedema, cutaneous hemorrhages, and symptoms of serum sickness.

(b) Chronic iodide administration can result in **iodism**. All of the symptoms usually resolve within a few days after the discontinuation of iodide.

(i) This is characterized by a brassy taste, increased salivation, and soreness of the teeth and gums. Swelling of the eyelids and symptoms resembling an upper respiratory tract infection may be observed.

(ii) Inflammation of the pharynx and larynx can occur, as can severe frontal headache.

(iii) Several types of skin lesions have been observed.

d. Radioactive iodine

(1) Pharmacokinetics

(a) The most commonly used isotope is **iodine-131 (^{131}I)**, which has a half-life of 8 days and emits both β particles and γ rays.

(b) Radioiodine is rapidly incorporated into the colloid of the thyroid follicles.

(2) Therapeutic uses

(a) Radioactive iodine is highly effective in the treatment of hyperthyroidism, especially in older patients with heart disease.

(b) It is the treatment of choice for recurrent hyperthyroidism after antithyroid drug therapy.

(c) It is also a useful diagnostic tool to delineate thyroid disorders.

(3) Preparations and route of administration. Sodium iodide labeled with either ^{131}I or iodine-125 (^{125}I) is available as a solution and as capsules and can be administered orally or intravenously.

(4) Adverse effects

(a) The treatment of hyperthyroidism with radioactive iodine is associated with a relatively high incidence of delayed hypothyroidism.

(b) Usually, there is a delayed onset in the control of hyperthyroidism.

(c) There is no conclusive evidence that radioiodine causes cancer in adults, but most physicians are hesitant to use it in patients younger than 30 years old, not only because of this possible risk but also because of potential unknown effects on future offspring.

(d) Radioiodine is contraindicated in pregnancy and in nursing mothers.

e. β-Adrenergic antagonists

(1) Therapeutic uses. β-Adrenergic antagonists alleviate the symptoms and signs of Graves' hyperthyroidism (e.g., tremor, anxiety, palpitations). The synthesis and secretion of thyroid hormone are not affected.

(2) Administration. β-Adrenergic antagonists are given when symptoms are moderate and discontinued when the patient is euthyroid.

F. Parathyroid hormones

1. General considerations

a. Physiologic role of parathyroid hormone (PTH, parathormone). PTH is a single peptide chain of 84 amino acids that **regulates the concentration of Ca^{2+} and phosphate levels in the extracellular fluid**. Plasma Ca^{2+} is the most important regulator of PTH secretion.

(1) PTH acts on various peripheral tissues to mobilize Ca^{2+} into the extracellular fluid and restore the concentration to normal when it has been lowered.

(2) PTH increases the active absorption of Ca^{2+} from the small intestine. This is a vitamin D–dependent process.

(3) PTH increases the rate of bone resorption of Ca^{2+} and phosphate.

(4) At physiologic doses, PTH increases the renal tubular reabsorption of Ca^{2+} and the excretion of phosphate. The effects on both bone and kidney are probably mediated via cAMP.

b. Pharmacokinetics. PTH has a plasma half-life of about 2–5 minutes and is rapidly removed by the liver and kidney.

c. Diseases of the parathyroid gland

(1) Hypoparathyroidism is one of many causes of **hypocalcemia**.

(a) Symptoms and signs include paresthesias of the extremities, tetany, laryngospasm, and eventually generalized convulsions. Spasms of smooth muscle can also occur. Electrocardiographic changes can include marked tachycardia.

(b) Treatment. Dietary supplementation of vitamin D and Ca^{2+} is the principal form of treatment.

    (2) Hyperparathyroidism
      (a) Etiology
        (i) The **primary form** of hyperparathyroidism is due to **parathyroid hyperplasia** or **adenoma** or to **tumors at other sites**.
        (ii) The **secondary form** is a result of **conditions producing a negative Ca^{2+} balance,** such as **malabsorption** or **renal disease**.
      (b) Symptoms and signs include hypercalciuria (which can result in a renal calculi), muscle weakness, constipation, nausea, and vomiting.
      (c) Treatment is usually by surgical resection, although long-term therapy with neutral phosphate, a low-calcium diet, and fluids may be given to those patients who are poor surgical candidates.

2. Calcitonin
  a. General considerations
    (1) Parafollicular C cells of the thyroid are the site of production and secretion of calcitonin. Parafollicular C cells are also found in the parathyroid and thymus.
    (2) The synthesis and secretion of calcitonin are regulated by the plasma Ca^{2+} concentration. cAMP, epinephrine, glucagon, gastrin, and cholecystokinin all stimulate calcitonin release after ingestion of Ca^{2+} salts.
    (3) By altering osteoclastic and osteocytic activity, calcitonin can directly inhibit bone resorption.
    (4) Calcitonin, in part by a cAMP–mediated reaction, increases kidney excretion of Ca^{2+}, phosphate, and sodium (Na^+).
  b. Therapeutic uses
    (1) The major uses of calcitonin are to decrease hypercalcemia and hyperphosphatemia in patients with:
      (a) Hyperparathyroidism
      (b) Idiopathic hypercalcemia of pregnancy
      (c) Vitamin D intoxication
      (d) Osteolytic bone metastases
    (2) Calcitonin may decrease the rate of bone loss in patients with postmenopausal osteoporosis.
    (3) Although calcitonin is effective for the treatment of Paget's disease of bone, patients may become resistant to therapy within several months.
  c. Preparations and route of administration
    (1) Salmon and human calcitonin are used clinically.
    (2) They are administered subcutaneously or intramuscularly. A nasal formulation is under development.
  d. Adverse effects include occasional edema and nausea and the stimulation of neutralizing antibody formation.

3. Sodium etidronate
  a. Mechanism of action. Sodium etidronate is thought to slow the formation and dissolution of hydroxyapatite crystals.
  b. Pharmacologic effects. Its advantages over calcitonin include oral efficacy and lack of antigenicity.
  c. Therapeutic uses. Sodium etidronate is used in the treatment of Paget's disease of bone.
  d. Route of administration. Etidronate disodium is given orally. Daily doses, given for not more than 6 months, may produce a long-lasting remission.

G. Corticotropin and adrenal corticosteroids

1. General considerations
  a. The **adrenal cortex** is a homeostatic organ, regulating reactions to stress.
  b. Corticosteroid pathway. The release of adrenal corticosteroids is controlled by a pathway (Figure 10-2) that includes the central nervous system (CNS). Corticosteroid secretion shows a diurnal rhythm; peak secretion occurs between 4 A.M. and 8 A.M.

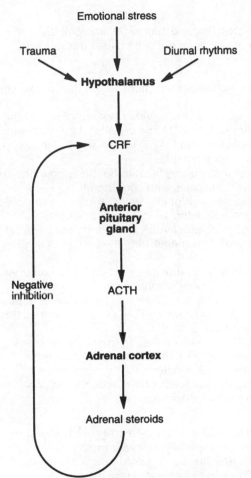

FIGURE 10-2. The pathway of adrenocorticotropic hormone (*ACTH*) and adrenal steroid secretion. *CRF* = corticotropin-releasing factor.

    (1) Corticotropin-releasing factor (CRF). A number of stimuli, including trauma, chemicals, diurnal rhythms, and emotion, can cause the hypothalamus to release CRF. CRF traverses the hypophyseal portal system and stimulates the anterior pituitary gland.

    (2) The **anterior pituitary gland,** in turn, is stimulated to release ACTH.

    (3) ACTH circulates in the bloodstream and stimulates the production of **glucocorticoids** from the adrenal cortex.

    (4) A **negative feedback pathway** maintains homeostasis. When the levels of endogenous corticosteroids increase, the **pituitary–adrenal axis** is suppressed, and the production of ACTH and CRF is reduced.

  c. Endogenous corticosteroids released by the adrenal cortex

    (1) Glucocorticoids chiefly affect carbohydrate and protein metabolism. In stressful situations, the amount of endogenous corticosteroids secreted daily can increase ten-fold.

      (a) Cortisol (hydrocortisone), 10–25 mg secreted daily

      (b) Cortisone, 0.5–2.0 mg secreted daily

      (c) Corticosterone, 30–150 µg secreted daily

    (2) Mineralocorticoids chiefly affect electrolyte and water metabolism.

(a) **Aldosterone** secretion is stimulated by serum angiotensin and serum potassium (K$^+$) levels.

(b) **Desoxycorticosterone**

2. Adrenocorticotropic hormone (ACTH)

a. Chemistry
(1) Human ACTH is a polypeptide hormone consisting of 39 amino acids.
(2) Synthetic derivatives have fewer amino acids but still possess the action of endogenous ACTH.

b. Mechanism of action
(1) ACTH is thought to stimulate specific protein receptor sites on the adrenal cortical cell membrane.
(2) This membrane receptor is believed to be linked with a system for generating cAMP. When the receptor is occupied by ACTH, the cAMP system is activated and the synthesis of corticosteroids is initiated. ACTH is thought to increase the amount of cholesterol entering the mitochondria.
(3) The binding of ACTH to the receptor stimulates the rate-limiting step in the corticosteroid synthetic pathway (which originates with cholesterol).
(4) Although ACTH is required for the synthesis of mineralocorticoids, it stimulates the synthesis of glucocorticoids more than that of mineralocorticoids.

c. Therapeutic uses.
The development of synthetic steroids limited the use of ACTH principally to serving as a **diagnostic tool** for distinguishing the two types of adrenal insufficiency.
(1) In **primary adrenal insufficiency (Addison's disease),** the administration of ACTH produces no effect because of the underlying adrenal cortex dysfunction.
(2) In **secondary adrenal insufficiency,** the dysfunction occurs in the anterior pituitary. If ACTH is administered, the adrenal cortex will respond by synthesizing and releasing the adrenocorticosteroids.

d. Route of administration.
Because ACTH is a polypeptide hormone, it must be administered parenterally, and most often is given intramuscularly. It is rapidly hydrolyzed in the tissues with a half-life of 15 minutes.

e. Adverse effects
are rare, but hypersensitivity reactions have occurred on occasion. Toxicity is dose-related and results from corticosteroid excess.

3. Adrenal corticosteroids

a. Structure–activity relationships.
The general structure of a corticosteroid is shown in Figure 10-3. Certain structural features are especially relevant to activity:
(1) Position 11: Oxygen or halogen is essential for corticoid function to exist.
(2) Position 17: The presence of OH or C = O increases corticoid activity.
(3) A double bond at position 1,2 increases glucocorticoid activity.
(4) Position 6 or 9: Halogenation increases activity.
(5) Position 6 or 16: The presence of an alkyl group increases glucocorticoid activity.

FIGURE 10-3. General structure of the adrenal corticosteroids.

b. Mechanism of action
   (1) The steroid receptor is nuclear.
   (2) Once the steroid traverses the cell membrane and binds to the receptor, the steroid–receptor complex in the cell nucleus then binds to chromatin.
   (3) The drug-receptor–chromatin complex stimulates the formation of messenger RNA (mRNA).
   (4) The mRNA stimulates the synthesis of enzymes that control rate-limiting reactions in the synthetic pathway of the steroids.

c. Pharmacokinetics
   (1) Adrenal corticosteroids are readily absorbed from the gastrointestinal tract.
   (2) Almost 90% of the dose binds to plasma proteins.
   (3) Steroids are metabolized in the liver and are often bioactivated by reduction reactions. The final or phase II metabolic reaction results in the conjugation of the steroid with sulfate or glucuronide, and the conjugate then is excreted by the kidney.

d. Glucocorticoid effects
   (1) Physiologic doses of cortisol are released into the circulation. Transport occurs via transcortin, which is a high-affinity, low-capacity carrier. Physiologic doses can result in:
      (a) Increased liver glycogen stores
      (b) Increased gluconeogenesis
      (c) Increased lipolysis
      (d) CNS effects, at times including euphoria
      (e) Maintenance of cardiovascular function by potentiation of norepinephrine
      (f) Maintenance of skeletal muscle function (in Addison's disease, there is wasting of skeletal muscle)
      (g) Increased hemoglobin synthesis, resulting in an elevation of the red blood cell count
   (2) Pharmacologic doses of cortisol bind to albumin, a low-affinity, high-capacity carrier. Pharmacologic doses can result in:
      (a) Anti-inflammatory and antiallergic effects, in which steroids:
         (i) Suppress leukocyte migration
         (ii) Stabilize lysosomal membranes
         (iii) Reduce the activity of fibroblasts, which are involved in collagen and tissue repair in inflamed areas
         (iv) Reverse the capillary permeability that is associated with histamine release
         (v) Suppress the immune response by inhibiting antibody synthesis
      (b) Inhibition of growth and cell division
   (3) The anti-inflammatory and antiallergic effects result from glucocorticoid inhibition of prostaglandin and leukotriene synthesis (see Chapter 8 V D 1; Figure 8-4).

e. Mineralocorticoid effects. Unlike the case with glucocorticoids, physiologic and pharmacologic doses of mineralocorticoids produce similar effects; it is the intensity of the effects that differs.
   (1) Mineralocorticoids cause retention of Na^+, phosphate, Ca^+, and bicarbonate (HCO_3^-) and reduction of serum K^+.
   (2) Control of serum Na^+ depends primarily on the juxtaglomerular apparatus; a low Na^+ level in the blood causes the release of renin from the kidney. Renin cleaves angiotensinogen to form angiotensin (see Chapter 8 III A); angiotensin II triggers aldosterone release.
   (3) Aldosterone acts on Na^+ and K^+ transport in the distal tubule of the kidney to enhance Na^+ reabsorption.

f. Route of administration. Corticosteroid dosing depends on the patient's condition.
   (1) Oral steroids are best taken around 8 A.M. to mimic the natural secretion of the adrenal cortex.
   (2) Suppression of the pituitary–adrenal axis must be avoided.
      (a) If the axis is suppressed, the adrenal cortex does not respond to stress by releasing steroids; the consequences can be fatal.

(b) Once the axis is suppressed, it may take more than 1 year for normal function to return.

(c) Less than 25 mg of prednisone per day (or equivalent; see Table 10-5) taken at 8 A.M. for fewer than 5–10 days usually does not suppress the pituitary–adrenal axis.

(d) To minimize the effects of pituitary–adrenal axis suppression, when steroid treatment ceases, doses should be tapered off rather than stopped abruptly.

(3) When steroids are used in children, alternate-day therapy is recommended. With this regimen, normal growth patterns can be maintained and suppression of the pituitary–adrenal axis by negative feedback is less likely.

g. **Preparations**

(1) **Systemic**

(a) **Mineralocorticoids**

(i) **Aldosterone** is an endogenous mineralocorticoid but is not available as a medicinal agent.

(ii) **Desoxycorticosterone** and **fludrocortisone** are the agents used as replacements for aldosterone in Addison's disease.

(b) **Glucocorticoids**

(i) **Hydrocortisone** and **cortisone** exhibit some mineralocorticoid activity (i.e., although they possess primarily glucocorticoid activity, they do cause some Na^+ retention). This becomes significant only in patients who are not able to tolerate the additional Na^+ load.

(ii) **Prednisone, prednisolone, methylprednisolone, triamcinolone, betamethasone,** and **beclomethasone** are semisynthetic analogues of the natural substances. They do not possess mineralocorticoid activity; therefore, an anti-inflammatory dose can be given without the adverse effect of Na^+ retention. Beclomethasone was the first corticosteroid available in inhalation form; it is used to treat acute bronchial asthma.

(c) Table 10-5 lists the commonly used corticosteroids, divided on the basis of their duration of action, with their anti-inflammatory potency, equivalent milligram potency, and Na^+ retention potential.

(2) **Topical** (Table 10-6)

(a) For mild pruritus or inflammation, or for maintenance treatment of some dermatoses, 1% topical hydrocortisone is adequate.

(b) For active acute dermatoses or resistant chronic dermatitis, a higher potency steroid may be more effective.

TABLE 10-5. Glucocorticoids: Anti-Inflammatory Potency, Relative Oral Potency, and Potential for Sodium Retention

Glucocorticoid	Anti-Inflammatory Potency	Equivalent Oral Potency (mg)	Sodium Retention
Short-acting (12 hr or less)			
Hydrocortisone	1.0	20	2+
Cortisone	0.8	25	2+
Intermediate-acting (12–24 hr)			
Prednisolone	5.0	5	1+
Prednisone	4.0	5	1+
Methylprednisolone	5.0	4	0
Triamcinolone	5.0	4	0
Long-acting (over 24 hr)			
Betamethasone	40.0	0.6	0
Dexamethasone	30.0	0.75	0

TABLE 10-6. Potency of Topical Steroids

(c) **Clobetasol propionate** is a high-potency topical steroid that appears to be effective for the treatment of psoriasis and other dermatoses. Clobetasol can cause adrenal suppression and, therefore, should be reserved for severe, refractory dermatoses.

(3) Inhaled

    (a) Mechanism of action. Inhaled glucocorticoids, which are highly lipophilic, bind to cystosolic receptors instead of nuclear receptors (see III G 3 b).

    (b) Pharmacologic effects. Inhaled glucocorticoids have anti-inflammatory effects on the bronchial mucosa in patients with asthma. Chronic administration reduces the number of mast cells, macrophages, T lymphocytes, and eosinophils in the bronchial epithelium and submucosa and reduces airway hyperresponsiveness.

(c) Pharmacokinetics
  (i) After inhalation, 80%–90% of the agent is deposited in the oropharynx and swallowed. Use of a spacer reduces oropharyngeal deposition. Ideally, inhaled agents have a high topical potency and low systemic bioavailability.
  (ii) The remainder of the dose enters the respiratory tract.
(d) Preparations. Beclomethasone, kudesonide, flunisolide, and **triamcinolone** are available as inhalation corticosteroids.
(e) Adverse effects. Local adverse effects include **dysphonia** and **oropharyngeal candidiasis**.

h. Therapeutic uses
  (1) Adrenal insufficiency
    (a) For **acute** adrenal insufficiency, cortisol (hydrocortisone) Na$^+$ succinate is given first by intravenous injection; it is then given in intravenous fluids.
    (b) For **chronic** adrenal insufficiency, cortisone acetate is taken on arising and in the late afternoon, and the mineralocorticoid fludrocortisone acetate is taken daily.
  (2) Rheumatoid arthritis
    (a) Before systemic steroids are used, therapy with nonsteroidal agents is tried (see Chapter 9 II). The patient also should be exhibiting progressive disability.
    (b) Steroids can also be administered by intra-articular injection for the temporary relief of especially painful joints.
  (3) Other uses. Corticosteroids are also widely used in the treatment of:
    (a) Rheumatic carditis
    (b) Renal diseases, including the nephrotic syndrome
    (c) Most collagen vascular diseases
    (d) Severe allergic reactions
    (e) Ocular disorders involving inflammation
    (f) Various skin diseases, usually by topical administration
    (g) Chronic ulcerative colitis
    (h) Cerebral edema
  (4) The use of corticosteroids in **cancer** patients is discussed in Chapter 11 V D.
  (5) Respiratory disorders. Inhaled glucocorticoids are used for:
    (a) Nocturnal asthma, including that in children
    (b) Seasonal and perennial allergic rhinitis
    (c) The management of chronic obstructive pulmonary disease (with minimal benefit)

i. Adverse effects
  (1) Prolonged therapy with corticosteroids can result in the following:
    (a) Suppression of pituitary–adrenal function. In the absence of previous or concomitant treatment with oral glucocorticoids, inhaled glucocorticoids in doses of 1500 mg/d or less in adults or 400 mg/d or less in children have little or no effect on pituitary–adrenal function.
    (b) Increased susceptibility to infection
    (c) Peptic ulceration, which may be the result of altered mucosal defense mechanisms
    (d) Myopathy characterized by proximal arm and leg weakness
    (e) Psychological disturbances, including suicidal tendencies or "steroid psychosis"
    (f) Posterior subcapsular cataracts, especially in children. There is little evidence that inhaled glucocorticoids increase the risk of cataracts or have clinically important metabolic effects.
    (g) Osteoporosis, which can lead to vertebral fractures
      (i) Glucocorticoids directly inhibit osteoblast formation as well as intestinal Ca^{2+} absorption.
      (ii) They also increase secretion of parathyroid hormone.
    (h) Hyperglycemia

(2) Glucocorticoids can arrest growth in small children receiving small doses. Both DNA synthesis and cell division are inhibited. Inhaled glucocorticoids have no significant effect on statural growth in doses up to 800 mg/d for up to 5 years of treatment.

4. **Adrenal steroid inhibitors. Metyrapone** reduces cortisol production by inhibiting the 11-β-hydroxylation reaction.
   a. It is used in diagnosing primary and secondary adrenal insufficiency. When cortisol production is blocked, negative feedback should increase ACTH and the production of precursors of cortisol if the pituitary and adrenal glands are functional.
   b. Metyrapone has also been used to treat hypercortisolism that results from adrenal neoplasms.

IV. DIABETES MELLITUS AND INSULIN THERAPY

A. General considerations

1. In 1921, Banting and Best extracted insulin from the pancreas and demonstrated its therapeutic effects in diabetic dogs and human subjects.

2. Diabetes mellitus involves not only a deficiency of insulin but also an excess of certain other hormones, such as growth hormone, glucocorticoids, and glucagon. Thus, not only the pancreas is involved in glucose homeostasis but also the anterior pituitary gland and the adrenal cortex.

3. **Etiology of diabetes mellitus**
   a. It is believed that the juvenile onset of diabetes mellitus [**insulin-dependent diabetes mellitus (IDDM)**] has a **chronic autoimmune etiology,** which usually exists for years in a preclinical phase.
   b. **Susceptibility** to IDDM **is inherited** and the main gene associated with predisposition is the major histocompatibility complex (MHC) on chromosome 6.

4. **Syndromes of diabetes mellitus**
   a. **Type I (IDDM) diabetes**
      (1) In this type I diabetes, there is no circulating insulin in the plasma and, thus, insulin replacement is required.
      (2) There is complete failure of pancreatic beta cell function. By contrast, alpha islet cells secreting glucagon, delta cells secreting somatostatin, and pancreatic polypeptide cells are preserved.
      (3) The patient is prone to both hyperglycemia and ketoacidosis, which occur late in the course of the disease after most beta cells are destroyed.
   b. **Type II [maturity-onset, non–insulin-dependent (NIDDM)] diabetes**
      (1) Type II diabetes may be due to a defect in the receptor on the pancreatic beta cell membrane.
      (2) In the earliest forms of the disease, there is a delay in the initial secretion of insulin after stimulation by glucose.
      (3) Also, less insulin than normal is secreted at any given glucose concentration.
      (4) The patient is not prone to ketoacidosis.
   c. In both types of diabetes mellitus, plasma immunoreactive glucagon concentrations are increased, especially during ketoacidosis. The normal suppression of glucagon by hyperglycemia is also impaired.
   d. The **pathognomonic finding of capillary basement membrane thickening** occurs early in the course of diabetes mellitus. It is this change that is probably responsible for the major **complications of diabetes,** including:
      (1) Microangiopathy
      (2) Nephropathy
      (3) Neuropathy

(4) Retinopathy
(5) Atherosclerosis
  (a) This disorder occurs more often in diabetics than in nondiabetics.
  (b) Tibial and peroneal artery sclerosis are almost the *sine qua non* of diabetes.

B. Chemistry of insulin

1. Insulin consists of two amino acid chains joined together by disulfide linkages; it has a molecular weight of about 6000.

2. Pancreatic beta cells form insulin from a single-chain precursor, proinsulin, which possesses little biologic activity.

3. Insulin can exist as a monomer, a dimer, or a hexamer consisting of three dimers.
   a. Two molecules of zinc are coordinated in the hexamer form, and it is this form that is stored in the granules of the beta cell.
   b. The biologically active form is thought to be the monomer.

4. There are species variations in the amino acid sequence of insulin.

C. Mechanism of action

1. The initial action of insulin is at the cell surface, where the hormone interacts with a highly specific receptor.

2. Exactly how insulin facilitates the transport of glucose and amino acids is not known.

D. Pharmacokinetics

1. **Regulation of insulin secretion**
   a. Insulin is synthesized in the beta cells of the islets of Langerhans as a single polypeptide precursor, preproinsulin, which is subsequently converted to proinsulin.
   b. **Proinsulin** is synthesized in the rough endoplasmic reticulum and packaged, through the Golgi apparatus, into secretory granules. Along the way, an enzymatic process converts proinsulin to insulin and C peptide.
   c. Stored granules containing many insulin molecules are released by **exocytosis**.
   d. **Stimuli for insulin secretion**
      (1) Oral **glucose** has a greater ability to stimulate insulin secretion than intravenously administered glucose. Fatty acids, amino acids, and ketone bodies all increase insulin secretion. Glucose-induced insulin release appears to occur in two phases:
         (a) An initial-burst phase, which peaks in minutes and then rapidly declines
         (b) A slow phase, which takes an hour to reach a peak
      (2) **Gastrointestinal hormones,** such as secretin, pancreozymin, and gastrin, can stimulate insulin secretion.
      (3) **Autonomic control of insulin secretion**
         (a) β-Adrenergic agonists increase insulin secretion by increasing intracellular cAMP.
         (b) cAMP plus Ca^{2+} may activate a microtubular–microfilament system that promotes the release of the insulin granule.

2. Most secreted insulin circulates in the blood and lymphatic system as the free hormone.

3. Although small quantities of insulin can be detected in the urine, the kidney normally filters and reabsorbs the hormone.

4. Both the liver and the kidney are of primary importance in the degradation of insulin by a proteolytic enzyme. Each is capable of destroying 40% of the insulin produced per day.

E. Metabolic effects of insulin deficiency

1. **Reduced rate of glucose transport.** When insulin is deficient, there is a reduction in the rate of transport of glucose across the membranes of certain cells, including muscle and

adipose cells. Insulin does not significantly influence the rate of glucose transport across liver cells, erythrocytes, or leukocytes, and the rate of entry of glucose into the brain is only affected in ketoacidosis.

2. **Reduced enzyme activity.** There is a reduction in the activity of the enzyme systems necessary for catalyzing glucose to glycogen.

3. **Hyperlipemia, ketonemia,** and **acidosis** can all occur with insulin deficiency. The lack of insulin allows hormone-sensitive lipase to mobilize fatty acids, which leads to elevated circulating levels of ketones, acetoacetate, and β-hydroxybutyrate.

4. **Azoturia.** Insulin deficiency combined with glucagon excess results in the conversion of large amounts of protein to glucose, resulting in an increased excretion of urea and ammonia.

F. Route of administration

1. The usual route of administration for all insulin preparations is subcutaneous. The limitation of the route is the variability on insulin absorption from the depot injection site.

2. Insulin is administered intravenously during emergency circumstances. If administration is via this route, the crystalline form is used. Recently, peritoneal infusion and intranasal administration with adjuvants have resulted in successful hormone replacement.

3. Intensified treatment regimens, including multiple daily injections and continuous subcutaneous infusion have been used to mimic the physiologic replacement of insulin.

4. Insulin is a protein and cannot be given orally because it would be digested.

G. Preparations. The types of insulin differ in their onset and duration of action. The potency of insulin is expressed in USP units.

1. **Crystalline zinc insulin (regular insulin)**
   a. Regular insulin is a short-acting, soluble insulin, which is prepared in a phosphate buffer with zinc at a pH of 3.5.
   b. Its peak action occurs in 2–4 hours and its duration is 5–7 hours.
   c. It can be administered subcutaneously or intravenously and is a good agent for controlling diabetic ketoacidosis rapidly.
   d. The frequency of injections (4–5/day) is not very convenient.

2. **Protamine zinc insulin**
   a. Adding the basic protein protamine to crystalline zinc insulin causes the formation of large crystals. This produces a compound that is less soluble.
   b. When injected, this formulation serves as a tissue depot, producing slow absorption into the bloodstream.
   c. The action of protamine zinc insulin peaks in 16–18 hours and lasts up to 36 hours.
   d. Fine control of hyperglycemia is difficult with such a long-acting preparation.

3. **Isophane insulin [neutral protamine Hagedorn (NPH)]**
   a. This intermediate-acting insulin is similar to protamine zinc insulin, but it contains only a small amount of protamine (0.5 mg/100 units of insulin). Therefore, NPH insulin has an earlier onset and earlier peak effects than protamine zinc insulin, but the duration of action is similar for both preparations.
   b. The effects of NPH insulin peak in 8–12 hours and have a duration of 24–48 hours.
   c. These effects are clinically equivalent to combining 2–3 units of crystalline zinc insulin with 1 unit of protamine zinc insulin.

4. **Lente insulins**
   a. Lente insulins do not contain protamine; their insolubility results from the addition of excess zinc in an acetate rather than a phosphate buffer.

b. The onset of action for the lente insulins depends on the physical state, the ambient zinc concentration, and the pH.

   (1) A microamorphous crystalline form, known as **prompt insulin zinc suspension (semilente insulin),** peaks in 4–8 hours and has a duration of action of 12–16 hours.

   (2) A large crystalline form with a high zinc content, known as **extended insulin zinc suspension (ultralente insulin),** has an onset and duration of action similar to those of protamine zinc insulin.

   (3) Combining 7 parts of ultralente with 3 parts of semilente produces **insulin zinc suspension (lente insulin),** which is similar to NPH insulin in its onset and duration of action.

5. Human insulins

   a. Human insulins are produced by semisynthetic and rDNA techniques.

   b. Since the human proinsulin gene was synthesized, human proinsulin has been produced on a large scale as the precursor to human insulin.

   c. The biologic activity and intravenous pharmacokinetics of human insulin are similar to porcine insulin. It is absorbed more quickly than porcine insulin after subcutaneous injection, thereby improving glycemic control after meals.

   d. Human insulins are useful for individuals with an allergy to insulin from animal sources.

H. | **Factors altering insulin requirements**

1. Other drugs. Salicylates inhibit the enzymes necessary for gluconeogenesis and accelerate their use. Anticoagulants tend to stimulate insulin secretion, thereby decreasing insulin requirements.

2. Hormones. Glucagon, epinephrine, and growth hormone all increase insulin requirements.

3. Exercise decreases insulin requirements by making muscle more permeable to glucose and releasing muscle-bound insulin.

4. Stress. Both physiologic (i.e., fever, infection, pregnancy) and psychological stress increase insulin requirements, possibly secondary to epinephrine release.

5. Eating patterns. Alterations in the diet or a change in eating time may increase or decrease insulin requirements.

6. Obesity increases insulin requirements, perhaps as the result of an increase in the number of insulin-binding sites on the greater surface area of the adipose tissue.

I. | **Adverse effects**

1. Hypoglycemia

   a. The worst sequela of hypoglycemia is **insulin shock,** characterized by abnormalities of the CNS, including hypoglycemic convulsions.

   b. Early symptoms of hypoglycemia, such as sweating, tachycardia, and hunger, are thought to be brought about by the compensatory secretion of epinephrine.

   c. Hypoglycemia is best treated by administering glucose intravenously, or by giving fruit juice or other soluble carbohydrates. Glucagon may be administered parenterally as an alternative to glucose.

2. Local reactions. Irritation at the site of insulin injection can lead to lipohypertrophy or lipoatrophy. Sites of injection should be rotated. Subcutaneous infusion can result in infection and local allergic reactions to components of the infusion system.

3. Antigenic response

   a. With the development of new, more highly purified animal insulins and the advent of human insulin, the production of insulin antibodies and the hypersensitivity reactions are less of a problem. Insulin antibodies may attenuate responses to regular insulin injected subcutaneously and delay recovery from hypoglycemia.

b. The order of antigenic potency, in descending order, is beef > pork > highly purified ("single-peak") pork > human insulin. Antigenicity increases as the duration of action of the insulin is increased. Thus, protamine zinc insulin is the most antigenic because of its long duration of action and because it contains a large amount of the basic protein protamine.

4. Growth-promoting properties of insulin may be a factor in the macrovascular complications of diabetes.

5. Weight gain is an undesirable effect of intensive insulin therapy.

V. ORAL HYPOGLYCEMIC AGENTS (SULFONYLUREAS)

A. Mechanism of action

1. In the absence of glucose, sulfonylureas stimulate insulin secretion from pancreatic beta cells without entering the cell.

2. Sulfonylureas may also sensitize the pancreatic beta cells to glucose and inhibit the efflux of K^+ from pancreatic beta cells.

3. Sulfonylureas induce increased activity of peripheral insulin intracellular receptors.

4. Sulfonylureas may act to reduce glucagon secretion.

5. High-affinity sulfonylurea receptors have been demonstrated on pancreatic beta cells. The order of potency of sulfonylurea in binding to beta cells approximates its potency in stimulating the release of insulin and inhibiting the effects of K^+.

B. Preparations and pharmacokinetics. All sulfonylurea agents are readily absorbed from the small intestine and are avidly bound by plasma proteins. The onset of action varies from 30 minutes to 3 hours. The duration of action also varies among agents. The general structure of a sulfonylurea is illustrated in Figure 10-4.

1. Tolbutamide
   a. The onset of action occurs in 30 minutes, while the duration of action is 6–12 hours.
   b. Tolbutamide is the shortest-acting and least potent sulfonylurea and is readily metabolized in the liver to inactive products. Excretion occurs via the kidney.

2. Acetohexamide
   a. Onset of action is rapid; effects peak in 3 hours and last for 12–18 hours.
   b. The major metabolite, **hydroxyhexamide,** is thought to possess most of the activity of this agent. It is excreted renally.

3. Tolazamide
   a. Tolazamide is slowly absorbed. Effects do not peak for 6 hours, and the drug has a duration of action of 24 hours.
   b. Its metabolic products are weaker hypoglycemics than the parent compound.
   c. Metabolic products are excreted by the kidney.

4. Glyburide and **glipizide** are second-generation sulfonylureas. They are the most potent sulfonylurea agents available. Both are metabolized by the liver to products with little activity. Both drugs have a duration of action of 24 hours.

5. Chlorpropamide
   a. Although rapidly absorbed, chlorpropamide has a duration of action of 24–60 hours because it binds to plasma proteins.
   b. It is metabolized in the liver and is excreted slowly by the kidney as unchanged drug and as metabolites.

FIGURE 10-4. Structure of sulfonylurea agents.

C. **Therapeutic uses**

1. The sulfonylureas are used in the treatment of patients who have NIDDM and who cannot be treated with diet alone or who are unwilling to take insulin if dietary control fails.

2. The findings of the University Group Diabetes Program (UGDP), although controversial, support the above statement, and many physicians have had success using the sulfonylurea agents. The UGDP study did suggest that use of these agents was associated with a higher cardiovascular mortality rate than that occurring with dietary control alone or with insulin therapy.

3. No study has demonstrated that sulfonylurea agents prevent the long-term complications of diabetes.

4. Combining a sulfonylurea with a suboptimal insulin regimen in patients with NIDDM may provide better glycemia control than the suboptimal insulin regimen alone or reduced insulin requirements.

D. **Adverse effects** are seen in 3%–5% of patients treated with a sulfonylurea agent.

1. **Hypoglycemia** can occur in elderly patients with hepatic or renal insufficiency because the agent will have a longer than expected duration of action. Its frequency is related to potency and duration of action of the drug. The highest incidence occurs with glyburide and chlorpropamide.

2. **Cutaneous reactions** include rashes and photosensitivity.

3. **Gastrointestinal reactions** include nausea and vomiting.

4. **Hematologic reactions**—leukopenia, agranulocytosis, thrombocytopenia, pancytopenia, and hemolytic anemia—have occurred.

5. **Transient cholestatic jaundice** occurs rarely.

6. **Inappropriate secretion of antidiuretic hormone** has been observed, especially with chlorpropamide, which can cause hyponatremia.

7. A **disulfiram-like reaction** has been reported with use of chlorpropamide.

E. **Drug interactions.** Other drugs may influence the hypoglycemic actions of sulfonylureas through pharmacodynamic and pharmacokinetic interactions. Because sulfonylureas are highly bound to plasma proteins, any drug that displaces them could enhance their hypoglycemic activity.

STUDY QUESTIONS

DIRECTIONS: Each of the numbered items or incomplete statements in this section is followed by answers or by completions of the statement. Select the **one** lettered answer or completion that is **best** in each case.

1. Which one of the following adrenocortical drugs is anti-inflammatory in pharmacologic doses?

(A) Desoxycorticosterone
(B) Aldosterone
(C) Cortisol
(D) Vasopressin
(E) Oxytocin

2. A poorly controlled diabetic patient is complaining of hunger, sweating, and palpitations. Examination reveals a moist, pale skin and hypothermia. Which one of the following can be deduced from this patient's symptoms?

(A) The patient's symptoms are caused by hyperglycemia
(B) The insulin dose is probably too low
(C) The patient is probably "spilling" sugar in her urine
(D) The symptoms are premonitory of insulin shock

3. Which of the following synthetic steroids shows predominantly mineralocorticoid action?

(A) Hydrocortisone
(B) Spironolactone
(C) Dexamethasone
(D) Fludrocortisone
(E) Cortisone

4. The primary reason for a physician to prescribe human insulin is that

(A) it has a faster onset of action than other insulins
(B) it has a shorter duration of action than other insulins
(C) it can be given to patients who have an allergy to animal insulins
(D) it is more effective in preventing the complications of diabetes than animal insulins
(E) it is cheaper than other insulins because it is produced by recombinant technology

5. A menopausal patient complains that the "hot flashes" are extremely disturbing. Which of the following drugs could relieve her symptoms?

(A) Ethinyl estradiol
(B) Ethynodiol
(C) Levonorgestrel
(D) Fluoxymesterone

6. Which one of the following statements about adrenal steroids is true?

(A) "Glucocorticoid activity" implies an effect on electrolyte homeostasis
(B) Adrenocorticotropic hormone (ACTH) and cortisol both have the basic steroid nucleus
(C) Pharmacologic doses of glucocorticoids cause few toxic effects
(D) Steroid receptors mediate the metabolic effects of steroids
(E) Aldosterone secretion is inhibited by serum angiotensin

DIRECTIONS: Each of the numbered items or incomplete statements in this section is negatively phrased, as indicated by a capitalized word such as NOT, LEAST, or EXCEPT. Select the ONE lettered answer or completion that is BEST in each case.

7. All of the following statements about growth hormone are true EXCEPT

(A) it may stimulate the synthesis or release of somatomedins
(B) low levels of insulin-like growth factor (IGF)-1 are associated with dwarfism
(C) Sheehan syndrome may result in growth hormone deficiency
(D) hyposecretion can result in acromegaly
(E) it is contraindicated in subjects with closed epiphyses

8. All of the following agents are correctly matched with the descriptive phrase that follows EXCEPT

(A) dopaminergic antagonist drug therapy—may result in hyperprolactinemia
(B) bromocriptine—restores ovulatory menses in women with hyperprolactinemia
(C) human chorionic gonadotropin (hCG)—peaks 2 weeks after conception
(D) sequential oral contraceptive preparations—associated with an increased incidence of endometrial tumors
(E) "minipill"—contains progestin alone

9. An elderly patient complains of urinary urgency and frequency. A diagnosis of benign prostatic hypertrophy is made, and finasteride is prescribed. All of the following statements are true about finasteride EXCEPT

(A) it is a specific inhibitor of steroid 5α-reductase
(B) the usual clinical response occurs within 48 hours
(C) if finasteride is discontinued, the prostate returns to its former size
(D) pregnant women should avoid direct contact with crushed tablets
(E) the libido of the patient is not adversely affected in most cases

10. All of the following statements about oral contraceptives are true EXCEPT

(A) the "combination pill" contains both estrogen and progestin
(B) ethinyl estradiol and mestranol are commonly used in oral contraceptives
(C) the "minipill" contains progestin alone
(D) the "triphasic pill" is a variant of the combination pill
(E) the triphasic pill contains estrogen, progestin, and luteinizing hormone (LH)

11. Correct statements about adrenocorticotropic hormone (ACTH) include all of the following EXCEPT

(A) endogenous ACTH is also called corticotropin
(B) ACTH stimulates the synthesis of corticosteroids
(C) release of ACTH can be inhibited by cortisol
(D) ACTH is most useful clinically as a diagnostic tool in adrenal insufficiency
(E) the oral route is the preferred route of administration

12. Correct statements about crystalline zinc (regular) insulin include all of the following EXCEPT

(A) it can serve as replacement therapy for juvenile-onset diabetes
(B) it can be administered intravenously
(C) it is a short-acting insulin
(D) it can be administered orally
(E) it is a good agent for the rapid control of diabetic ketoacidosis

13. Endogenous corticosteroids released by the adrenal cortex include all of the following EXCEPT

(A) cortisol
(B) cortisone
(C) beclomethasone
(D) aldosterone
(E) corticosterone

14. Effects of physiologic doses of cortisol (glucocorticoids) include all of the following EXCEPT

(A) an increase of liver glycogen stores
(B) maintenance of normal cardiovascular function
(C) changes in mood and behavior
(D) increased lipogenesis from protein
(E) increased hemoglobin synthesis

15. Prolonged therapy with corticosteroids can lead to all of the following adverse effects EXCEPT

(A) suppression of the pituitary–adrenal axis
(B) increased susceptibility to infection
(C) peptic ulceration
(D) muscle hypertrophy
(E) psychological disturbances

DIRECTIONS: The group of questions below consists of lettered choices followed by several numbered items. For each numbered item select the **one** lettered choice which it is **most** closely associated. Each lettered choice may be used once, more than once, or not at all.

Questions 16–18

For each indication listed below, select the drug that is most appropriate.

(A) Levothyroxine
(B) Propylthiouracil
(C) Iodide
(D) Parathyroid hormone
(E) Calcitonin

16. Useful in the treatment of hyperparathyroidism

17. Useful in conjunction with radioiodine therapy

18. Useful in the treatment of myxedema

1. The answer is C *[I A 2; III G 1 c, 3 d (2) (a), g (1) (b); Table 10-5]*. Adrenocorticotropic hormone (ACTH) and cortisol possess anti-inflammatory properties, ACTH because it stimulates glucocorticoid synthesis and cortisol because it is a glucocorticoid. Both desoxycorticosterone and aldosterone are mineralocorticoids and, thus, have no anti-inflammatory effects. Vasopressin and oxytocin are produced by the hypothalamus and have no anti-inflammatory properties.

2. The answer is D *[IV I 1]*. The patient described in the question has symptoms of hypoglycemia, not hyperglycemia, and is rapidly approaching insulin shock. The insulin dose is probably too high. Because of the low glucose level, the patient would not be "spilling" sugar into the urine. Early symptoms of hypoglycemia can be treated with soluble oral carbohydrates (e.g., fruit juice). Insulin shock calls for emergency treatment with intravenous glucose or parenteral glucagon.

3. The answer is D *[III G 3 g (1) (a) (ii); Ch 6 IX B]*. Hydrocortisone and cortisone are short-acting glucocorticoids with some mineralocorticoid activity. Spironolactone is an aldosterone antagonist. Dexamethasone has no Na+-retaining potency. Fludrocortisone shows predominantly mineralocorticoid action.

4. The answer is C *[IV G 5 d]*. The major advantage of human insulin is that it can be administered to patients who are allergic to insulin made from animal sources. Clinically available human insulins are produced by semisynthetic and recombinant DNA techniques. They are more expensive than the traditional insulin preparations. Some forms of human insulin may have a faster onset of action and shorter duration than conventional preparations, but this may or may not be advantageous. Human insulins are no more effective in preventing the complications of diabetes than any other insulin preparation.

5. The answer is A *[III D 2 a (1) (a) (i), 4 c (1)]*. Estrogens are used during and after menopause to relieve vasomotor symptoms such as hot flashes. Ethinyl estradiol and mestranol are estrogens. Ethynodiol and levonorgestrel are progestins, and fluoxymesterone is an androgen.

6. The answer is D *[III G 1 c (2), 2 a (1), 3 b, i]*. Steroid receptors mediate the metabolic effects of steroids. Mineralocorticoids, not glucocorticoids, affect electrolyte homeostasis. Adrenocorticotropic hormone (ACTH) does not have a basic steroid nucleus; it is a polypeptide with 39 amino acids. Pharmacologic doses of glucocorticoids often result in a number of adverse effects. Aldosterone secretion is stimulated by serum angiotensin.

7. The answer is D *[III A 1 f, 2 a (1), b, 3]*. Acromegaly and gigantism result from hypersecretion, not hyposecretion, of growth hormone. Over 90% of cases are caused by growth hormone–secreting adenomas. Growth hormone may stimulate the synthesis or release of somatomedins. Low levels of insulin-like growth factor (IGF)-1 are associated with dwarfism. Sheehan's syndrome may cause growth hormone deficiency. Growth hormone is contraindicated in subjects with closed epiphyses.

8. The answer is C *[III B 2 a, b (2), D 1 b (2), 2 a (2), (4)]*. Human chorionic gonadotropin (hCG) levels peak after 6 weeks, not 2 weeks, after conception and stabilize at a lower level during pregnancy. Hyperprolactinemia may result from dopaminergic antagonist drug therapy, infiltrating disorders of the hypothalamus or pituitary, hypothyroidism, use of oral contraceptives, and prolactin-secreting tumors. Bromocriptine, an ergot alkaloid derivative and dopaminergic agonist, is often used to treat pituitary adenomas. Sequential preparations (estrogen for 14–16 days followed by 5–6 days of combined estrogen and progestin) were removed from the market following reports of an increased incidence of endometrial tumors. The "minipill" contains progestin alone, which acts by thickening the consistency of cervical mucus, creating a barrier to sperm.

9. The answer is B *[III D 7 b (2)]*. Six to twelve months of administration are usually necessary to determine the patient's response to finasteride. Finasteride is a specific inhibitor of steroid 5α-reductase, which catalyzes the conversion of testosterone to dihydrotestosterone. Unless finasteride is continued indefinitely, the prostate will return to its previous size. A developing fetus may be adversely affected if the mother has direct contact with crushed finasteride tablets or the semen of a man taking the drug. Finasteride does not interfere with testosterone-dependent functions, such as potency and libido.

10. The answer is E *[III D 2 a]*. The "triphasic pill," a variation on the combination pill, does not contain luteinizing hormone (LH). It provides estrogen in constant dosage and a progestin in varying dosage to reflect the changing progesterone levels of the normal menstrual cycle. The "combination pill" contains both estrogen and progestin. Ethinyl estradiol and mestranol are commonly used estrogens in oral contraceptives. The "minipill" contains only progestin.

11. The answer is E *[III G 1 b (1)–(4), 2 c, d]*. Adrenocorticotropic hormone (ACTH) cannot be administered orally. Because it is a polypeptide hormone, it must be administered parenterally, most often intramuscularly. Endogenous ACTH, also called corticotropin, stimulates the synthesis of corticosteroids. Release of ACTH can be inhibited by cortisol. ACTH is most useful clinically as a diagnostic tool in adrenal insufficiency.

12. The answer is D *[IV F, G 1]*. Crystalline zinc (regular) insulin is a short-acting insulin that can serve as a replacement therapy in juvenile-onset diabetes. However, its early onset of action and the fact that it can be given intravenously are particularly advantageous when rapid control is important, as in diabetic ketoacidosis. Crystalline zinc insulin, like any insulin preparation, can only be administered parenterally because it is a protein and would be digested in the gastrointestinal tract. It is the only form of insulin that can be given intravenously as well as by the usual subcutaneous route.

13. The answer is C *[III G 1 c, 3 g (1) (b) (ii)]*. Cortisol, cortisone, aldosterone, and corticosterone are endogenous corticosteroids released by the adrenal cortex. Beclometha-sone was the first steroid available in a form suitable for inhalation and is used to treat acute bronchial asthma.

14. The answer is D *[III G 3 d (1)]*. Glucocorticoids facilitate the conversion of protein to carbohydrate and facilitate the effect of adipokinetic peptides, causing lipolysis and triglycerides in adipose tissue. Glucocorticoids produce a dose-dependent increase in liver glycogen with consequent hyperglycemia. Glucocorticoids participate in blood pressure homeostasis by maintaining normal blood volume and peripheral vascular reactivity. They can affect thought processes and central nervous system (CNS) metabolism. Glucocorticoids can increase hemoglobin synthesis, resulting in an elevation of the red blood cell count.

15. The answer is D *[III G 3 i]*. Corticosteroids, especially when used for long periods, can result in a variety of unwanted effects. Some of these include suppression of the pituitary–adrenal axis, increased susceptibility to infection, peptic ulceration, osteoporosis, and psychological disturbances including suicidal tendencies. Muscle hypertrophy is not an adverse effect of prolonged corticosteroid therapy. Rather, a myopathy can occur that is characterized by proximal arm and leg weakness.

16–18. The answers are: 16-E *[III F 2 b]*, **17-B** *[III E 6 b (2)]*, **18-A** *[III E 3]*. Calcitonin is chiefly used therapeutically to decrease hypercalcemia and hyperphosphatemia in patients with hyperparathyroidism and other disorders associated with hypercalcemia.

Propylthiouracil may be used with radioiodine to control the effects of hyperthyroidism until the benefits of radiation take effect. Unlike iodide, which blocks thyroidal uptake of the radioiodine, propylthiouracil interferes with the synthesis of thyroid hormone.

Levothyroxine is used for the treatment of hypothyroidism, including myxedema coma and neonatal hypothyroidism.

Chapter 11

Cancer Chemotherapy

I. INTRODUCTION

A. **General considerations.** Cancer, or neoplastic disease, is characterized by uncontrolled cell division, invasion, and metastasis. Most of the current clinical antineoplastic agents act on the proliferating population of cells; none acts primarily to influence tumor cell invasion or metastases.

1. There may be as many as 100 different types of cancer, each with its own response rate to a given drug. The sensitivity of a given cancer to a given drug depends on its location, its degree of differentiation, its size, and, presumably, other biochemical factors that are poorly understood.

2. Most tumors are **clonal,** arising from a single altered cell. Tumor progression frequently results from a series of acquired genetic changes within the neoplastic clone, giving rise to subpopulations of tumor cells with increasingly aggressive characteristics. This evolution may occur, in part, because the genetic apparatus of tumor cells is abnormally unstable. A new class of "tumor suppressor" genes is presumed to inhibit the growth of tumors; thus, the loss of function in a cell, by a combination of inherited and somatic deletions or other mechanisms, allows abnormal proliferation.

B. **Combination therapy**

1. Combinations of anticancer agents with different mechanisms of action are often used to destroy all of the malignant cells. Acronyms for these combinations are frequently used; for example, **MOPP** stands for mechlorethamine, vincristine (Oncovin), procarbazine, and prednisone.

2. Antineoplastic agents kill a **constant fraction** of the tumor cells **rather than a fixed number** of cells. To eliminate all of the malignant cells, cancer chemotherapeutic agents are often administered as an **adjunct** to surgery or irradiation.

C. **Cell cycle and anticancer therapy**

1. **Tumor growth** is a function of the:
   a. Fraction of the total cell population that is proliferating
   b. Time required for an individual cell to divide (cell cycle time)
   c. Rate of cell loss

2. **Cell cycle**
   a. Both normal and malignant cells that are proliferating pass through four discrete phases (Figure 11-1):
      (1) Mitosis, or M phase
      (2) Gap 1, or G_1 phase
      (3) DNA synthesis, or S phase
      (4) Gap 2, or G_2 phase
   b. G_0 is a resting phase in which the cells are not proliferating.
   c. Interphase is any period between episodes of mitosis.

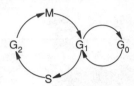

FIGURE 11-1. The cell cycle. M = mitosis; G_1 = gap 1 phase; S = DNA synthesis phase; G_2 = gap 2 phase; G_0 = resting phase.

3. **Antitumor therapies**
   a. Some antitumor therapies, such as irradiation, carmustine, or mechlorethamine, are cytotoxic to proliferating and nonproliferating cells. These **proliferation-independent agents** kill both normal and malignant cells.
   b. Most antitumor agents are preferentially toxic to proliferating cells.
      (1) There are two general classes:
         (a) **Phase-specific agents** act at specific phases of the cell cycle. For example, hydroxyurea and cytarabine kill only cells in the S phase.
         (b) **Phase-nonspecific agents** kill proliferating cells preferentially but do not act on cells at a specific phase in the cell cycle. Examples of these drugs are 5-fluorouracil and cyclophosphamide.
      (2) Some agents exert their major cytotoxic action in one phase of the cell cycle but also have a more limited activity in other phases.
      (3) Some agents are **self-limiting** because they are not only phase-specific but also block the cell in another phase of the cell cycle. For example, methotrexate kills cells in the S phase, but also inhibits RNA synthesis in the G_1 and G_2 phases, thereby limiting its own cytotoxicity.

D. Toxicity

1. Antineoplastic agents generally have a slight selectivity for tumor cells as opposed to normal tissues. Therefore, many of the clinically used antineoplastic agents cause severe toxicity to the patient's normal tissues.

2. Because rapidly proliferating cells are likely to be the ones most severely affected, the common side effects are:
   a. Myelosuppression
   b. Gastrointestinal bleeding and ulcers, nausea, and vomiting
   c. Alopecia
   d. Nephrotoxicity
   e. Teratogenesis, abortion
   f. Immunosuppression

3. Anticancer agents can also be carcinogenic.

E. Dosage calculations. The doses of antineoplastic agents are usually calculated on the basis of the patient's body surface area (in square meters) rather than body weight.

F. Classification. The major classes of antineoplastic agents are grouped primarily by chemical structure, source, or mechanism of action. The five major groups are:

1. **Alkylating agents**

2. **Antimetabolites**

3. **Natural products**

4. **Hormones and antagonists**

5. **Miscellaneous agents**

II. | ALKYLATING AGENTS

A. | General considerations

1. Alkylating agents have or can form an alkyl group that becomes covalently bound to cellular constituents.

2. All alkylating agents are phase-specific. In addition to killing rapidly proliferating cells, these drugs also kill nonproliferating cells as a result of alkylation of RNA, DNA, and essential proteins. Thus, some nitrogen mustards are proliferation-independent.

3. **Alkylation of DNA** is responsible for the cytotoxic antitumor activity of most alkylating agents.
   a. The 7-nitrogen and 6-oxygen of guanine are the most favored sites in DNA for alkylation.
   b. Once one of these sites has been alkylated, several events may follow:
      (1) **Cross-linking. Bifunctional alkylating agents** (those which have two chloroethyl moieties) may form a second covalent bond with an adjacent DNA substituent, a protein, or RNA, resulting in inhibition of DNA replication.
      (2) **Mispairing of bases.** Alkylated guanine forms base pairs with thymine rather than cytosine. This leads to miscoding of the gene and the possible production of defective proteins.
      (3) **Depurination of DNA.** Alkylation of the 7-nitrogen in guanine causes cleavage of the imidazole ring, which leads to a weakened sugar–phosphate backbone of DNA and strand breakage.

4. Enzymes involved in DNA repair may limit the responsiveness of some tumors to the alkylating agents.

5. The major classes of alkylating agents are:
   a. **Nitrogen mustards**
   b. **Nitrosoureas**
   c. **Alkyl sulfonates**
   d. **Triazenes**

B. | Nitrogen mustards

1. **Chemistry.** The basic structure of the nitrogen mustards is shown in Figure 11-2.

2. **Mechanism of action**
   a. One chloroethyl moiety undergoes cyclization with the release of a chloride ion.
   b. The resulting highly reactive carbonium ion can attack nucleophilic groups on protein, DNA, RNA, and other cell constituents.
   c. The nitrogen mustards are phase-nonspecific as are all alkylating agents.
   d. **Tumor cell resistance** to nitrogen mustards can occur due to an increased cellular capacity for DNA repair with resulting cross-resistance to other alkylating agents.

3. **Mechlorethamine** is the prototype of the nitrogen mustards.
   a. **Chemistry.** In the mechlorethamine structure, R = CH_3 (see Figure 11-2).
   b. **Pharmacokinetics**
      (1) Mechlorethamine was the first clinically used nitrogen mustard.

$$R - N \begin{cases} CH_2 - CH_2 - Cl \\ CH_2 - CH_2 - Cl \end{cases}$$

FIGURE 11-2. Basic structure of the nitrogen mustards.

(2) It is highly reactive with a chemical and biologic half-life in plasma of 10 minutes.

(3) It is proliferation-independent.

c. Therapeutic uses

(1) It is used to treat Hodgkin's disease and non-Hodgkin's lymphomas.

(2) In the treatment of Hodgkin's disease, mechlorethamine is combined with vincristine, procarbazine, and prednisone to form the MOPP regimen.

(3) It has also been used topically for the treatment of mycosis fungoides.

d. Route of administration

(1) Because it causes severe tissue damage when given by other routes, mechlorethamine **must be given intravenously** in a rapidly flowing infusion of saline.

(2) Care must be taken to avoid extravasation during administration.'

e. Adverse effects

(1) Myelosuppression

(2) Nausea and vomiting

(3) Alopecia

(4) Menstrual irregularities

4. Cyclophosphamide is an essential part of many effective drug combinations.

a. Pharmacokinetics

(1) Cyclophosphamide is well absorbed orally. It must be activated in the liver by the mixed-function oxidase system.

(2) The metabolites **phosphoramide mustard** and **acrolein** are believed to be the final cytotoxic species.

(3) Alkylating activity levels in the blood remain high for 2–10 hours.

(4) Cyclophosphamide and its metabolites are eliminated primarily by the kidneys; thus, renal failure greatly increases their retention.

b. Therapeutic uses

(1) Cyclophosphamide is used alone or in combination with other agents in the treatment of a variety of neoplastic disorders, including:

(a) Hodgkin's disease

(b) Burkitt's lymphoma

(c) Ovarian and breast carcinomas

(d) Oat cell lung cancer

(e) Neuroblastoma

(2) Cyclophosphamide has also been used as an immunosuppressing agent for organ transplants.

c. Route of administration

(1) Cyclophosphamide is administered orally or intravenously.

(2) The total leukocyte count is monitored, and the dose is adjusted accordingly.

d. Adverse effects

(1) Unlike other nitrogen mustards, cyclophosphamide rarely induces thrombocytopenia.

(2) Alopecia occurs frequently but is modest.

(3) Up to 10% of treated patients develop a sterile hemorrhagic cystitis, which is probably caused by chemical irritation of the bladder mucosa by the metabolite acrolein. A liberal fluid intake dilutes the urinary concentration of acrolein and decreases this side effect.

(4) Prolonged cyclophosphamide treatment can occasionally produce interstitial pulmonary fibrosis.

(5) Prolonged use has also resulted in fatal cardiomyopathy, especially when cyclophosphamide was used with other cardiotoxic drugs.

5. Melphalan (L-sarcolysin)

a. Pharmacokinetics and therapeutic uses

(1) Melphalan is well absorbed from the gastrointestinal tract.

(2) Its major use is in the treatment of multiple myeloma, but it is also used in treatment of breast and ovarian cancer.

b. Route of administration. Melphalan is administered orally. Close hematologic monitoring is essential.

c. Adverse effects
   (1) Like other alkylating agents, melphalan causes prominent myelosuppression.
   (2) Nausea, vomiting, and alopecia are rare.

6. Chlorambucil
   a. Pharmacokinetics
      (1) Like melphalan, chlorambucil is well absorbed from the gastrointestinal tract.
      (2) It is completely metabolized.
      (3) It is the slowest-acting nitrogen mustard.
   b. Therapeutic uses
      (1) Chronic lymphocytic leukemia
      (2) Waldenström's macroglobulinemia
      (3) Hodgkin's disease and non-Hodgkin's lymphomas
   c. Adverse effects include myelosuppression, nausea, and vomiting.

C. **Nitrosoureas**

1. Chemistry
   a. The basic structure of nitrosoureas is shown in Figure 11-3.
   b. In general, the nitrosoureas are chemically unstable and decompose rapidly.

2. Mechanisms of action
   a. In aqueous environments, the nitrosoureas decompose to alkylating and carbamylating intermediates.
   b. The therapeutic and toxic effects of the nitrosoureas are due to both the alkylation of DNA and other nucleophiles and the carbamylation of lysine residues on proteins.
   c. The consequences of DNA alkylation by the nitrosoureas are similar to those seen with other alkylating agents (see II A 3).
   d. The **high lipid solubility** of some of the nitrosoureas allows penetration of the blood–brain barrier and are useful in the treatment of malignancies of the central nervous system (CNS).
   e. The nitrosoureas are proliferation-independent.

3. Carmustine
   a. Chemistry
      (1) Carmustine is 1,3-bis(2-chloroethyl)-1-nitrosourea (**BCNU**).
      (2) Both R_1 and R_2 in Figure 11-3 have the same structure: R_1 and $R_2 = CH_2CH_2Cl$.
   b. Pharmacokinetics
      (1) Carmustine is administered intravenously due to its rapid tissue uptake and metabolism.
      (2) The plasma half-life is about 90 minutes.
      (3) The major degradation and metabolic products are excreted in the urine.
   c. Therapeutic uses
      (1) Hodgkin's disease and non-Hodgkin's lymphomas
      (2) Meningeal leukemia
      (3) Tumors of the brain
      (4) Multiple myeloma
      (5) Malignant melanoma

FIGURE 11-3. Basic structure of the nitrosoureas.

d. Adverse effects
(1) Delayed hematopoietic depression
(2) Nausea and vomiting
(3) CNS toxicity
(4) Pulmonary fibrosis

4. Lomustine
a. Chemistry. Lomustine is 1-(2-chloroethyl)-3-cyclohexyl-1-nitrosourea (**CCNU**).
b. Pharmacokinetics
(1) Lomustine, which is given orally, is rapidly absorbed from the gastrointestinal tract and metabolized.
(2) The metabolites have a long half-life (over 16 hours).
(3) The metabolites can enter the cerebrospinal fluid (CSF).
c. Therapeutic uses
(1) Hodgkin's disease and non-Hodgkin's lymphoma
(2) Primary neoplastic disease of the brain, kidney, stomach, colon, and lung
d. Adverse effects include myelosuppression, nausea, and vomiting.

D. Alkyl sulfonates

1. Chemistry. The prototypic agent is **busulfan**.

2. Mechanism of action. Cleavage of the alkyl–oxygen bond in busulfan produces an electrophile, which forms intrastrand DNA cross-links.

3. Pharmacokinetics
a. Busulfan is well absorbed after oral administration.
b. Almost all of the drug is eliminated in the urine as methanesulfonic acid.

4. Therapeutic uses include chronic granulocytic leukemia and Waldenström's macroglobulinemia.

5. Adverse effects
a. Myelosuppression is common.
b. Endocrine dysfunction, including impotence, sterility, and amenorrhea, can occur.
c. Hyperuricemia can result from rapid purine catabolism.
d. Skin pigmentation and pulmonary fibrosis have been noted.

E. Triazenes

1. Chemistry. The prototype agent is **dacarbazine,** the chemical formula of which is 5-(3,3-dimethyl-1-triazeno)-imidazole-4-carboxamide (**DTIC**).

2. Mechanism of action
a. Dacarbazine is *N*-demethylated by liver microsomal enzymes and then functions as an alkylating agent.
b. The active species has a methyl carbonium ion that can methylate DNA and RNA and inhibits the synthesis of DNA, RNA, and protein.

3. Therapeutic uses
a. Dacarbazine is one of the most active agents against malignant melanoma.
b. It is also used for soft-tissue sarcomas and Hodgkin's disease.

4. Adverse effects include nausea, vomiting, myelosuppression, and neurotoxicity.

III. ANTIMETABOLITES

A. General considerations

1. Antimetabolites are compounds that bear a structural similarity to a naturally occurring substance, such as a vitamin, nucleoside, or amino acid.

2. The antimetabolite competes with the natural substrate for the active site on an essential enzyme or for an important receptor.

3. Some antimetabolites can be incorporated into DNA or RNA and, thus, can disrupt cellular function.

4. Most antimetabolites are phase-specific and act during DNA synthesis (the S phase; see Figure 11-1).

5. There are three major classes of antimetabolites:
   a. **Folic acid analogues** (primarily methotrexate)
   b. **Purine analogues** and related inhibitors
   c. **Pyrimidine analogues**

B. Methotrexate

1. Mechanism of action
   a. Methotrexate is a folic acid analogue that competitively inhibits dihydrofolate reductase, the enzyme that catalyzes the formation of tetrahydrofolate from dihydrofolate.
   - (1) Normally, tetrahydrofolate is converted to a variety of coenzymes that are necessary for one-carbon transfer reactions involved in the synthesis of purines, thymidylate, methionine, and glycine.
   - (2) Therefore, methotrexate inhibits the formation of these coenzymes.
   b. The primary cause of cell death is the blockade of the biosynthesis of thymidylate and purines required for DNA synthesis. Thus, methotrexate kills cells in S phase.
   c. Because methotrexate also inhibits RNA and protein synthesis, the drug slows the rate of entry of cells into S phase; therefore, it is a **self-limiting** S-phase–specific drug.
   d. The blockade caused by methotrexate can be circumvented.
   - (1) Substances such as **leucovorin** (also called citrovorum factor or folinic acid) and **thymidine** can be converted to the required tetrahydrofolate coenzymes or to thymidylate even in the presence of methotrexate.
   - (2) This allows the **"rescue"** of nonmalignant cells with a consequent reduction in toxicity from methotrexate.

2. Pharmacokinetics
   a. Methotrexate is well absorbed after oral administration.
   b. It is eliminated primarily by the kidneys without extensive metabolism and is approximately 50% bound to plasma proteins.
   - (1) Weak acids, such as salicylates and sulfonamides, can increase methotrexate toxicity by inhibiting renal tubular secretion and displacing methotrexate from plasma proteins.
   - (2) High doses of methotrexate can cause oversaturation of the renal acid secretory system with the formation of 7-hydroxy-methotrexate. This may be the etiology of nephrotoxicity (see III B 6 e).
   c. Cellular uptake of the drug is by carrier-mediated active transport.
   d. After an intravenous injection of methotrexate, plasma decay kinetics are triphasic with a half-life of 45 minutes for the first (distributional) phase, 3.5 hours for the second (renal clearance) phase, and 27 hours for the third (final excretion) phase.
   e. Methotrexate does not penetrate the blood–brain barrier well, but it is one of a few agents that can be administered intrathecally for cerebral leukemia.

3. Tumor cell resistance. Tumor cells may become resistant to methotrexate because:
   a. Their cellular transport is impaired.
   b. An altered form of dihydrofolate reductase is formed.
   c. The tumor cells generate an increased concentration of dihydrofolate reductase through **gene amplification**. This is the major mechanism of tumor cell resistance.

4. Therapeutic uses
   a. Methotrexate is used in combination with other agents to treat acute lymphoblastic leukemia, Burkitt's lymphoma, trophoblastic choriocarcinoma, and carcinomas of the breast, cervix, lung, head, and neck.

b. The drug is also useful in the treatment of mycosis fungoides and psoriasis.

c. There is no good rationale for high-dose methotrexate therapy.

d. At low, pulsed doses, this agent has been used experimentally in the treatment of rheumatoid arthritis.

5. Route of administration. Methotrexate can be administered intravenously, intra-arterially, intrathecally, or orally.

6. Adverse effects

a. Myelosuppression is significant with leukopenia and thrombocytopenia occurring 1–2 weeks after administration.

b. Gastrointestinal toxicity is manifested by ulcerative stomatitis and diarrhea and can disrupt therapy.

c. Nausea and vomiting are common acute adverse effects.

d. Prolonged low-dose methotrexate therapy can cause **hepatic dysfunction,** culminating in cirrhosis of the liver if drug treatment is not terminated.

e. Renal failure can occur with high doses of methotrexate as a result of precipitation of the drug in the renal tubules. Large volumes of alkaline urine must be maintained to prevent this toxicity. The drug is not administered to individuals with poor renal function.

f. Methotrexate may cause dermatitis.

g. There have been reports of necrotizing leukoencephalopathy when methotrexate was given with concomitant radiation therapy.

C. Purine analogues

1. 6-Mercaptopurine

a. Chemistry. 6-Mercaptopurine is a structural analogue of hypoxanthine.

b. Mechanism of action

(1) 6-Mercaptopurine must be converted intracellularly to the nucleotide 6-mercaptopurine ribose phosphate by hypoxanthine–guanine phosphoribosyl transferase (HGPRT). 6-Mercaptopurine also can be converted to 6-methylmercaptopurine ribonucleotide.

(2) 6-Mercaptopurine ribose phosphate and the methylated nucleotide are cytotoxic primarily because they inhibit de novo purine biosynthesis. Both block the aminotransferase that is responsible for the first step in purine biosynthesis, namely, the formation of 5-phosphoribosylamine, by feedback inhibition.

(3) In addition, 6-mercaptopurine ribose phosphate inhibits both adenylosuccinate synthetase, the enzyme that converts inosinic acid to adenylosuccinic acid, and inosinate dehydrogenase, the enzyme that converts inosinac acid to xanthylic acid.

c. Pharmacokinetics

(1) 6-Mercaptopurine is well-absorbed orally, and 50% is found in the urine in 24 hours, principally as 6-thiouric acid and inorganic sulfate.

(2) After an intravenous injection, the plasma half-life is approximately 1 hour.

(3) The drug is 20% bound to plasma protein and does not cross the blood–brain barrier.

(4) 6-Mercaptopurine can be metabolically inactivated by desulfuration and by oxidation via xanthine oxidase to form 6-thiouric acid.

d. Tumor cell resistance. Tumor cells may become resistant to 6-mercaptopurine due to either a decreased drug activation by HGPRT or an increased inactivation by alkaline phosphatase.

e. Therapeutic uses

(1) 6-Mercaptopurine is used in the maintenance therapy of acute lymphocytic and acute lymphoblastic leukemia.

(2) It is also useful in the treatment of acute and chronic myelogenous and granulocytic leukemia.

f. Route of administration. 6-Mercaptopurine is administered orally.

g. Adverse effects
  (1) 6-Mercaptopurine causes myelosuppression, but this is more gradual in onset than the suppression caused by methotrexate.
  (2) 6-Mercaptopurine also causes anorexia and nausea.
  (3) One-third of treated patients may develop jaundice associated with biliary stasis and hepatic necrosis. Discontinuation of therapy usually reverses this adverse effect.
  (4) Hyperuricemia and hyperuricosuria may occur with 6-mercaptopurine therapy.
    (a) This is caused by the destruction of cells and the release of purines that are metabolized by xanthine oxidase.
    (b) Allopurinol, an inhibitor of xanthine oxidase, can block the hyperuricemia and hyperuricosuria (see Chapter 9 IV E), but it also prevents the inactivation of 6-mercaptopurine.
    (c) Therefore, the dose of 6-mercaptopurine must be reduced when a patient is receiving concurrent allopurinol to prevent significant toxicity.

2. 6-Thioguanine
  a. Chemistry. 6-Thioguanine is a structural analogue of guanine in which a sulfhydryl replaces a hydroxyl group in the 6 position.
  b. Mechanism of action
    (1) Like 6-mercaptopurine, 6-thioguanine is converted by HGPRT to the nucleotide, in this case, 6-thioguanine ribose phosphate.
    (2) The cytotoxicity of 6-thioguanine may be due to feedback inhibition of purine biosynthesis by 6-thioguanine ribose phosphate.
    (3) Alternatively, the cytotoxicity of 6-thioguanine may be due to conversion of 6-thioguanine to the deoxynucleoside triphosphate, which is incorporated into tumor cell DNA and RNA.
  c. Pharmacokinetics
    (1) 6-Thioguanine is only slowly absorbed orally, and less than 50% of the administered dose is found in the urine in 24 hours, all in the form of metabolites.
    (2) 6-Thioguanine is not a good substrate for xanthine oxidase, in contrast to 6-mercaptopurine, and only small amounts of 6-thiouric acid are detected. Therefore, no dose reduction is required with concurrent allopurinol use.
  d. Tumor cell resistance. The proposed mechanisms for tumor cell resistance to 6-thioguanine are the same as those for 6-mercaptopurine.
  e. Therapeutic uses. 6-Thioguanine is used primarily in the treatment of acute myelogenous leukemia.
  f. Route of administration. 6-Thioguanine is administered orally.
  g. Adverse effects
    (1) Myelosuppression is a common side effect.
    (2) 6-Thioguanine causes mild nausea.
    (3) Hepatotoxicity is less common with 6-thioguanine than with 6-mercaptopurine.

3. Pentostatin is a purine analogue that is a potent inhibitor of adenosine deaminase. Pentostatin also interferes with the synthesis of nicotinamide adenine dinucleotide, resulting in DNA strand breakage. Pentostatin has been used for the treatment of hairy cell leukemia, mycosis fungoides, and chronic lymphocytic leukemia.

D. Pyrimidine analogues

1. 5-Fluorouracil
  a. Chemistry. 5-Fluorouracil is a fluorine-substituted analogue of uracil. Its structure is shown in Figure 11-4.
  b. Mechanism of action
    (1) Like the purine antimetabolites, 5-fluorouracil must be metabolically activated to a nucleotide, in this case 5-fluoro-2′-deoxyuridine-5′-monophosphate (FdUMP).

FIGURE 11-4. 5-Fluorouracil.

There are three general pathways for FdUMP formation:
- **(a)** 5-Fluorouracil can be metabolized to the deoxyribonucleoside with subsequent phosphorylation by thymidine kinase.
- **(b)** 5-Fluorouracil can be converted to 5-fluorouridine-5'-phosphate by pyrimidine phosphoribosyltransferase and then to the deoxyribonucleoside by ribonucleotide reductase.
- **(c)** FdUMP can also be formed by the conversion of 5-fluorouracil to fluorouridine, which is subsequently phosphorylated by uridine kinase to form 5-fluorouridine-5'-phosphate and ultimately FdUMP.

(2) The cytotoxicity of 5-fluorouracil is due primarily to inhibition of DNA synthesis caused by a FdUMP-produced blockage of thymidylate synthetase.

(3) Thymidylate synthetase normally transfers a methylene group from reduced folic acid to deoxyuridylate monophosphate (dUMP) to form thymidylate, which is essential for DNA synthesis.

(4) Cytotoxicity may also be due to incorporation of 5-fluorouridine triphosphate into RNA, which leads to "fraudulent" RNA formation.

(5) 5-Fluorouracil is **phase-nonspecific,** killing cells not only in S phase but throughout the cell cycle, perhaps due to its RNA actions.

c. Pharmacokinetics

(1) 5-Fluorouracil is administered intravenously and is catabolized by the liver.

(2) The first, and rate-limiting, hepatic enzyme involved in 5-fluorouracil catabolism is dihydrouracil dehydrogenase. After cleavage of the pyrimidine ring, the final degradation products are ammonia, urea, 2-fluoro-3-alanine, and carbon dioxide.

(3) 5-Fluorouracil is distributed throughout the body, including the CSF.

d. Tumor cell resistance may result from any of several causes:

(1) An increased synthesis of thymidylate synthetase

(2) An altered affinity of thymidylate synthetase for FdUMP

(3) An increased rate of 5-fluorouracil catabolism

(4) The deletion of enzymes that convert 5-fluorouracil to the active nucleotide

(5) An increase in the pool of deoxyuridylic acid

e. Therapeutic uses

(1) 5-Fluorouracil is used in combination with other agents for the treatment of breast cancer.

(2) It has palliative activity in gastrointestinal adenocarcinoma. Preliminary data suggest that adjuvant treatment with levamisole (an old antiparasitic drug) plus 5-fluorouracil may increase remissions and possibly prolong survival in some patients with resectable colon cancer.

(3) It is also used to treat carcinomas of the cervix, bladder, and prostate.

(4) Topical application of the drug has been useful for the treatment of premalignant keratoses of the skin and superficial basal cell carcinoma.

f. Route of administration. 5-Fluorouracil is usually administered intravenously.

g. Adverse effects

(1) Myelosuppression, especially leukopenia, frequently occurs.

(2) Stomatitis, diarrhea, nausea, and alopecia are seen.

(3) Neurologic toxicity occurs in 1%–2% of treated patients.

2. **Cytarabine** (cytosine arabinoside, ara-C, 1-β-D-arabinofuranosylcytosine)
   a. **Chemistry.** Cytarabine is an analogue of cytidine in which the ribose moiety has been replaced with an arabinose.
   b. **Mechanism of action**
      (1) Cytarabine must be activated by pyrimidine nucleoside kinase to the nucleotide triphosphate, ara-cytosine triphosphate.
      (2) The nucleotide triphosphate competitively inhibits DNA polymerase, thus blocking DNA synthesis and causing cell death.
      (3) Cytarabine nucleotides can be incorporated into DNA and RNA, but the biologic significance of this remains to be established.
      (4) It is an **S-phase–specific** agent.
   c. **Pharmacokinetics**
      (1) Cytarabine is poorly absorbed after oral administration.
      (2) It is rapidly metabolized in the liver and other tissues by cytidine deaminase.
      (3) It has an extremely short plasma half-life of 10 minutes.
   d. **Tumor cell resistance** may be due to:
      (1) Depressed levels of the kinase required for activation
      (2) Enhanced levels of the deaminase that inactivate the drug
   e. **Therapeutic uses.** Cytarabine is used to treat acute myelogenous leukemia in combination with an anthracycline (see IV B 2) or 6-thioguanine. It is also used to treat acute granulocytic and acute lymphocytic leukemias.
   f. **Route of administration**
      (1) Cytarabine is given by intravenous, intramuscular, or subcutaneous injection.
      (2) Because it is a phase-specific agent and rapidly inactivated, continuous infusion is the preferred mode of administration.
   g. **Adverse effects** include severe myelosuppression, nausea, and mucosal inflammation.

IV. NATURAL PRODUCTS

A. General considerations

1. Unlike the other classes of antitumor agents, membership in this group is determined by the source of the drug.

2. The natural products used in cancer chemotherapy are extracted from a variety of plants and lower organisms.

3. Most of the natural products have complex chemical structures.

4. The major classes of natural products are:
   a. **Antibiotics**
   b. **Vinca alkaloids**
   c. **Biologic response modifiers**
   d. **Enzymes**
   e. **Epipodophyllotoxins**
   f. **Western yew tree extract**

B. Antibiotics

1. **Dactinomycin (actinomycin D)**
   a. **Chemistry**
      (1) Dactinomycin is isolated from a *Streptomyces* species.
      (2) It contains two cyclic polypeptides that are linked by a chromophore moiety.
   b. **Mechanism of action**
      (1) Dactinomycin binds noncovalently to double-stranded DNA and inhibits DNA-directed RNA synthesis.
      (2) It is a phase-nonspecific agent.

c. Pharmacokinetics

(1) Dactinomycin is rapidly cleared from the plasma but is retained in the body for prolonged periods. Only 30% of the drug is recovered in the urine and stool after 7 days.

(2) It does not cross the blood–brain barrier.

d. Tumor cell resistance is due to decreased ability of tumor cells to take up or retain the drug.

e. Therapeutic uses

(1) Dactinomycin is used in combination with other agents to treat Wilms' tumor, Ewing's sarcoma, rhabdomyosarcoma, Kaposi's sarcoma, and soft-tissue sarcomas.

(2) Due to its lympholytic effects, dactinomycin is immunosuppressive and has been used in renal transplantation.

f. Route of administration. Dactinomycin is administered intravenously.

g. Adverse effects

(1) Dactinomycin produces myelosuppression, nausea, and vomiting.

(2) Skin damage can occur in areas of previous irradiation.

2. Anthracyclines

a. Chemistry

(1) Doxorubicin is the prototypic agent. Isolated from *Streptomyces,* it contains an amino sugar and an anthracycline ring.

(2) Daunorubicin is structurally almost identical to doxorubicin, lacking only a hydroxyl moiety.

(3) Mitoxantrone is a synthetic anthracene related to the anthracyclines.

b. Mechanism of action

(1) The aglycone portion of the drug molecule intercalates with DNA and RNA.

(2) The ionic sugar portion of the molecule bonds ionically to stabilize the intercalation.

(3) As a result, DNA and RNA are distorted during synthesis.

(4) This action is phase-nonspecific.

(5) There may be some free radical production, which may play a role in tissue cytotoxicity. Mitoxantrone causes less free radical formation and lipid peroxidation than doxorubicin and theoretically should cause less cardiotoxicity.

c. Pharmacokinetics

(1) Doxorubicin and daunorubicin are rapidly taken up by all tissues except the brain.

(2) They are extensively bound to cellular components, which is responsible for their long plasma half-life.

(3) Both drugs are metabolized primarily to hydroxylated and conjugated species.

(4) Mitoxantrone is extensively bound to plasma proteins and tissues following intravenous administration. The plasma half-life is highly variable (3 hours to 12 days). The highest concentrations are found in the thyroid, liver, and heart. Mitoxantrone is metabolized in the liver.

d. Tumor cell resistance to doxorubicin or daunorubicin appears to result from reduced cellular uptake of the drug or a more rapid removal of the intracellular drug.

e. Therapeutic uses

(1) Doxorubicin is one of the most effective agents against solid tumors. It is also effective against acute leukemias and malignant lymphoma.

(2) Daunorubicin is most effective against acute lymphocytic and granulocytic leukemia. It has little activity against solid tumors.

(3) Mitoxantrone appears to be as effective as daunorubicin but may be less toxic when combined with cytarabine for the initial treatment of acute nonlymphocytic leukemia. It may also be effective in some patients with advanced breast cancer.

f. Route of administration

(1) Doxorubicin is administered intravenously. Because it causes severe tissue necrosis, doxorubicin **cannot be injected subcutaneously or intramuscularly,** and special care must be taken to avoid extravasation during intravenous infusions or injections.

(2) Cumulative doses of doxorubicin appear to be important in the development of cardiac damage, and a maximum total dose of 550 mg/m² of body surface area is recommended to avoid cardiotoxicity.

(3) Daunorubicin is administered similarly.

(4) Mitoxantrone produces a lower frequency of severe local reactions after inadvertent extravasation compared with doxorubicin and daunorubicin.

g. Adverse effects

(1) Doxorubicin, daunorubicin, and mitoxantrone cause both **acute** and **chronic cardiomyopathy**. The depression of cardiac function resulting from repeated doses limits the total amount of drug that can be administered.

(2) Myelosuppression, especially leukopenia, occurs in most patients.

(3) Alopecia is a common side effect.

(4) Both drugs also cause nausea and vomiting.

(5) Dermatitis at the site of previous irradiation can occur.

3. Bleomycin

a. Chemistry

(1) Clinically used, bleomycin is a group of glycopeptides extracted from a *Streptomyces* species.

(2) Each bleomycin molecule has a planar end and an amine end. Different types of bleomycins differ in their terminal amine moieties.

b. Mechanism of action

(1) The planar end of the bleomycin molecule intercalates with DNA.

(2) The other end binds ferrous ion and facilitates its oxidation to ferric ion, thereby generating a free radical.

(3) The free radical oxygen cleaves DNA, acting specifically at purine-guanosine-cytosine-pyrimidine sequences.

(4) Cells in G_0 and G_2 phases are most sensitive.

c. Pharmacokinetics

(1) Bleomycin has a plasma half-life of approximately 1 hour.

(2) More than half of the drug is eliminated unchanged in the urine within 24 hours.

(3) Bleomycin is inactivated in most tissues, except skin and lungs, by an enzyme, bleomycin hydrolase. Toxicity in a specific organ occurs if the organ is lacking in enzyme activity.

d. Tumor cell resistance

(1) Tumor cells may fail to respond because of high levels of bleomycin hydrolase activity.

(2) Tumor cells may mutate, altering the sequences that are sensitive to bleomycin intercalation.

(3) Resistance may also result from poor cellular accumulation of bleomycin or rapid drug removal.

e. Therapeutic uses

(1) Bleomycin is used only in combination with other agents.

(2) It is effective with cisplatin and vinblastine for the treatment of testicular carcinoma.

(3) It is also used for Hodgkin's disease and non-Hodgkin's lymphomas and for squamous cell carcinomas of the head and neck, cervix, and skin.

f. Route of administration

(1) Bleomycin is administered intravenously or intramuscularly.

(2) It is sold in **units of activity**. The units are based on the toxicity to bacteria; 1 unit equals approximately 1.7 mg.

(3) A maximum total cumulative dose of 400 units is recommended to avoid pulmonary toxicity.

g. Adverse effects

(1) Bleomycin causes an age-related and cumulative-dose–related pulmonary toxicity. This consists of a pneumonitis, which can progress to fatal pulmonary fibrosis.

(2) Bleomycin does not produce significant bone marrow toxicity.

4. Mitomycin (mitomycin C)

a. Chemistry. Isolated from *Streptomyces,* mitomycin contains an aziridine ring as well as a urethane and a quinone moiety.

b. Mechanism of action

(1) Mitomycin is reduced intracellularly by a reduced nicotinamide adenine dinucleotide phosphate (NADPH)–dependent reductase, and then alkylates DNA. Thus, it can also be classified as an **alkylating agent**.

(2) Because oxygen-derived free radicals can be formed, single-strand DNA lesions also can occur.

c. Pharmacokinetics

(1) After intravenous administration, mitomycin disappears rapidly from the blood.

(2) Mitomycin does not penetrate the CNS.

(3) It is extensively metabolized by the liver.

(4) Is is not absorbed through the bladder mucosa when given intravesically.

d. Therapeutic uses

(1) Mitomycin has limited use in the treatment of carcinomas of the stomach and cervix.

(2) It is also used to treat superficial carcinoma of the bladder.

e. Route of administration

(1) Mitomycin is administered in a rapidly flowing intravenous infusion.

(2) For superficial bladder carcinoma, it can also be given by intravesical infusion. Systemic side effects are lessened with intravesical administration.

f. Adverse effects

(1) Myelosuppression is a major complication with intravenous administration.

(2) Dermal, pulmonary, renal, and gastrointestinal toxicity may occur.

(3) Extravasation can result in severe local injury.

C. **Vinca alkaloids**

1. Chemistry

a. The two prominent agents in this group, **vincristine** and **vinblastine,** are derived from the periwinkle plant.

b. Both are structurally complex compounds, and vincristine differs from vinblastine only in having an aldehyde moiety.

c. Despite their similarity in chemical structure, the two alkaloids are different in their therapeutic applications and toxicities.

2. Mechanism of action

a. Both alkaloids bind to tubulin, thereby interfering with the assembly of spindle proteins during mitosis.

b. Both agents are M-phase–specific, blocking proliferating cells as they enter metaphase.

3. Pharmacokinetics

a. Both agents are extensively bound to tissue components. Less than 30% of a dose of vinblastine or its metabolites, for example, is recovered during a 6-day period after injection.

b. Only a small amount of either of these vinca alkaloids penetrates the brain or enters the CSF.

c. Both agents are metabolized by the liver and excreted in the bile.

4. Tumor cell resistance

a. It is believed that resistance to both agents is caused by a reduced ability of tumor cells to retain the drugs.

b. Although cross-resistance between vinblastine and vincristine has been observed in experimental murine tumors, cross-resistance does not appear to occur in human tumors.

5. Therapeutic uses

a. Vinblastine is used in combination with bleomycin and cisplatin for the treatment of testicular carcinoma. It is also effective against lymphomas, neuroblastoma, and Letterer-Siwe disease.

b. Vincristine

    (1) Vincristine is effective against acute lymphoblastic leukemia, Hodgkin's disease, and non-Hodgkin's lymphomas.

    (2) It is also useful in the treatment of solid tumors in children and tumors of the breast, lung, and cervix in adults.

    (3) Vincristine is less likely to cause myelosuppression and is preferred over vinblastine for use in combination with myelosuppressive agents in the therapy of lymphomas.

    (4) Vincristine is used in combination with the corticosteroid prednisone, procarbazine, and an alkylating agent (e.g., mechlorethamine) in the MOPP regimen for treating Hodgkin's disease.

    (5) The combination of vincristine with prednisone is considered the treatment of choice for inducing remission in childhood leukemia.

6. Route of administration

    a. Vinblastine is administered intravenously with particular caution being taken not to produce subcutaneous extravasation.

    b. Vincristine is also administered intravenously with avoidance of extravasation.

7. Adverse effects

    a. Vinblastine causes leukopenia within 4–10 days after treatment. Minimal nausea, paresthesias, and jaw pain have been reported.

    b. Vincristine is significantly neurotoxic with paresthesias and motor weakness being the most prominent effects. These neurologic manifestations are minimized by stopping or reducing the dose at the earliest onset of symptoms.

D. **Biologic response modifiers** are agents that act directly on tumor cells or indirectly by enhancing the immunologic response to neoplastic cells. Examples include:

1. Interleukin-2 (IL-2), which is a cytokine secreted by T cells that enhance natural killer cell activity. It is being tested alone and in combination for treatment of melanoma and renal cell cancer.

2. Interferons (alpha, beta, gamma). Alpha-interferons have been approved for the treatment of hairy cell leukemia and Kaposi's sarcoma in patients with AIDS. Additionally, it is effective for condylomata acuminata.

E. **Enzymes.** L-Asparaginase catalyzes the hydrolysis of asparagine to aspartic acid and ammonia. Depriving the malignant cell of asparagine results in cessation of protein synthesis and cellular death. It has exhibited modest success in the treatment of acute lymphocytic leukemia.

F. **Epipodophyllotoxins (etoposide and teniposide)** are semisynthetic glycosides of the active podophyllotoxin (extracted from the mandrake plant) that show activity in several human neoplasms.

1. Mechanism of action

    a. At low concentrations, epipodophyllotoxins block cells at the $S-G_2$ interface.

    b. At high concentrations, they cause G_2 arrest.

    c. They stimulate DNA topoisomerase II to cleave DNA.

2. Pharmacokinetics

    a. Etoposide can be administered orally and intravenously. It has a terminal half-life of 8 hours. Forty percent is excreted in the urine.

    b. Teniposide is administered intravenously with a terminal half-life of 10–40 hours. As much as 80% is recovered as metabolite.

3. Therapeutic uses

    a. Etoposide is used for testicular tumors and in combination with cisplatin for small cell carcinoma of the lung. It is active against a variety of other carcinomas, including non-Hodgkin's lymphoma, breast carcinoma, and AIDS-related Kaposi's sarcoma.

    b. Teniposide is being investigated for the treatment of refractory acute lymphoblastic leukemia.

4. Adverse effects
    a. Etoposide causes dose-limiting leukopenia.
    b. Teniposide causes myelosuppression.

G. **Paclitaxel (Taxol)** is a natural product extracted in small amounts from the inner bark of the western yew tree. A fungus growing on the Pacific yew was also found to produce paclitaxel.

1. Mechanism of action
    a. Paclitaxel causes formation of stable microtubule bundles, interfering with the late G_2 (mitotic) phase of the cell cycle and inhibiting cell replication.
    b. Paclitaxel inhibits the G_2 phase, thus inhibiting cell replication.

2. Pharmacokinetics
    a. Following intravenous administration, paclitaxel is widely distributed; however, it is not found in the CSF.
    b. Small amounts are found in urine, and high concentrations of the parent and hydroxylated metabolites are found in bile.

3. Therapeutic uses
    a. Paclitaxel produces a temporary partial response in up to 33% of previously treated patients with metastatic ovarian cancer, including some who are resistant to platinum drugs.
    b. Preliminary studies indicate paclitaxel has activity in metastatic breast cancer, advanced non–small cell lung cancer, malignant melanoma, and head and neck cancer.

4. Adverse effects
    a. Severe hypersensitivity reactions can occur and are thought to be caused by the castor oil vehicle. A slower infusion rate and pretreatment with corticosteroids and histamine blockers decrease the frequency and severity of the reactions.
    b. The major dose-limiting toxicity is granulocytopenia, which is reduced with the concurrent use of granulocyte colony-stimulating factor (G-CSF).
    c. Dose-related peripheral neuropathy, arthralgia, and myalgia can occur.
    d. Bradycardia is common but does not require treatment; second- and third-degree heart block have also occurred and require therapy.
    e. Complete hair loss usually occurs but is reversible when paclitaxel therapy is stopped.

5. Drug interactions. Concurrent use of **ketoconazole** might increase paclitaxel toxicity.

V. HORMONES AND ANTAGONISTS

A. **General considerations**

1. Hormonal therapy relies on the presence of receptors for endogenous hormones required for cell proliferation.

2. Unlike agents in the other classes of antineoplastic drugs, members of this class generally do not cause severe toxicity.

B. **Tamoxifen**

1. Chemistry. Tamoxifen is a nonsteroidal compound containing a triphenylethylene moiety (Figure 11-5).

2. Mechanism of action
    a. Some tumors, notably breast carcinomas, require estrogen for cell proliferation.
        (1) Estrogen binds to a cytoplasmic protein receptor, and the receptor–hormone complex translocates into the nucleus, inducing RNA synthesis.
        (2) Estrogen receptors are found in two thirds of the breast tumors that occur in postmenopausal women.

FIGURE 11-5. Tamoxifen.

   b. Tamoxifen, an estrogen receptor antagonist, is useful in women whose tumors contain estrogen receptors.
     (1) Tamoxifen competes with estrogen for the cytoplasmic receptor, although it has little or no estrogenic activity.
     (2) The **antiestrogen action** of tamoxifen blocks the growth-promoting effects of estrogen in estrogen-dependent tumors.

3. Pharmacokinetics
   a. Tamoxifen is absorbed when given orally.
   b. It concentrates in tissues with estrogen receptors, such as the ovaries and breast tissue, as well as in tumors that contain these receptors.
   c. Tamoxifen undergoes extensive hepatic metabolism.
   d. It undergoes enterohepatic recirculation and then is found as metabolites in the stool.

4. Therapeutic uses. Tamoxifen is used for palliative treatment of advanced breast carcinoma in the postmenopausal woman.
   a. Although the response rate has been favorable in both estrogen receptor-rich and receptor-poor forms of breast carcinoma, the response is more favorable in the receptor-rich variant.
   b. The tumor reappears upon withdrawal of the drug.

5. Route of administration. Tamoxifen is administered orally.

6. Adverse effects
   a. Hot flashes, mild fluid retention, and nausea occur frequently.
   b. With high doses, corneal and retinal opacities have been observed.
   c. Hypercalcemia can occur.

C. Androgens and antiandrogens

1. Androgens have been used in the treatment of breast carcinoma in postmenopausal women.
   a. The **mechanism of action** is not completely understood.
   b. A number of androgens are available, such as **fluoxymesterone, dromostanolone,** and **testosterone**. All are equally active and usually produce a response within 2 months.
   c. Common side effects are masculinization and fluid retention.

2. Antiandrogens (flutamide)
   a. Flutamide is an oral antiandrogen used concurrently with an analogue of luteinizing hormone–releasing hormone, such as leuprolide for the treatment of metastatic prostate cancer.
   b. Flutamide prevents adrenal androgens from binding to androgen receptors in the prostate gland and in prostate cancer cells.
   c. Flutamide frequently causes gynecomastia and may cause hepatitis.

D. **Adrenal corticosteroids**

1. Corticosteroids inhibit cellular protein synthesis and attach to specific corticosteroid binding proteins associated with leukemia cells. (See Chapter 10 III G for further information about their intracellular mechanism of action.)

2. **Prednisone,** a glucocorticoid, has been used successfully in combination with cytotoxic agents in the treatment of lymphoblastic and chronic lymphocytic leukemia.

3. Prednisone is also active in combination with other cytotoxic agents in the treatment of Hodgkin's disease (e.g., a component of the MOPP regimen), non-Hodgkin's lymphomas, and multiple myeloma.

4. Because of their ability to suppress androgen production by suppressing the adrenal cortex, corticosteroids (e.g., prednisolone) have also been used in the treatment of breast carcinoma.

E. **Progestins**

1. Progestins bind to cytosolic progesterone receptors and cause maturation of the endometrium to a nonproliferating secretory state. Thus, progestins are sometimes used in the therapy of metastatic endometrial carcinoma that can no longer be treated with irradiation or surgery.

2. The progestins most commonly used as antitumor agents are **medroxyprogesterone,** which is given intramuscularly, and **megestrol,** which is given orally.

3. Progestins also have some limited use in the treatment of metastatic renal cell carcinoma. The mechanism of action in this tumor type is unclear.

4. The progestins cause mild fluid retention and vaginal bleeding.

VI. MISCELLANEOUS AGENTS

A. **Hydroxyurea**

1. **Chemistry.** Hydroxyurea is a derivative of urea.

2. **Mechanism of action**
   a. Hydroxyurea inhibits ribonucleotide reductase. This enzyme is crucial to the biosynthesis of deoxyribonucleotides that are essential for the formation of DNA.
   b. Hydroxyurea is specific for the S phase of the cell cycle.

3. **Pharmacokinetics**
   a. Hydroxyurea is rapidly absorbed from the gastrointestinal tract.
   b. Twenty percent of a dose is metabolized in the liver, while the remainder is excreted via the kidney.

4. **Therapeutic uses**
   a. Hydroxyurea is an alternative to busulfan (see II D) in the treatment of chronic myelogenous leukemia.
   b. Hydroxyurea reduces high white blood cell counts in patients with acute myelogenous leukemia.
   c. Other uses include treatment of polycythemia vera, essential thrombocytosis, and hypereosinophilic syndrome.

5. **Route of administration**
   a. Hydroxyurea can be administered orally or intravenously.
   b. Because of its renal elimination, administration in patients with impaired renal function must be conducted with caution.

6. Adverse effects

a. Reversible myelosuppression is the major adverse effect.

b. Gastrointestinal and cutaneous disturbances occasionally occur.

B. Procarbazine

1. Chemistry. Procarbazine is a substituted hydrazine derivative with a structure similar to that of some monoamine oxidase (MAO) inhibitors.

2. Mechanism of action

a. Procarbazine undergoes auto-oxidation and forms hydrogen peroxide, leading to the degradation of DNA.

b. It also inhibits DNA, RNA, and protein synthesis.

c. It also can transmethylate DNA at the 7-nitrogen position of guanine.

3. Pharmacokinetics

a. Procarbazine is rapidly absorbed from the gastrointestinal tract.

b. It readily equilibrates between the plasma and the CSF.

c. It is rapidly metabolized, and about 40% is excreted in the urine within 24 hours, chiefly as a metabolite.

4. Therapeutic uses

a. The major use of procarbazine is in combination with mechlorethamine, vincristine, and prednisone (i.e., in the MOPP regimen) in the treatment of Hodgkin's disease.

b. Procarbazine also has some activity in the treatment of oat cell carcinomas.

5. Route of administration. Procarbazine is administered orally until the desired response occurs or limiting toxicity is seen.

6. Adverse effects

a. Leukopenia and thrombocytopenia occur commonly.

b. Gastrointestinal adverse effects as well as potentiation of other CNS-dependent drugs can occur.

c. Because procarbazine is a weak MAO inhibitor, hypertensive reactions can occur when sympathomimetics, tricyclic antidepressants, or foods with a high tyramine content are ingested concomitantly.

C. Mitotane (o,p′-DDD)

1. Chemistry. Mitotane is a derivative of the insecticide DDT.

2. Mechanism of action

a. Mitotane selectively destroys normal and neoplastic adrenocortical cells by an unknown mechanism.

b. It rapidly lowers adrenocorticosteroid levels.

3. Pharmacokinetics

a. Mitotane is partially (40%) absorbed from the gastrointestinal tract.

b. Blood levels persist for up to 9 weeks after cessation of therapy.

c. Mitotane is widely distributed, with fat being the primary site of storage.

4. Therapeutic uses. Mitotane is used as palliative treatment for inoperable adrenal carcinoma.

5. Route of administration. Mitotane is administered orally.

6. Adverse effects

a. Gastrointestinal disturbances, lethargy, and dermatitis occur.

b. If patients have Addison's disease, or if shock or trauma occur during mitotane therapy, adrenocorticosteroid replacement is indicated.

D. Cisplatin

1. Chemistry. Cisplatin (*cis*-diamminedichloroplatinum) is an inorganic platinum coordination complex with a planar configuration (Figure 11-6). Only the *cis* isomer is active.

NH$_3$ Cl$^-$

    Pt^{2+}

NH$_3$ Cl$^-$

FIGURE 11-6. Cisplatin.

2. Mechanism of action
   a. Cisplatin binds to DNA, causing both interstrand and intrastrand cross-linking similar to the actions of the bifunctional alkylating agents.
   b. It also binds extensively to nuclear and cytoplasmic proteins.
   c. Cisplatin is a phase-nonspecific agent.

3. Pharmacokinetics
   a. After intravenous administration, 90% becomes protein-bound.
   b. Cisplatin has a long terminal half-life of greater than 2 days.
   c. It penetrates the CNS poorly.

4. Therapeutic uses
   a. Cisplatin is one of the most effective agents against solid tumors.
   b. It is effective alone and in combination with bleomycin and vinblastine in the treatment of testicular tumors.
   c. Cisplatin is also useful in the treatment of ovarian carcinoma.

5. Route of administration.
Cisplatin is administered intravenously with vigorous hydration and mannitol diuresis to avoid renal toxicity.

6. Adverse effects
   a. Dose-dependent impairment of renal tubular function can occur; therefore, cisplatin should not be used in patients with impaired renal function.
   b. High-frequency hearing loss can occur.
   c. Severe nausea and vomiting are almost inevitable.
   d. Anaphylaxis has occurred.

E. Carboplatin

1. Chemistry.
Carboplatin is chemically related to cisplatin.

2. Mechanism of action.
Like cisplatin, it binds to DNA and causes interstrand and intrastrand cross-links.

3. Pharmacokinetics
   a. The drug is eliminated primarily by the kidney.
   a. Sixty percent of a single dose is found in the urine within the first 24 hours.

4. Therapeutic uses
   a. Carboplatin can be used as a single agent in patients with persistent or recurrent ovarian cancer.
   b. The therapeutic response is slightly higher in patients not previously treated with cisplatin and much lower in those whose disease did not respond to cisplatin.

5. Route of administration.
Carboplatin is also given by intravenous infusion, but unlike cisplatin, forced hydration or diuresis is not required.

6. Adverse effects
   a. Carboplatin induces less nausea and vomiting compared with cisplatin.
   b. There is less nephrotoxicity, neurotoxicity, and ototoxicity compared with cisplatin.
   c. There is greater likelihood of dose-dependent bone marrow suppression, especially thrombocytopenia, compared with cisplatin.
   d. Allergic reactions have been reported.

F. Interleukin-2 (IL-2)

1. **Recombinant IL-2** is a lymphokine that stimulates growth of T lymphocytes. Its use is still considered experimental.

2. **Mechanism of action.** The incubation of peripheral T lymphocytes with IL-2 produces lymphocyte-activated killer cells that lyse several types of tumor cells in vitro. IL-2 plus the killer cells has caused regression of metastatic tumors in animals.

3. **Therapeutic uses.** IL-2 may offer some benefit to a small number of patients with metastatic renal cancer or melanoma.

4. **Route of administration.** IL-2 has been given by intravenous bolus or continuous infusion.

5. **Adverse effects** include:
   a. Fever
   b. Fluid retention leading to pulmonary edema
   c. Hypotension; capillary leak syndrome
   d. Cardiac arrhythmias
   e. Disorientation

VII. ANTIEMETICS FOR CANCER PATIENTS

A. General considerations

1. Chemotherapeutic agents may induce emesis by stimulating dopamine, serotonin, and opiate receptors in the vomiting center, the chemotrigger zone (CTZ).

2. **Effectiveness of the antiemetic agents** varies with:
   a. Route of administration
   b. Time of administration
   c. Anticancer agent used
   d. Dose of anticancer agent
   e. Mechanism of action

B. Ondansetron

1. **Mechanism of action.** Ondansetron is a $5HT_3$ receptor antagonist acting on the afferent vagal nerve terminals in the upper gastrointestinal tract and in the CTZ. Unlike metoclopramide or prochlorperazine, it does not have antidopaminergic activity and will not cause extrapyramidal effects.

2. **Pharmacokinetics.** Ondansetron is metabolized in the liver, and the metabolites are excreted in the urine.

3. **Administration**
   a. Ondansetron is more effective than metoclopramide alone when administered intravenously.
   b. Adding dexamethasone increases the effectiveness of ondansetron, but how dexamethasone prevents vomiting is unclear.

4. **Adverse effects.** Headache and constipation are the most common adverse effects.

C. Granisetron

1. **Mechanism of action.** Granisetron is a $5HT_3$ receptor antagonist with a mechanism of action similar to that of ondansetron.

2. **Pharmacokinetics.** Granisetron is metabolized in the liver and excreted in the urine and feces. It has a half-life of 9 hours.

3. **Administration.** Granisetron is available in the United States by intravenous administration only, although an oral form does exist. The addition of dexamethasone appears to increase the effectiveness of granisetron.

4. **Adverse effects** are similar to those of ondansetron.

D. Metoclopramide

1. **Mechanism of action.** Metoclopramide is a dopamine antagonist.

2. **Administration.** Metoclopramide is administered intravenously or orally.
   a. It should not be given concurrently with other dopamine antagonists (e.g., phenothiazines, butyrophenones) because doing so could precipitate acute dystonic reactions.
   b. Given alone, it is less effective than intravenous ondansetron and granisetron. Combining it with dexamethasone and lorazepam increases its effectiveness.

3. **Adverse effects** include somnolence and extrapyramidal reactions (e.g., parkinsonian syndrome).

E. Dronabinol is an oral tetrahydrocannabinol that is used in patients who have failed to respond to conventional antiemetic therapy. Adverse effects include xerostomia, orthostatic hypotension, sedation, ataxia, and dysphoria.

F. Phenothiazines and butyrophenones (haloperidol) are effective when administered intravenously. They can cause acute dystonic reactions, extrapyramidal symptoms, and hypotension.

DIRECTIONS: Each of the numbered items or incomplete statements in this section is followed by answers or by completions of the statement. Select the **one** lettered answer or completion that is **best** in each case.

1. Which of the following statements about the cancer chemotherapeutic agent mitomycin is true?

(A) It can be given orally
(B) It can be given intravesically
(C) It penetrates the central nervous system (CNS)
(D) It is useful in treating breast cancer
(E) It is effective for the treatment of prostate carcinoma

2. Drugs correctly matched with the drug category to which they belong include which of the following?

(A) Mechlorethamine—an alkylating agent
(B) Methotrexate—a natural product
(C) 5-Fluorouracil—a natural product
(D) Vinblastine—a purine analogue

DIRECTIONS: Each of the numbered items or incomplete statements in this section is negatively phrased, as indicated by a capitalized word such as NOT, LEAST, or EXCEPT. Select the ONE lettered answer or completion that is BEST in each case.

3. All of the following drugs are components of the MOPP cancer chemotherapy regimen EXCEPT

(A) procarbazine
(B) vincristine
(C) mechlorethamine
(D) pentostatin
(E) prednisone

4. Proliferation-independent agents include all of the following EXCEPT

(A) vincristine
(B) carmustine
(C) cyclophosphamide
(D) mechlorethamine
(E) melphalan

5. All of the following adverse effects are commonly associated with cancer chemotherapy EXCEPT

(A) alopecia
(B) teratogenesis
(C) myelosuppression
(D) nausea
(E) exfoliative dermatitis

6. All of the following agents have been used for cancer chemotherapy EXCEPT

(A) alkylating agents
(B) antimetabolites
(C) vitamin D derivatives
(D) plant alkaloids
(E) hormonal agents

7. True statements regarding alkylating agents include all of the following EXCEPT

(A) they are phase-nonspecific
(B) they kill rapidly proliferating cells
(C) acquired resistance can occur
(D) they are structurally similar to naturally occurring endogenous substances
(E) they kill nonproliferating cells

8. Alkylating nitrogen mustards often produce all of the following side effects EXCEPT

(A) aplasia of the bone marrow
(B) renal toxicity
(C) alopecia
(D) menstrual irregularities
(E) nausea and vomiting

9. Cyclophosphamide can be used to treat all of the following neoplastic disorders EXCEPT

(A) Hodgkin's disease
(B) Burkitt's lymphoma
(C) choriocarcinoma
(D) ovarian carcinoma
(E) breast carcinoma

10. Characteristics of methotrexate include all of the following EXCEPT

(A) it can be used in the treatment of psoriasis
(B) it is eliminated by the kidneys
(C) it is a self-limiting S-phase–specific drug
(D) it penetrates the blood–brain barrier
(E) it competitively inhibits dihydrofolate reductase

11. All of the following statements about the purine analogue 6-mercaptopurine are correct EXCEPT

(A) it is a structural analogue of hypoxanthine
(B) it decreases the synthesis of 5-phosphoribosylamine
(C) it interferes with the formation of adenylosuccinic acid
(D) its metabolism is stimulated by allopurinol
(E) it is used in the maintenance therapy of acute lymphoblastic leukemia

12. All of the following statements regarding biologic response modifiers are true EXCEPT

(A) they can act directly on tumor cells
(B) they can act indirectly by enhancing the immunologic response to neoplastic cells
(C) interleukin-2 (IL-2) may have a role in the treatment of renal cell carcinoma
(D) they can deprive malignant cells of aspar-agene, resulting in the cessation of protein synthesis
(E) alpha-interferon is useful for the treatment of hairy cell leukemia

13. All of the following statements about the epipodophyllotoxins, which show activity in several human neoplasms, are true EXCEPT

(A) at high concentrations, they cause G_2 arrest
(B) they stimulate RNA topoisomerase II
(C) etoposide can be used for testicular tumors
(D) etoposide can cause dose-limiting leukopenia
(E) teniposide is being investigated for the treatment of refractory acute lymphoblastic leukemia

14. Bleomycin is an antitumor agent that has all of the following characteristics EXCEPT

(A) it intercalates with DNA
(B) it acts by generating a free radical
(C) it requires ferrous ion for its action
(D) it kills cells in G_0 and G_2 phases
(E) it is a useful single agent for testicular carcinoma

15. A patient is placed on leuprolide plus flutamide, an oral antiandrogen. All of the following statements about flutamide are true EXCEPT that this agent

(A) prevents adrenal androgens from binding to androgen receptors in the prostate gland
(B) frequently causes gynecomastia
(C) can cause hepatitis
(D) is effective against metastatic prostate cancer, when used with leuprolide
(E) decreases plasma concentrations of luteinizing hormone (LH) and testosterone

DIRECTIONS: The group of items in this section consists of lettered options followed by a set of numbered items. For each item, select the **one** lettered option that is most closely associated with it. Each lettered option may be selected once, more than once, or not at all.

Questions 16–18

Match each antiemetic agent with the statement that best describes it.

(A) Ondansetron
(B) Metoclopramide
(C) Nabilone
(D) Prochlorperazine
(E) Dexamethazone

16. This agent is a $5HT_3$ receptor antagonist.

17. This agent is a nonphenothiazine dopamine antagonist.

18. Ondansetron increases this agent's effectiveness.

ANSWERS AND EXPLANATIONS

1. The answer is B *[IV B 4 c–e]*. Mitomycin is not absorbed into the bloodstream through the bladder wall, and therefore, it can be given by intravesical infusion to treat superficial carcinoma of the bladder. Mitomycin is also used to treat carcinomas of the stomach and cervix for which it is given by intravenous infusion. It is not used to treat breast cancer or prostate carcinoma. Mitomycin cannot be given orally and does not penetrate the central nervous system (CNS).

2. The answer is A *[II B 3; III B, D 1; IV C]*. Mechlorethamine, an alkylating agent, will produce DNA cross-linking, mispairing of bases, and depurination of DNA because of the highly reactive carbonium ion produced from mechlorethamine. This is true of all alkylating agents. Methotrexate is not a natural product but a folic acid antagonist and an antimetabolite. Vinblastine is a plant alkaloid, not a purine analogue. 5-Fluorouracil is a fluorine-substituted analogue of uracil and, thus, a pyrimidine analogue.

3. The answer is D *[I B 1]*. The MOPP regimen combines mechlorethamine, vincristine (Oncovin), procarbazine, and prednisone. It is used primarily for the treatment of Hodgkin's disease. Cancer chemotherapy often employs a combination of drugs that have different mechanisms of action, chiefly because of the discovery that individual tumors are made up of heterogeneous subpopulations of neoplastic cells with differences that cause them to vary in their susceptibility to anticancer drugs. The aim is to destroy all of these cells by a multiple approach without an increase in toxic effects.

4. The answer is A *[I C 3; II A 2, B 3 b, 4, 5, C 2 e; IV C 2 b]*. Proliferation-independent agents are toxic to both proliferating and nonproliferating cells. Examples include carmustine, mechlorethamine, cyclophosphamide, melphalan, and irradiation. The vinca alkaloids, such as vincristine, bind to tubulin and are M-phase–specific, blocking cells as they enter metaphase.

5. The answer is E *[I D 2]*. Exfoliative dermatitis is not a common adverse effect of chemotherapy. Many cancer chemotherapeutic agents cause alopecia, induce bone marrow suppression, and are teratogenic. Gastrointestinal tract toxicity (i.e., nausea, diarrhea) is also common.

6. The answer is C *[I F]*. Vitamin D derivatives have not been effective as cancer chemotherapeutic agents. A good diet, of course, is always important for the patient. The alkylating agents, antimetabolites, plant alkaloids, and hormonal agents are major classes of antineoplastic agents available for clinical use.

7. The answer is D *[II A 2–4, B 2 d; III A 1]*. Antimetabolites, not alkylating agents, are substances with structural similarity to endogenous substances. All alkylating agents are phase-nonspecific. In addition, cell death also occurs during interphase, and thus, they can be proliferation-independent. Both acquired resistance and cross-resistance can occur. They kill both rapidly proliferating and nonproliferating cells.

8. The answer is B *[II B 3 e, 4 d, 6 c]*. Nitrogen mustards can produce nausea, menstrual irregularities, alopecia, and myelosuppression. Renal toxicity is not a common problem with the alkylating agents but is a serious side effect of cisplatin.

9. The answer is C *[II B 4 b; III B 4 a]*. Cyclophosphamide is used alone or in combination for the treatment of Hodgkin's disease and Burkitt's lymphoma and for ovarian and breast carcinomas, but not for choriocarcinoma. The latter is most effectively treated with methotrexate. When used for lymphomas, cyclophosphamide is frequently used with vincristine and prednisone. Cyclophosphamide has also been used as an immunosuppressive agent during organ transplantation.

10. The answer is D *[III B 1 a, c, 2 b, e, 4 b]*. Methotrexate competitively inhibits dihydrofolate reductase and has been used in the treatment of psoriasis to suppress the proliferation of epidermal cells. It is a folic acid antagonist, which is eliminated unmetabolized, primarily via the kidneys. It slows the rate of entry of cells into S phase but kills cells in S phase. Thus, it can be labeled a self-limiting S-phase–specific drug. Methotrexate does not cross the blood–brain barrier well, but it can be administered intrathecally.

11. The answer is D *[III C 1]*. Allopurinol blocks, rather than stimulates, the metabolism of 6-mercaptopurine. Therefore, to prevent significant toxicity, the dose of 6-mercaptopurine must be reduced when a patient is also receiving allopurinol. Allopurinol is used in conjunction with 6-mercaptopurine because allopurinol blocks the formation of uric acid from hypoxanthine and xanthine. 6-Mercaptopurine decreases the synthesis of 5-phosphoribosyl-amine and interferes with the formation of adenylosuccinic acid. It is used in the maintenance therapy of acute lymphoblastic leukemia.

12. The answer is D *[IV D 1–2]*. The enzyme L-asparaginase deprives the malignant cells of asparagene, which results in cell death. L-Asparaginase has exhibited modest success in the treatment of acute lymphocytic leukemia. Biologic response modifiers [e.g., interleukin-2 (IL-2) and the interferons (alpha, beta, gamma)] act directly on tumor cells or indirectly by enhancing the immunologic response to neoplastic cells. IL-2 may be effective against renal cell carcinoma. Alpha interferon is useful for the treatment of hairy cell leukemia.

13. The answer is B *[IV F 1, 3, 4]*. Epipodophyllotoxins are semisynthetic glycosides of the active podophyllotoxin that show activity in several neoplasms. They stimulate DNA (not RNA) topoisomerase II to cleave DNA. At high concentrations, they cause G_2 arrest. Etoposide is used to treat testicular tumors; adverse effects include dose-limiting leukopenia. Teniposide is under investigation for the treatment of refractory acute lymphoblastic leukemia.

14. The answer is E *[IV B 3 b, e]*. Bleomycin is a natural product that intercalates with DNA and generates a free radical, which cleaves DNA at purine-guanosine-cytosine-pyrimidine sequences. Ferrous ion is required to produce the free radicals necessary for the DNA strand breaks. The most sensitive cells are cells in G_0 and G_2 phases of the cell cycle. Bleomycin is used only in combination with other agents. It is effective for testicular carcinoma, but only in combination with cisplatin and vinblastine.

15. The answer is E *[V C 2]*. The oral antiandrogen, flutamide, plus leuprolide is effective in treating metastatic prostate cancer. It prevents adrenal androgens from binding to androgen receptors in the prostate gland. It also blocks the inhibitory action of testosterone on luteinizing hormone (LH) production, resulting in increased plasma concentrations of LH and testosterone. Flutamide can cause gynecomastia and hepatitis.

16–18. The answers are: 16-A *[VII B]*, **17-B** *[VII D]*, **18-E** *[VII B 3 b]*. Ondansetron is a $5HT_3$ receptor antagonist that does not have antidopaminergic activity and will not cause extrapyramidal symptoms. It is more effective than metoclopramide alone when given intravenously.

Metoclopramide is a dopamine antagonist, which can be administered intravenously or orally. It should not be given concurrently with other dopamine antagonists because they could precipitate acute dystonic reactions.

Dexamethasone enhances the antiemetic activity of ondansetron, metoclopramide, and nabilone.

Chapter 12

Anti-Infective Agents

I. INTRODUCTION

A. Definitions

1. **Antimicrobial agents** are chemical substances that can kill or suppress the growth of microorganisms.

2. **Antibiotics** are soluble compounds that are derived from certain microorganisms and that inhibit the growth of other microorganisms.

B. Types of infections and their treatment

1. **Bacterial infections** are readily treated in most instances by a wide variety of agents. Some antibacterial drugs are **bacteriostatic;** that is, they inhibit the growth of susceptible bacteria. Other antibacterials are truly **bactericidal;** that is, they kill susceptible bacteria.
   a. The **minimal inhibitory concentration (MIC)** is the minimum amount of a drug required to inhibit the growth of bacteria.
   b. The **minimal bactericidal concentration (MBC)** is the minimum amount of a drug required to kill bacteria.

2. **Fungal infections,** in contrast to bacterial infections, generally are quite resistant to chemotherapy, and the number of useful agents for these infections is somewhat restricted. Fungal infections often occur as **superinfections;** that is, secondary infections superimposed on the original infection as a result of changes in the host's flora (e.g., as a result of antibacterial therapy).

3. **Mycobacterial infections,** in the past, often required treatment in specialized centers; today most therapy is conducted on an outpatient basis.
   a. **Tuberculosis** is one of the few diseases that requires a combination of antimicrobial drugs, which are used to prevent the appearance of resistant strains of the infecting organism. The emergence of resistant strains of tuberculosis, particularly in AIDS patients, has created a major health problem.
   b. **Leprosy** is a disease whose course has been remarkably altered by chemotherapy.
   c. **Infections with atypical mycobacteria** (e.g., *Mycobacterium avium* complex) are seen in patients with AIDS.

4. **Helminthiasis** may now affect as many as 1 billion people each year, and its incidence is increasing with increased agricultural use of land and increased travel. With the advent of several new, highly selective anthelmintic drugs, older agents used to treat parasitic worm infections have become obsolete.

5. **Protozoal infections,** such as amebiasis and various trypanosomal infections, are treated by a wide variety of agents. Metronidazole is directly trichomonacidal and also is the agent of choice for several other protozoal infections.

6. **Viral infections** are difficult to treat because viruses are intracellular parasites, requiring the active participation of a host cell's metabolic processes, and few pharmacologic agents are selective enough to kill a virus without injuring the involved host cell.

C. **General principles of anti-infective therapy**

1. Selection of an appropriate anti-infective agent
   a. Identification of the infecting organism should precede antimicrobial therapy when possible.
   (1) The patient's condition may require **empiric therapy** before the infecting organism is known.
   (2) In this case, **"umbrella" therapy** is often used. A broad-spectrum antimicrobial agent or a combination of agents is chosen that will be effective against the likeliest causative pathogens.
   b. The **organism's susceptibility to antimicrobial agents** should be determined, if a suitable test exists.
   c. Factors that influence the choice of an anti-infective agent or its dosage include:
   (1) The patient's **age**
   (2) The patient's **renal and hepatic function**
   (3) The patient's **pregnancy status**
   (4) The **site of infection**

2. Route of administration
   a. Oral administration is used for mild infections.
   (1) It is especially useful for outpatient therapy.
   (2) Timing of administration is important if food impairs absorption.
   b. Parenteral administration is used for serious infections, especially when high serum levels are required.
   c. Intrathecal administration is used for meningeal infections when the appropriate agent does not cross the blood–brain barrier.

3. Antimicrobial combination therapy
   a. Applications. Therapy with two or more antimicrobial agents has several purposes:
   (1) To **provide broad coverage** (e.g., when infections are due to more than one organism)
   (2) For **initial (blind) therapy** when the patient is seriously ill and results of cultures are pending
   (3) To **provide synergism** when organisms are not effectively eradicated with a single agent alone; for example, in enterococcal endocarditis, both penicillin and an aminoglycoside are given because their combined effect is greater than the sum of their independent activities
   (4) To **prevent the emergence of resistance,** as in the treatment of tuberculosis
   b. Inappropriate use of combinations could result in:
   (1) Antagonism between the antimicrobial agents
   (2) An increase in the number or severity of adverse reactions
   (3) Increased cost

4. Drug resistance. The emergence of bacteria that are resistant to several drugs is the major cause of failure in the treatment of infectious diseases (Table 12-1).

II. **AGENTS USED FOR TREATMENT OF BACTERIAL INFECTIONS**

A. **Sulfonamides**

1. Chemistry. The sulfonamides are derivatives of **sulfanilamide** (Figure 12-1).

2. Mechanism of action. Sulfonamides are **bacteriostatic**.
   a. Sulfonamides **prevent the incorporation of para-aminobenzoic acid (PABA) into folic acid,** which in the reduced form is necessary in purine biosynthesis for the transfer of one-carbon units.

TABLE 12-1. Mechanisms of Resistance to Antimicrobial Agents

Mechanism of Resistance	Antimicrobial Agent
Reduced uptake by microorganism	Chloramphenicol
Active transport out of microorganism	Tetracycline
Modification of receptor, leading to inability or reduced ability of the agent to bind to the receptor	Beta-lactams, erythromycin, lincomycin
Hydrolysis of agent via enzymes produced by microorganism	Beta-lactams, erythromycin
Production of altered enzymes that are less affected by agent	Sulfonamides
Sequestration of agent by protein binding	Beta-lactams, fusidic acid
Development of alternate metabolic pathway that renders reaction inhibited by the drug obsolete	Sulfonamides, trimethoprim
Binding of specific immunity protein to agent	Bleomycin
Overproduction of the target (titration)	Trimethoprim

Modified with permission from Davies J: Inactivation of antibiotics and the dissemination of resistance genes. *Science* 264:375, 1994.

   b. Susceptible bacteria are those that need PABA because they are incapable of using folic acid directly.
   c. Human cells use exogenous folic acid exclusively, and thus, a lack of PABA does not affect them.

3. Pharmacokinetics
   a. Sulfonamides are absorbed within minutes following oral administration.
   b. They diffuse readily into cerebrospinal fluid.
   c. They are metabolized by acetylation of the para-NH_2, which negates the antibacterial activity but not the adverse effects.
   d. Excretion is chiefly via the urine within 24 hours of administration. The urinary solubility of the various sulfonamides varies widely.

4. Pharmacologic effects
   a. Sulfonamides are effective against many gram-positive bacteria, including group A *Streptococcus pyogenes* and *Streptococcus pneumoniae*.
   b. Many gram-negative bacteria are resistant to sulfonamides, but some, such as *Haemophilus influenzae, Escherichia coli* (the organism most often suspect in acute urinary tract infections), *Shigella, Yersinia enterocolitica,* and *Proteus mirabilis,* often are sensitive.
   c. Other susceptible organisms include *Bacillus anthracis, Nocardia, Actinomyces,* and *Chlamydia trachomatis,* the agent responsible for trachoma, lymphogranuloma venereum, and inclusion conjunctivitis.

5. Therapeutic uses
   a. Sulfonamides are the preferred agents for treatment of:
      (1) Acute uncomplicated urinary tract infections
      (2) Nocardiosis

H_2N

SO_2NH_2

FIGURE 12-1. Sulfanilamide.

b. They are effective for treatment of toxoplasmosis when used in combination with pyrimethamine.

c. They are used in trachoma and inclusion conjunctivitis as an alternative to tetracycline.

d. Aside from acute urinary tract infections, the use of sulfonamides alone in many infections has been replaced by more effective and safer drugs.

6. Preparations. Commonly used sulfonamides include:

  a. Trimethoprim–sulfamethoxazole

   (1) Sulfamethoxazole and trimethoprim inhibit two separate steps in folate metabolism.

    (a) Trimethoprim is a highly selective inhibitor of the dihydrofolate reductase of lower organisms.

    (b) In combination, the two drugs act synergistically.

   (2) Trimethoprim–sulfamethoxazole is useful for treating *Pneumocystis carinii* pneumonia, an opportunistic infection seen in patients with AIDS (see X C).

  b. Sulfisoxazole

  c. Sulfadiazine

   (1) Sulfadiazine is now used less often for urinary tract infections.

   (2) It is useful for treating nocardiosis.

7. Adverse effects

  a. Approximately 75% of untoward effects involve the skin, with sensitization often being responsible. Conditions produced include:

   (1) Exfoliative dermatitis

   (2) Stevens-Johnson syndrome (fever, malaise, erythema multiforme)

  b. Drug fever can occur and probably results from sensitization.

  c. Blood dyscrasias are rare but can occur. Sulfonamide therapy is stopped immediately if any hematologic conditions develop to a serious extent. **Acute hemolytic anemia,** which is often, but not solely, the result of an erythrocytic deficiency of glucose-6-phosphate dehydrogenase activity, is particularly likely to develop in blacks and children.

  d. Eosinophilia may accompany other manifestations of hypersensitivity.

  e. Crystalluria is a condition that was seen with the older sulfonamides but rarely occurs with the newer, more soluble agents such as sulfisoxazole, although some renal damage is still possible.

  f. Kernicterus can occur in the newborn because of displacement of bilirubin from plasma albumin.

B. | **Beta-lactam antibiotics** (Figure 12-2)

1. Overview

  a. Chemistry. A **beta-lactam ring** is a four-membered ring in which an amide linkage joins a carbonyl group and a nitrogen. This ring is the **key structural feature** of the beta-lactam antibiotics.

  b. Mechanism of action. The beta-lactam antibiotics are **bactericidal**.

   (1) The beta-lactam antibiotics **inhibit key enzymes in bacterial cell wall synthesis**.

   (2) They also appear to activate one or more cell-wall autolytic enzymes, causing lysis of the bacterium.

  c. Bacterial resistance

   (1) Beta-lactamases, enzymes produced by many different bacteria, hydrolyze the beta-lactam ring, inactivating the antibiotic. **Penicillinase** (see II B 2 c) and **cephalosporinase** are beta-lactamases with narrow substrate specificities.

    (a) Initially sensitive bacterial strains can become permanently resistant to a particular antibiotic by acquiring plasmids or R (resistance) factors carrying the genetic code for a beta-lactamase.

    (b) The penicillins and the other beta-lactam antibiotics differ in their sensitivity to the beta-lactamases.

   (2) Beta-lactamase inhibitors are substances that can irreversibly bind and, thus, inactivate bacterial beta-lactamases (see Figure 12-2).

Figure 12-2. Overview of the beta-lactam antibiotics, which act by inhibiting cell wall synthesis. Beta-lactamase inhibitors are also shown. Beta-lactamases are enzymes produced by many bacteria that render beta-lactam antibiotics ineffective.

FIGURE 12-3. Structure of the penicillins. R = side chain; *1* = thiazolidine ring; *2* = beta-lactam ring.

2. **Penicillins** (see Figure 12-2)
   a. **Chemistry**
      (1) The structure of the penicillins (Figure 12-3) consists of a thiazolidine ring connected to a beta-lactam ring, which is attached to a side chain.
      (2) All penicillins are derived from 6-aminopenicillanic acid.
      (3) The various penicillins differ in their side chain structure.
   b. **Mechanism of action**
      (1) Penicillins inhibit the synthesis of bacterial cell walls and are considered **bactericidal**.
      (2) They combine with and inactivate transpeptidase, which normally is responsible for cross-linking the linear glycopeptide strands of bacterial cell walls. Loss of cell wall rigidity in the presence of normal high intracellular osmotic pressure causes lysis of the bacterial membrane.
   c. **Bacterial resistance** (see II B 1 c)
      (1) **Penicillinase** is a beta-lactamase that is produced by a number of bacteria. It can hydrolyze the beta-lactam ring of penicillin to form penicilloic acid, a substance that has no antibacterial activity.
      (2) Microorganisms that are capable of producing penicillinase include:
         (a) *Staphylococcus aureus*
         (b) *Bacillus* species
         (c) *Bacteroides* species
         (d) *E. coli*
         (e) *Proteus* species
         (f) *Pseudomonas aeruginosa*
         (g) *Mycobacterium tuberculosis*
   d. **Pharmacokinetics of penicillins G and V**
      (1) **Absorption**
         (a) **Oral administration**
            (i) Because gastric acid inactivates **penicillin G,** only 30% of an oral dose is absorbed from the duodenum. **Penicillin V** is more stable in an acidic environment; an equivalent oral dose leads to plasma levels two to five times higher than those obtained with penicillin G.
            (ii) Because food interferes with absorption, penicillin G or V should be administered at least 1 hour before meals and at least 2–3 hours after meals.
            (iii) Peak plasma concentrations occur 30–60 minutes after administration.
         (b) **Subcutaneous or intramuscular administration**
            (i) Following injection of crystalline penicillin G, peak plasma concentrations occur in 15 minutes, then rapidly decline.
            (ii) The simultaneous administration of **probenecid** prolongs the duration of penicillin in the body because probenecid blocks the transport of penicillin in the proximal tubule. **Repository penicillin preparations** [see II B 2 g (1) (b)] provide an alternative means for maintaining high plasma levels of penicillin.
      (2) **Distribution**
         (a) Penicillins G and V are distributed widely throughout the body with approximately 60% reversibly bound to plasma albumin.

(b) They penetrate poorly into ocular, pericardial, and cerebrospinal fluids.

(c) Significant amounts of the drug appear in the liver, intestine, and kidney, as well as in bile, semen, and lymph.

(3) Excretion

    (a) From 60%–90% of an intramuscular dose of penicillin G is excreted within 1 hour.

    (b) Up to 99% of the dose is eliminated via the kidney; that is, about 90% by tubular secretion and 10% by glomerular filtration.

e. Pharmacologic effects and therapeutic uses. The various types of penicillin differ in their spectrum of activity and in their degree of efficacy against particular species or strains. In general, microbial sensitivity should be verified whenever possible.

(1) Penicillins G and V

    (a) Gram-positive coccal (streptococcal, staphylococcal) infections (Table 12-2)

    (b) Gram-negative coccal (meningococcal, gonococcal) infections

        (i) For **gonococcal infections,** ceftriaxone is considered the drug of first choice because strains have become increasingly resistant to penicillin G.

        (ii) In **penicillin-resistant strains,** procaine penicillin G, ampicillin, or amoxicillin is used, usually given with probenecid [see II B 2 d (1) (b) (ii)].

    (c) Syphilis. Penicillin G is the most effective treatment for all stages of syphilis, because *Treponema pallidum* is very sensitive to penicillin G.

    (d) Other microbial infections responding to penicillin G

        (i) Penicillin G is active against many oral anaerobes and is still widely used for **oral, dental, pulmonary,** and **soft tissue infections caused by organisms normally found in the oral flora.**

        (ii) Penicillin G is also the drug of first choice in **gas gangrene** (usually due to *Clostridium*). However, subdiaphragmatic anaerobic infections (e.g., resulting from *Bacteroides fragilis*) are generally resistant to penicillins with the exception of the "antipseudomonas" penicillins [see Figure 12-2 and II B 2 e (3)].

TABLE 12-2. Use of Penicillins G and V in the Treatment of Gram-positive Coccal Infections

Type of Infection	Causative Agent	Therapy
Streptococcal infections		
Pneumococcal infections	*Streptococcus pneumoniae*	
Pneumococcal pneumonia		Penicillin G or V
Pneumococcal meningitis		Penicillin G intravenously*
Suppurative arthritis		Penicillin G
Mastoiditis		Penicillin G
Endocarditis		Penicillin G
Osteomyelitis		Penicillin G
Other infections	Group A, *S. pyogenes*	
Streptococcal pharyngitis, scarlet fever		Penicillin V orally
Otitis media		Penicillin V
Endocarditis		Penicillin G[†]
Arthritis		Penicillin G
Meningitis		Penicillin G
Staphylococcal infections	*Staphylococcus aureus*	Penicillin G[‡]

*For pneumococcal meningitis, intrathecal administration is sometimes used, but arachnoiditis and encephalopathy can complicate this form of therapy.
[†]α-Hemolytic streptococci often are the cause of subacute endocarditis and, in this case, occasionally are resistant to penicillins G and V, necessitating the use of a semisynthetic penicillin such as nafcillin.
[‡]Approximately 20% of strains of *S. aureus* are resistant because of penicillinase activity; the penicillinase-resistant penicillins oxacillin, cloxacillin, dicloxacillin, methicillin, and nafcillin are highly effective against these strains.

    (iii) Most strains of *Corynebacterium diphtheriae* are sensitive to penicillin G, which is used in diphtheria to eliminate the acute and chronic carrier states. Specific antitoxin is used for treatment of diphtheria.

    (iv) Penicillin G is also the drug of first choice in **anthrax** (the majority of *B. anthracis* strains are sensitive), **actinomycosis,** and *Listeria* infections.

(2) Broad-spectrum penicillins are effective against gram-positive organisms, some strains of *E. coli, H. influenzae, Salmonella,* and *Shigella,* and some *Proteus* species. When strains are sensitive, ampicillin and amoxicillin are used to treat:

    (a) Some forms of gonorrhea

    (b) Sinusitis and otitis media resulting from *H. influenzae,* pneumococci, or *S. pyogenes*

    (c) Urinary tract infections resulting from *E. coli* or *P. mirabilis*

    (d) Meningitis resulting from *H. influenzae,* meningococci, or pneumococci

(3) "Antipseudomonas" penicillins are chiefly used to treat serious infections (bacteremia, pneumonia, burn infections) resulting from gram-negative organisms, particularly *P. aeruginosa,* indole-positive *Proteus,* and *Enterobacter.*

    (a) Carbenicillin and **ticarcillin** have a spectrum of activity similar to that of ampicillin and, in addition, are effective against indole-positive *Proteus* and *Pseudomonas.*

    (b) Azlocillin, mezlocillin, and **piperacillin** are known collectively as the **ureidopenicillins**.

        (i) Azlocillin and piperacillin are active against *Pseudomonas* organisms.

        (ii) Mezlocillin and piperacillin are active against *Klebsiella.*

    (c) When a *Pseudomonas* infection is life-threatening, an antipseudomonas penicillin is often used in combination with gentamicin, amikacin, or tobramycin.

(4) Combinations of a penicillin and a beta-lactamase inhibitor

    (a) Clavulanic acid is a beta-lactamase inhibitor that is structurally related to the penicillins.

        (i) Clavulanic acid extends the antibacterial spectrum of beta-lactam antibiotics by irreversibly binding and, thus, inhibiting many bacterial beta-lactamases.

        (ii) The combination of **amoxicillin and clavulanate** is used to treat infections caused by beta-lactamase–producing strains of *H. influenzae, B. catarrhalis, S. aureus, E. coli, Klebsiella,* and *Enterobacter.*

    (b) Sulbactam is a penicillanic acid sulfone with limited antibacterial activity. Its principal action is to inactivate bacterial beta-lactamases, thereby enhancing the antibacterial spectrum of ampicillin. The combination of **ampicillin and sulbactam** has been useful in treating intra-abdominal and gynecologic infections.

f. Prophylactic uses. Penicillins G and V have been shown to be effective prophylactically in the following conditions:

(1) Streptococcal infections

(2) Rheumatic fever recurrences

(3) Gonorrheal ophthalmia in neonates for which conjunctival instillation of penicillin G solution is effective

(4) Surgical procedures in patients who have valvular heart disease

    (a) When undergoing dental extractions, tonsillectomy, or genitourinary or intestinal operations, such patients often receive penicillin prophylactically.

    (b) Bacteremia is not totally prevented by using prophylactic penicillin.

g. Preparations and administration

(1) Penicillins G and V

    (a) Soluble forms

        (i) Penicillin G (benzylpenicillin) sodium and potassium salts are used intramuscularly, intravenously, and orally.

        (ii) Penicillin V (phenoxymethyl penicillin) is a soluble form that is resistant to acid; it is used orally.

(b) Repository forms are insoluble salts that allow the slow absorption of penicillin from the site of injection, providing a duration of action lasting 12–24 hours. These forms are used intramuscularly only and include:

  (i) Procaine penicillin G

  (ii) Benzathine penicillin G (This drug has a low solubility, and effective blood levels often are present for a week.)

(2) Penicillinase-resistant penicillins

  (a) Methicillin

    (i) This drug has one-twentieth the potency of penicillin G.

    (ii) It is not administered orally because of poor absorption via this route.

  (b) Oxacillin

    (i) This drug is acid-stable and, therefore, can be given orally as well as intravenously and intramuscularly.

    (ii) It is highly protein-bound in the plasma.

    (iii) It is up to eight times as potent as methicillin.

  (c) Cloxacillin has pharmacologic and pharmacokinetic properties that are similar to those of oxacillin.

  (d) Nafcillin can be given orally, intravenously, or intramuscularly.

  (e) Dicloxacillin, because it is highly resistant to penicillinase and acid hydrolysis, is very effective when administered orally.

(3) Broad-spectrum penicillins

  (a) Ampicillin is given orally, intravenously, or intramuscularly. It is acid-stable but not penicillinase-resistant.

  (b) Amoxicillin is given orally only.

    (i) It attains higher blood levels than ampicillin.

    (ii) It is thought to cause a lower incidence of diarrhea than ampicillin.

(4) Antipseudomonas penicillins

  (a) Azlocillin is given intravenously.

  (b) Carbenicillin, ticarcillin, mezlocillin, and **piperacillin** are given intravenously or intramuscularly.

  (c) Carbenicillin indanyl is acid-stable and is administered orally.

(5) Combinations of penicillin and a beta-lactamase inhibitor

  (a) Amoxicillin with clavulanate is given orally.

  (b) Ticarcillin with clavulanate is given intravenously.

  (c) Ampicillin with sulbactam is given intravenously or intramuscularly.

h. Adverse effects

(1) Hypersensitivity reactions to the penicillins occur in 5%–20% of patients receiving these drugs, and all forms of penicillin can cause hypersensitivity reactions. A reaction can occur in the absence of prior therapeutic penicillin administration.

  (a) The reaction can range from a mild rash to life-threatening anaphylaxis and may persist 1–2 weeks after discontinuation of therapy. Hypersensitivity reactions include:

    (i) Skin rashes of all types. In severe cases, the Stevens-Johnson syndrome can occur. The highest incidence of skin rash (about 9%) occurs after ampicillin administration. Skin tests using benzylpenicilloyl polylysine or minor determinant mixture can be used to identify penicillin-allergic individuals.

    (ii) Fever, which disappears within 36 hours after termination of administration

    (iii) Eosinophilia

    (iv) Angioedema

    (v) Serum sickness

    (vi) Anaphylactic reactions. One in 50,000 patients treated with penicillin dies from an anaphylactic reaction, which is most common after parenteral administration, but can occur after oral ingestion and with minute quantities of penicillin.

    (b) Recurrent reactions and cross-sensitivity
        (i) A hypersensitivity reaction to one form of penicillin places the affected patient at high risk of reaction to that form or to any other penicillin.
        (ii) The risk of cross-reactions with other beta-lactams is less clear. Penicillin-allergic individuals occasionally have allergic reactions to cephalosporins.
        (iii) In penicillin-allergic patients, serious infections resulting from gram-positive organisms are often treated with vancomycin. Alternatives for other infections include erythromycin, trimethoprim–sulfamethoxazole, aminoglycosides, and ciprofloxacin.
  (2) Other adverse effects
    (a) Gastrointestinal upset is more likely with orally administered preparations; an example is ampicillin-associated diarrhea.
    (b) Nephrotoxicity is very rare and usually occurs only in patients with compromised renal function.
    (c) Superinfection results from alterations in intestinal flora.
        (i) A low incidence occurs with penicillin G administration.
        (ii) A higher incidence occurs with broad-spectrum penicillins, such as ampicillin and carbenicillin.

3. Cephalosporins. The cephalosporins are typically classified by "generations" (see Figure 12-2), which roughly parallel their chronologic development and their antimicrobial spectrum.
  a. Chemistry
    (1) The cephalosporins (Figure 12-4) are derivatives of 7-aminocephalosporanic acid and are closely related in structure to penicillin.
    (2) They have a six-membered sulfur-containing ring adjoining a beta-lactam ring.
    (3) They are relatively stable in dilute acid.
  b. Mechanism of action. Cephalosporins, like the penicillins, inhibit bacterial cell wall synthesis and are considered **bactericidal**.
  c. Bacterial resistance
    (1) The cephalosporins are highly resistant to penicillinase.
    (2) Some bacteria elaborate a beta-lactamase called **cephalosporinase** that acts on the cephalosporin nucleus to destroy its antibacterial activity. However, many cephalosporins are resistant to the enzyme.
  d. Pharmacokinetics
    (1) Most cephalosporins are administered parenterally; some, however, are well absorbed from the gastrointestinal tract and can be given orally.
    (2) The cephalosporins become widely distributed throughout body tissues and fluids. The majority do not penetrate the blood–brain barrier and, thus, are not effective in the treatment of central nervous system (CNS) infections.
    (3) The half-life and the degree of serum protein binding vary widely from agent to agent.
    (4) Although some cephalosporins are excreted via the bile, most are excreted in the urine via renal tubular secretion. **Probenecid** blocks the tubular secretion of cephalosporins, often resulting in an increased half-life and elevated plasma concentration.

FIGURE 12-4. Structure of the cephalosporins. 1 = sulfur-containing ring; 2 = beta-lactam ring; R_1, R_2 = variable side chains.

e. Pharmacologic effects. All cephalosporins are active against most gram-positive cocci, including penicillinase-producing staphylococci and many strains of gram-negative bacilli. The cephalosporins are in general ineffective against enterococci.

f. Therapeutic uses (Table 12-3)

   (1) Diseases produced by *S. aureus,* both penicillin-sensitive and penicillin-resistant, including skin infections, osteomyelitis, and endocarditis, respond favorably to the cephalosporins.

   (2) Cephalosporins are the drugs of first choice for *Klebsiella pneumoniae* infections.

   (3) These drugs are used successfully in the treatment of pneumococcal pneumonia and in infections caused by *S. pyogenes.*

   (4) Some of the parenteral cephalosporins are efficacious in the treatment of gonococcal disease that is resistant to other agents.

   (5) Diseases caused by a number of gram-negative bacteria, including respiratory and urinary tract infections, respond well.

   (6) The expanded-spectrum activity of the cephalosporins includes effectiveness against *Proteus, B. fragilis, Serratia, Enterobacter,* and some activity against *Pseudomonas.* These agents are effective for the treatment of meningitis caused by susceptible strains.

g. Prophylactic cephalosporin therapy plays an important role in reducing perioperative infection.

h. Preparations and administration (see Table 12-3)

i. Adverse effects

   (1) Hypersensitivity reactions occur in approximately 5% of patients receiving cephalosporin therapy.

   (a) Cephalosporins, like penicillins, elicit a spectrum of reactions that range from mild skin rash to anaphylaxis.

   (b) A **cross-sensitivity reaction** to the cephalosporins occasionally occurs in individuals who are allergic to penicillin.

   (c) Patients receiving large doses of cephalosporin often have a positive direct Coombs' reaction.

   (2) Renal damage, although rare with normal doses of cephalosporins, can occur.

   (3) Local tissue reactions can occur with parenteral administration. Intravenous administration can cause thrombophlebitis.

   (4) Superinfections caused by gram-negative bacteria or yeasts can occur following administration of the cephalosporins.

4. Imipenem is a beta-lactam antibiotic derived from thienamycin. Like other beta-lactam antibiotics, it acts by interfering with the synthesis of the bacterial cell and is **bactericidal**.

a. Pharmacokinetics

   (1) Imipenem is given in combination with **cilastatin,** a dipeptidase inhibitor that inhibits the renal tubular metabolism of imipenem and prevents the formation of potentially nephrotoxic compounds.

   (2) The serum elimination half-life of both imipenem and cilastatin is 1 hour.

   (3) Imipenem is filtered and secreted by the kidney, and if given alone, it is inactivated by a dipeptidase enzyme in the kidney, which opens the beta-lactam ring.

b. Pharmacologic effects. Imipenem has the broadest antimicrobial spectrum of all the beta-lactam antibiotics.

   (1) It is active against both gram-positive and gram-negative cocci (except methicillin-resistant staphylococci), Enterobacteriaceae, *P. aeruginosa,* and anaerobic bacteria, including *B. fragilis.*

   (2) Gonococci and *H. influenzae* strains that are resistant to both penicillin and ampicillin are susceptible to imipenem.

c. Therapeutic uses

   (1) Use of imipenem is limited to the treatment of serious hospital-acquired infections resulting from susceptible organisms. It is given intravenously.

   (a) It is used in urinary tract, respiratory tract, skin, and soft tissue infections.

TABLE 12-3. Properties of Cephalosporins

Drug	Spectrum of Activity	Route of Administration	Half-life	Route of Excretion
First generation	Most gram-positive and some gram-negative organisms; *Klebsiella; Escherichia coli*; penicillin- and sulfonamide-resistant urinary tract infections; surgical prophylaxis			
Cephalothin		IV; IM is painful	0.5–0.9 hour	Renal tubular secretion
Cefazolin		IV; IM	1.4–2.2 hours	Primarily renal glomerular filtration; secondarily, renal tubular secretion and biliary secretion
Cephalexin, cefadroxil		Oral (capsules, suspensions, pediatric drops)	0.9–1.3 hours	> 90% excreted unchanged in urine, also excreted into bile
Second generation				
Cefamandole	Indole-positive *Proteus;* beta-lactamase–producing *Haemophilus influenzae*	IV only	1 hour	Renal
Cefoxitin	Indole-positive *Proteus; Bacteroides fragilis;* less effective against gram-positive organisms	IV	0.8 hour	Renal
Cefaclor	Similar to cephalexin; also effective against beta-lactamase–producing *H. influenzae*	Oral	1.5 hours	Secondary hepatic elimination
Cefonicid	Similar to cefamandole	IV	4 hours	Renal
Cefuroxime	Serious *H. influenzae* infections, particular respiratory tract infections and otitis media	IV; oral	1.5–2.2 hours	Renal
Cefotetan	In-vitro spectrum similar to cefoxitin; less active against some anaerobes	IV	2.8–4.6 hours	Renal

Drug	Description	Route	Half-life	Elimination
Cefprozil	Alternative to cefaclor and cefuroxime in the treatment of otitis media and bronchitis	Oral	1.3 hours	Renal
Third generation				
Cefotaxime	Highly resistant to beta-lactamases; effective against many gram-positive and gram-negative bacteria	IV	1.5 hours	Secondary hepatic elimination
Ceftizoxime	In-vitro spectrum similar to cefotaxime	IV	1.7 hours	Not metabolized; excreted in urine
Ceftriaxone	Particularly effective against penicillinase-producing strains of *Neisseria gonorrhoeae*	IV; IM	8 hours	Renal
Cefoperazone	*Pseudomonas aeruginosa*	IV	1.6–2.4 hours	Hepatic
Ceftazidime	*P. aeruginosa*	IV; IM	1.8 hours	Renal
Cefixime	Beta-lactamase–producing strains of *H. influenzae*	Oral	3–4 hours	Renal
Cefpodoxime	Similar to cefixime	Oral	2.5 hours	Renal

IM = intramuscular; IV = intravenous.

    (b) It is effective for the treatment of osteomyelitis, septic arthritis, bacteremia, and gynecologic and intra-abdominal infections.

   (2) Its usefulness in staphylococcal endocarditis has been established, but not in CNS infections.

  d. Adverse effects

   (1) *P. aeruginosa* may become resistant during imipenem therapy.

   (2) Allergic reactions may occur, as with other beta-lactam antibiotics. Patients allergic to penicillin should be considered allergic to imipenem.

   (3) Nausea, vomiting, and diarrhea have occurred.

 5. Aztreonam

  a. Chemistry. Aztreonam, a monobactam, differs from penicillins and cephalosporins in having a monocyclic rather than a bicyclic beta-lactam nucleus.

  b. Mechanism of action. Like other beta-lactams, aztreonam interferes with the synthesis of the bacterial cell wall; however, its action results from a high affinity for bacterial penicillin-binding protein 3.

  c. Pharmacokinetics

   (1) The bioavailability of an intramuscular dose is 100%.

   (2) The serum elimination half-life is 1.7 hours.

   (3) Two-thirds of a dose appears in the urine within 24 hours.

  d. Pharmacologic effects

   (1) Aztreonam is highly resistant to beta-lactamases.

   (2) It is highly active against aerobic gram-negative bacteria, including *P. aeruginosa* and penicillinase-producing strains of *H. influenzae* and gonococci.

   (3) It shows poor activity against gram-positive cocci and anaerobic bacteria.

  e. Therapeutic uses

   (1) Aztreonam has been substituted for aminoglycosides in the treatment of urinary tract, lower respiratory tract, and skin and soft tissue infections. Additionally, osteomyelitis, gonorrhea, and gynecologic and intra-abdominal infections resulting from susceptible pathogens have been successfully treated.

   (2) Because of its narrow spectrum, aztreonam is often used in combination with another antimicrobial agent.

   (3) Aztreonam is administered parenterally.

  f. Adverse effects

   (1) Colonization and superinfection with gram-positive cocci can occur.

   (2) Pseudomembranous colitis has been reported.

   (3) Aztreonam shows little or no immunologic cross-reactivity with other beta-lactams.

 6. Loracarbef

  a. Chemistry. Loracarbef is a beta-lactam and chemically identical to cefaclor; it is classified as a carbacephem rather than a cephalosporin because a methylene group replaces the sulfur atom, forming a tetrahydropyridine ring.

  b. Mechanism of action. Like other beta-lactams, loracarbef interferes with the synthesis of the bacterial cell wall.

  c. Pharmacokinetics. Loracarbef is well absorbed from the gastrointestinal tract, is excreted unchanged in the urine, and has a half-life of approximately one hour.

  d. Pharmacologic effects. Loracarbef's antibacterial activity is similar to that of cefaclor, cefprozil, and cefuroxime.

  e. Therapeutic uses. Loracarbef can be used for the treatment of respiratory, urinary tract, and skin infections.

  f. Adverse effects. Loracarbef is comparable in tolerability to similar spectrum antimicrobials.

C. **Aminoglycosides** (Figure 12-5)

 1. Chemistry

  a. The aminoglycosides are compounds containing characteristic amino sugars joined to a hexose nucleus in glycosidic linkage.

INHIBITORS OF PROTEIN SYNTHESIS

AMINOGLYCOSIDES
- Streptomycin
- Neomycin
- Gentamicin
- Tobramycin
- Amikacin
- Netilmicin
- Kanamycin

TETRACYCLINES
- Tetracycline
- Demeclocycline
- Methacycline
- Minocycline
- Doxycycline
- Chlortetracycline
- Oxytetracycline

MACROLIDES
- Erythromycin
- Clarithromycin
- Azithromycin

• Chloramphenicol • Clindamycin

FIGURE 12-5. Overview of the aminoglycosides, which work by inhibiting protein synthesis.

    b. They are polycations, and their polarity accounts for their pharmacokinetic properties.

2. Mechanism of action
    a. The aminoglycosides **inhibit protein biosynthesis by acting directly on the ribosome**.
        (1) They interfere with the proper attachment of messenger RNA to ribosomes in the initiation of protein synthesis.
        (2) They also cause misreading of the genetic code and, hence, cause decreased or abnormal protein synthesis.
    b. The aminoglycosides also appear to **disrupt the bacterial cytoplasmic membrane**.
    c. The rapid **bactericidal** effect of the aminoglycosides is not, however, adequately explained by any of their known actions.

3. Pharmacokinetics
    a. All of the aminoglycosides are poorly absorbed after oral administration because of their polycationic structure.
    b. They are absorbed rapidly after intramuscular or subcutaneous administration.
        (1) They are distributed in all extracellular fluids, but tissue concentrations are low except in the kidney and ear.
        (2) They cross the blood–brain barrier only if the meninges are inflamed.
        (3) They are excreted by glomerular filtration.
    c. All the aminoglycosides are more active in an alkaline environment.

4. Microbial resistance can result from several bacterial enzymes that inactivate the aminoglycoside molecule.
    a. Plasmids and R (resistance) factors have spread the genetic codes for these enzymes, so that many initially sensitive microbes have become resistant to the aminoglycosides.
    b. Synergism between beta-lactam antibiotics and aminoglycosides against enterococci can also be lost by this mechanism.
    c. Cross-resistance between the aminoglycosides can occur.
    d. Amikacin and netilmicin are not affected by most aminoglycoside-inactivating enzymes that cause bacterial resistance in some species.

5. Pharmacologic effects (Table 12-4). Anaerobic microorganisms are generally resistant to the aminoglycosides.

6. Therapeutic uses (see Table 12-4)
    a. Streptomycin. Because of the frequent development of bacterial resistance (see II C 4), streptomycin is used alone to treat only two infections—tularemia and plague.
    b. Gentamicin, tobramycin, amikacin, and netilmicin
        (1) Many infections can be treated successfully with these agents, but their toxicity restricts their use to situations involving life-threatening infections caused by:
            (a) *P. aeruginosa*, *Serratia*, *Enterobacter*, and *Klebsiella*
            (b) Methicillin-resistant staphylococci that are sensitive to gentamicin

TABLE 12-4. Aminoglycosides

Drug	Spectrum of Activity
Streptomycin*	Alone: Organisms that cause plague (*Yersinia pestis*), tularemia (*Francisella tularensis*) With penicillin G: Subacute bacterial endocarditis caused by *Streptococcus viridans*, gram-positive enterococci
	With tetracycline: Severe cases of brucellosis
	Used with other agents to treat severe forms of *Mycobacterium tuberculosis*
Neomycin	Many gram-negative organisms Many gram-positive organisms (e.g., *S. aureus*) Some activity against *M. tuberculosis*
Gentamicin	Many gram-negative organisms, including indole-positive *Proteus, Pseudomonas aeruginosa, Enterobacter, Klebsiella,* and *Serratia* Some strains of *Staphylococcus*
Tobramycin	Similar to gentamicin; may be slightly more effective against *Pseudomonas*
Amikacin	Similar to gentamicin; effective against certain gentamicin-resistant pathogens Some activity against *M. tuberculosis*
Netilmicin	Similar to gentamicin; effective against certain gentamicin-resistant pathogens
Kanamycin	More limited than gentamicin; effective against some gram-negative organisms (with the exception of *Pseudomonas*) Some activity against *M. tuberculosis*

*High concentrations of streptomycin are bactericidal; low concentrations are bacteriostatic.

      (2) These agents are sometimes used as part of an initial "blind therapy" for serious infections of unknown etiology, in which case a penicillinase-resistant penicillin or a cephalosporin is administered in combination with an aminoglycoside.
   c. Neomycin, because of its serious toxic effects when absorbed systemically, is used most frequently in dermatologic and ophthalmic ointments. In addition, neomycin can be used orally as a bowel preparation for surgery or for the management of hepatic coma.

  7. Preparations and administration. All of the aminoglycosides have a narrow therapeutic index that limits their parenteral usage.
   a. Streptomycin
      (1) Intramuscular injection is the most common route of administration.
      (2) To avoid the development of bacterial resistance, streptomycin therapy rarely is extended beyond 10 days (except in tuberculosis and subacute bacterial endocarditis).
   b. Gentamicin
      (1) This drug can be administered intramuscularly, intravenously, or as an ointment or cream.
      (2) When renal function is impaired, peak and trough serum concentrations of gentamicin are measured intermittently to allow optimal guidance for adjusting dosage, and renal function is monitored by means of the serum creatinine level.
   c. Tobramycin, amikacin, and **netilmicin** can be given intramuscularly or intravenously.
   d. Neomycin
      (1) This drug is available in the form of creams, ointments, and sprays, both alone and in combination with polymyxin, bacitracin, other antibiotics, and corticosteroids.
      (2) It is also available for oral and parenteral administration, although it is rarely used parenterally.

  8. Adverse effects
   a. Ototoxicity and nephrotoxicity are the most serious side effects.
      (1) Ototoxicity. Both labyrinthine damage and vestibular disturbances can occur.
         (a) Permanent damage occurs in a small percentage of patients.

(b) The incidence is directly related to daily dose and duration of therapy. The high-frequency sound range is first to be affected.

(c) Ototoxicity occurs more commonly when renal failure is present.

(d) The simultaneous administration of ethacrynic acid or furosemide increases the risk of ototoxicity.

(2) Nephrotoxicity

(a) Gentamicin is the most nephrotoxic of the aminoglycosides. It can produce acute renal insufficiency and tubular necrosis.

(b) When renal failure of any degree is present, serum creatinine and aminoglycoside levels must be measured and drug dosage adjusted accordingly.

b. Neuromuscular junction blockade may result when an aminoglycoside is given at high doses and in combination with curariform drugs. This apparently results from a decreased sensitivity of the postjunctional membrane to acetylcholine and decreased presynaptic release of the transmitter.

c. Hypersensitivity reactions can occur. Up to 8% of patients develop a skin rash when neomycin is applied topically.

D. Tetracyclines (see Figure 12-5)

1. **Chemistry.** Tetracycline (Figure 12-6) and its congeners are derivatives of the polycyclic naphthacenecarboxamide.

2. **Mechanism of action.** Tetracyclines are primarily **bacteriostatic,** inhibiting protein synthesis by binding to 30S ribosomes.

3. **Pharmacokinetics**

a. Tetracyclines are adequately but incompletely absorbed from the gastrointestinal tract, particularly from the stomach and upper small intestine.

(1) **Absorption is impaired by food,** especially milk and milk products, by aluminum hydroxide gels, and by calcium and magnesium salts. The cations in these substances chelate with tetracycline, preventing gastrointestinal absorption.

(2) **Minocycline** and **doxycycline are exceptions** in that they chelate poorly with calcium, and food does not interfere with their absorption. However, like other tetracyclines, they do chelate with iron to form insoluble complexes.

b. The tetracyclines diffuse readily into body fluids and bind to plasma proteins to varying degrees, depending on the particular preparation. Concentrations in the cerebrospinal fluid are about 20% of serum levels unless the meninges are inflamed.

c. The tetracyclines are removed from the blood by the liver and are excreted into the intestine by way of the bile. They undergo enterohepatic circulation.

d. Excretion occurs primarily via the kidney, although there is some fecal excretion. Renal clearance of these drugs is by glomerular filtration.

4. **Bacterial resistance**

a. Gram-positive bacteria often become resistant to the tetracyclines, limiting the usefulness of these drugs.

b. Complete cross-resistance among the tetracycline preparations occurs.

FIGURE 12-6. Tetracycline.

5. Pharmacologic effects
   a. Tetracyclines are effective against many gram-positive and gram-negative bacteria.
   b. The tetracyclines are effective against *Mycoplasma, Borrelia, Chlamydia,* and rickettsial species.
   c. They are useful secondary drugs against *Leptospira* and *Treponema* species.
   d. In high concentrations, the tetracyclines inhibit the growth of the protozoan *Entamoeba histolytica.*

6. Therapeutic uses
   a. The use of tetracyclines for treatment of infectious disease has declined because of increasing bacterial resistance and the development of newer, more effective antimicrobial agents.
   b. Tetracyclines are used in the treatment of the following conditions.
      (1) Rickettsial infections. Tetracyclines are the drugs of first choice for these diseases, which include:
         (a) Rocky Mountain spotted fever
         (b) Brill's disease
         (c) Murine and scrub typhus
         (d) Rickettsialpox
         (e) Q fever
      (2) Chlamydial infections
         (a) Lymphogranuloma venereum
         (b) Psittacosis
         (c) Inclusion conjunctivitis
         (d) Trachoma
      (3) Mycoplasmal infections
      (4) Bacillary infections
         (a) Brucellosis
         (b) Tularemia
         (c) Cholera
         (d) Some *Shigella* and *Salmonella* infections
      (5) Venereal infections
         (a) Gonorrhea
         (b) Syphilis
         (c) Chancroid
         (d) Granuloma inguinale
         (e) Chlamydial urethritis or cervicitis
      (6) Amebic infections (amebiasis)
      (7) Spirochetal infections. Lyme disease, a multisystem inflammatory disorder, is caused by the spirochete *Borrelia burgdorferi,* which is transmitted by ticks. Oral tetracycline or doxycycline for 10–20 days shortens the duration of symptoms and often prevents the development of more serious sequelae.
   c. In urinary tract infections, the use of tetracyclines is limited because of the increasing number of resistant microorganisms.
   d. Tetracyclines may be beneficial in the treatment of acne.

7. Preparations and administration. Tetracyclines are available in formulations suitable for oral, intravenous, and intramuscular administration. They are also available for topical use, including ophthalmic solutions.
   a. Demeclocycline has a greater acid and alkaline stability and slower rate of excretion than most tetracyclines; therefore, it produces higher and more prolonged blood levels.
   b. Methacycline is absorbed rapidly.
   c. Minocycline absorption is not impaired by food or calcium ion.
   d. Doxycycline
      (1) Increased absorption of doxycycline allows once-daily administration after the first day.
      (2) As with minocycline, food and calcium ions do not affect absorption.

(3) As opposed to the other tetracyclines, 90% of this drug is excreted in the feces; therefore, it does not accumulate in the blood of patients with compromised renal function. Thus, it is one of the safest tetracyclines for use against extrarenal infections in patients with renal dysfunction.

8. **Adverse effects**
   a. **Hypersensitivity reactions,** including skin rash and drug fever, can occur. Cross-sensitivity among the various tetracyclines is common.
   b. When tetracyclines are administered orally, **gastrointestinal irritation** is common.
   c. The intravenous administration of tetracyclines often produces **thrombophlebitis** resulting from local irritation. Intramuscular injections are painful, cause local irritation, and result in poor absorption of the drugs.
   d. Demeclocycline, and less often the other tetracyclines, can produce a **phototoxic reaction,** resulting in severe skin lesions in patients exposed to sunlight.
   e. High doses of tetracyclines can produce **hepatic dysfunction**. This reaction is exacerbated during pregnancy.
   f. Children receiving tetracycline may develop yellow-brown **discoloration of the teeth** and suffer **depressed bone growth**.
      (1) The drugs are deposited in the teeth and bones, where they form a tetracycline–calcium orthophosphate complex because of their chelating properties.
      (2) The tooth discoloration is related to the total dose and the time of ingestion.
         (a) The risk of discoloration is greatest when tetracyclines are given to infants prior to their first dentition. Discoloration of the permanent teeth can result, however, from the administration of tetracycline at any time between the ages of 2 months and 7 years, the period of tooth calcification.
         (b) Tetracycline treatment during pregnancy can produce discoloration of the teeth in the offspring.
   g. The ingestion of outdated and degraded tetracycline can result in a form of the **Fanconi syndrome** (renal tubular dysfunction, which can lead to renal failure).
   h. **Vestibular toxicity** can occur following minocycline therapy.
   i. **Superinfection** by strains of resistant bacteria and yeasts is a significant problem that can result in staphylococcal enterocolitis, intestinal candidiasis, and pseudomembranous colitis.

E. | **Chloramphenicol**

1. **Chemistry.** Chloramphenicol (Figure 12-7) is a nitrobenzene derivative.

2. **Mechanism of action**
   a. Chloramphenicol inhibits protein synthesis by acting on the 50S ribosomal subunit, a site of action shared with macrolide antibiotics and clindamycin.
   b. This drug is primarily **bacteriostatic,** although it may be bactericidal to some strains.

NO_2

CHOH

CH — NH — C — $CHCl_2$

CH_2OH

FIGURE 12-7. Chloramphenicol.

3. Pharmacokinetics

a. Chloramphenicol is absorbed rapidly from the gastrointestinal tract.

b. It is widely distributed in body fluids and reaches therapeutic levels in cerebrospinal fluid. It also is present in bile, milk, and aqueous humor.

c. Chloramphenicol is metabolized in the liver by glucuronyl transferase.

d. Its metabolites are excreted in the urine.

4. Pharmacologic effects

a. Chloramphenicol has a fairly wide spectrum of antimicrobial activity, including:

   (1) Many gram-negative organisms (e.g., it is bactericidal for *H. influenzae*)

   (2) Anaerobic organisms, such as *Bacteroides* species (e.g., *B. fragilis*)

   (3) Some strains of *Streptococcus* and *Staphylococcus* (at high antibiotic concentration)

   (4) Species of *Clostridium, Chlamydia,* and *Mycoplasma*

   (5) Rickettsiae, in which it suppresses growth

b. *P. aeruginosa* is resistant.

5. Therapeutic uses. Potentially severe toxicity limits the use of chloramphenicol to those infections that cannot be treated effectively with other antibiotic agents.

a. Chloramphenicol is the drug of choice for **typhoid fever**.

b. **Bacterial meningitis** caused by *H. influenzae* is effectively treated. When children are affected, the combination of ampicillin and chloramphenicol is recommended for initial therapy.

c. Most **anaerobic infections** respond to chloramphenicol.

d. **Rickettsial diseases** and **brucellosis** can be treated with chloramphenicol; however, tetracyclines are the preferred agents.

6. Preparations and administration

a. Chloramphenicol and its palmitate salt are given orally.

b. Chloramphenicol sodium succinate is given intravenously. It has no antibacterial activity until it has been hydrolyzed to chloramphenicol. Levels do not peak for 1 hour.

c. Ophthalmic solutions and ointments are also available.

7. Adverse effects

a. **Hypersensitivity reactions** can occur.

b. The most important effect, which may be related to hypersensitivity, is **bone marrow depression,** resulting in **pancytopenia**.

   (1) The incidence of this reaction is not dose-related.

   (2) It is usually associated with prolonged therapy and more than one episode of treatment with chloramphenicol.

   (3) It occurs in 1 in 40,000 patients given chloramphenicol and often is fatal.

c. Dose-dependent, **reversible blood dyscrasias** may also occur.

d. **Superinfections** can occur, including oropharyngeal candidiasis and acute staphylococcal enterocolitis.

e. **Gray-baby syndrome** is seen in neonates, especially premature infants, who have been given relatively large doses of chloramphenicol.

   (1) Cyanosis, respiratory irregularities, vasomotor collapse, abdominal distention, loose green stools, and an ashen-gray color characterize this often fatal syndrome.

   (2) The condition develops because of the immature hepatic conjugating mechanism and the inadequate mechanism for renal excretion in neonates.

F. Macrolides (see Figure 12-5)

1. Chemistry. Macrolides contain a lactone ring and one or more deoxy sugars.

a. **Clarithromycin** is 6-methoxy-erythromycin.

b. **Azithromycin** has a nitrogen group added to the 14-member macrolide ring of erythromycin.

2. Mechanism of action. The macrolides inhibit bacterial protein synthesis by binding to 50S ribosomal subunits of sensitive microorganisms; they are usually **bacteriostatic** but can be bactericidal in some situations.

3. Pharmacokinetics

a. Erythromycin

(1) All forms of erythromycin are absorbed following oral administration and diffuse into most body tissues and fluids except cerebrospinal fluid.

(a) The **base** is absorbed from the upper part of the small intestine. It is destroyed by gastric juice.

(b) The **estolate** is resistant to gastric inactivation. In children, the estolate appears to be more bioavailable than the ethylsuccinate.

(2) Erythromycin is concentrated in the liver and is excreted primarily in bile and feces.

b. Clarithromycin

(1) Clarithromycin is well absorbed from the gastrointestinal tract with or without food.

(2) Clarithromycin penetrates tissues and cells including macrophages and polymorphonuclear leukocytes (PMNs).

(3) Clarithromycin is metabolized in the liver and 40% is recovered in urine.

c. Azithromycin

(1) Azithromycin results in very low blood levels after oral administration and food decreases bioavailability.

(2) Azithromycin concentrates in tissues, macrophages, and PMNs.

(3) Only 6% is recovered in the urine, and its terminal half-life is 68 hours.

4. Pharmacologic effects

a. Erythromycin

(1) This drug is effective against gram-positive organisms including some strains of *S. aureus* that are penicillin G-resistant.

(2) *Neisseria* species, some strains of *H. influenzae,* and *Bordetella, Legionella, Treponema,* and *Mycoplasma* species are sensitive to erythromycin.

b. Clarithromycin

(1) Clarithromycin is two to four times more active than erythromycin against streptococci and staphylococci. When these organisms are resistant to erythromycin, they are resistant to clarithromycin.

(2) It is more active than erythromycin against *Moraxella, Legionella, Mycoplasma, Chlamydia,* and *B. burgdorferi.*

c. Azithromycin

(1) Azithromycin is two to four times less active than erythromycin against staphylococci and streptococci.

(2) Its spectrum is slightly broader than that of clarithromycin, in that azithromycin is active against some aerobic and facultative gram-negative bacilli (e.g., *Salmonella*).

5. Therapeutic uses

a. Erythromycin

(1) This drug is useful for patients who are allergic to penicillin when the infecting organism is sensitive to erythromycin, particularly in cases of infection with group A *S. pyogenes* and *S. pneumoniae.*

(2) Pneumonia due to *Mycoplasma* organisms is effectively treated.

(3) Legionnaires' disease is treated with erythromycin.

(4) Topical erythromycin preparations are used to treat acne.

b. Both **clarithromycin** and **azithromycin** are expensive alternatives to erythromycin. Both show promise for the treatment of *M. avium* and other infections associated with AIDS (e.g., toxoplasmosis, cryptosporidiosis)

6. Preparations and administration

a. Erythromycin

(1) Erythromycin base and several salts are available in various forms for oral administration.

(2) Sterile erythromycin gluceptate is available for parenteral administration.

(3) Erythromycin base is available in topical formulations.

b. Both **clarithromycin** and **azithromycin** are available in various forms for oral administration.

7. Adverse effects

    a. Erythromycin has a very low incidence of serious side effects.

        (1) Cholestatic hepatitis has occurred in adults treated for a week or longer with the estolate form. Hepatitis can also occur with the ethylsuccinate and possibly with the stearate. The hepatitis is uncommon and is reversible.

        (2) Epigastric distress can occur.

        (3) A high incidence of **thrombophlebitis** occurs when erythromycin is administered intravenously, even when the drug is dissolved in a large fluid volume.

        (4) Erythromycin can interfere with the hepatic metabolism of theophylline compounds, leading to **toxic accumulation**. It can also increase the effects and toxicity of oral anticoagulants, carbamazepine, and digoxin.

    b. Both **clarithromycin** and **azithromycin** are well-tolerated and cause little nausea or diarrhea compared with erythromycin. **Reversible dose-related hearing loss** can occur with both drugs when high doses are used to treat *M. avium* infections.

G. Clindamycin

1. Chemistry. Clindamycin is the 7-deoxy,7-chloro derivative of the **parent drug, lincomycin,** which it has essentially replaced.

2. Mechanism of action. Like the macrolide antibiotics, clindamycin **inhibits bacterial protein synthesis** by binding to 50S ribosomal subunits of sensitive microorganisms. Clindamycin is usually **bacteriostatic** but can be bactericidal in certain situations.

3. Pharmacokinetics

    a. Although it is well absorbed following oral administration, clindamycin most often is administered parenterally because pseudomembranous colitis is less likely to follow parenteral administration.

    b. The drug is widely distributed in body fluids and tissues but does not pass readily into cerebrospinal fluid.

    c. Most of the drug is metabolized to the inactive sulfoxide form, which then is excreted in the urine and bile.

4. Pharmacologic effects. Clindamycin is effective against:

    a. Gram-positive organisms, including anaerobic streptococci

    b. Many other anaerobic bacteria, especially *B. fragilis*

5. Therapeutic uses

    a. Clindamycin is the drug of first choice against *Bacteroides,* especially *B. fragilis,* which often is the cause of anaerobic abdominal infections. Anaerobic infections of the brain are treated more effectively with chloramphenicol because clindamycin shows poor CNS penetration.

    b. Topical clindamycin preparations are used to treat acne.

6. Preparations and administration. Clindamycin is available in oral, parenteral, and topical forms.

7. Adverse effects. Pseudomembranous colitis can occur, resulting in diarrhea, abdominal pain, fever, and mucus and blood in the stools. This potentially fatal condition, caused by *Clostridium difficile,* can be treated with vancomycin (see II H).

H. Vancomycin

1. Chemistry. Vancomycin is a complex glycopeptide.

2. Mechanism of action. Vancomycin inhibits synthesis of the bacterial cell wall. Thus, unlike erythromycin and clindamycin, vancomycin is clearly **bactericidal.**

3. Pharmacokinetics. Vancomycin is absorbed poorly after oral administration, and intravenous administration is, therefore, preferred.

    a. It is widely distributed and passes into the cerebrospinal fluid when the meninges are inflamed.

    b. Most of the compound is excreted via the kidney.

FIGURE 12-8. Nalidixic acid.

4. Pharmacologic effects. Vancomycin is active primarily against gram-positive bacteria.

5. Therapeutic uses
   a. Vancomycin is very effective against penicillin-resistant staphylococci, streptococci of the viridans group, and serious enterococcal infections, such as staphylococcal enterocolitis and pseudomembranous colitis caused by *C. difficile*. Recently vancomycin-resistant enterococci have been reported.
   b. Toxicity limits its use to serious infections.

6. Preparations and administration
   a. Because it is reserved for severe infections, vancomycin is most often administered intravenously.
   b. Oral use is limited to the treatment of susceptible enteric infections.

7. Adverse effects
   a. Ototoxicity can lead to deafness.
   b. Nephrotoxicity can occur.

I. Quinolones

1. Chemistry. These synthetic antimicrobials are structurally related to the **older quinolone, nalidixic acid** (Figure 12-8). The newer quinolones (Table 12-5) are **fluoroquinolone** antimicrobial agents.

2. Mechanism of action. The quinolones **act on DNA gyrase,** an enzyme involved in DNA replication. They are **rapidly bactericidal**.

3. Pharmacokinetics
   a. Ofloxacin, enoxacin, and lomefloxacin are almost completely absorbed orally; ciprofloxacin is 67% orally absorbed.
   b. Serum concentrations reach peak in 1–3 hours. The fluoroquinolones are widely distributed throughout the body, but concentrations in the cerebrospinal fluid are low.

TABLE 12-5. Therapeutic Uses of Fluoroquinolones

Drug	Therapeutic Use
Norfloxacin	Urinary tract infections
Lomefloxacin	Urinary tract infections; bronchitis
Ciprofloxacin	Uncomplicated and complicated urinary tract infections; infectious diarrhea; soft tissue infections; infections of the bones, joints, skin, and lower respiratory tract
Ofloxacin	Same as ciprofloxacin; uncomplicated gonorrhea (single dose); chlamydial infections
Enoxacin	Urinary tract infections; uncomplicated urethral or cervical gonorrhea

  c. Half-lives of elimination from serum are 7–8 hours for lomefloxacin, 5 hours for ofloxacin and enoxacin, and 3–4 hours for ciprofloxacin and norfloxacin.

  d. Renal clearance is the primary method of clearance; therefore, the dosage must be adjusted according to renal function.

4. Pharmacologic effects

  a. All fluoroquinolones are active against *Neisseria gonorrhea, H. influenzae, Moraxella catarrhalis,* and against most organisms causing bacterial gastroenteritis.

  b. Ciprofloxacin is highly active against *P. aeruginosa.* The other fluoroquinolones are less effective against this microorganism.

  c. Pneumococci and group A streptococci are resistant to enoxacin. In general, penicillins and cephalosporins are more active than fluoroquinolones against streptococci and staphylococci.

  d. Although fluoroquinolones are effective against some other sexually transmitted diseases, no fluoroquinolone inhibits *T. pallidum.*

5. Therapeutic uses (see Table 12-5). Emergence of resistance is occurring and is significant, especially concerning the treatment of conditions caused by *S. aureus* and *P. aeruginosa.*

6. Preparations and administration

  a. Ciprofloxacin and ofloxacin are available for both oral and parenteral use.

  b. Norfloxacin and lomefloxacin are available for oral use only.

7. Adverse effects. Fluoroquinolones are generally well-tolerated.

  a. Seizures and **hypersensitivity reactions,** including photosensitivity, have been reported.

  b. Fluoroquinolones cause erosions of cartilage in young dogs; therefore, they are not recommended for use in patients younger than 18 years of age or for pregnant or nursing women.

III.   AGENTS USED FOR TREATMENT OF FUNGAL INFECTIONS

A.   **Agents used for superficial fungal infections**

1. Nystatin

  a. Chemistry. Nystatin is a polyene antibiotic.

  b. Mechanism of action

   (1) The drug is **fungistatic** and **fungicidal**.

   (2) It binds to sterols, especially ergosterol, which is enriched in the membrane of fungi and yeasts. As a result of this binding, the drug appears to form channels in the membrane that allow small molecules to leak out of the cell.

  c. Pharmacokinetics

   (1) Nystatin is not absorbed appreciably from the gastrointestinal tract.

   (2) It is not absorbed from the skin or mucous membranes.

   (3) It is not employed parenterally.

  d. Therapeutic uses

   (1) Nystatin is used to treat *Candida* infections of the skin, mucous membranes, and intestinal tract.

   (2) Thrush (oral candidiasis) and vaginitis are treated by topical application, whereas intestinal candidiasis is treated by oral administration.

  e. Preparations. Nystatin is supplied as an ointment, oral suspension, oral tablets, drops, and powder.

  f. Adverse effects. Occasional gastrointestinal disturbances occur with oral administration.

2. Griseofulvin

  a. Chemistry. The drug is produced by *Penicillium griseofulvum.* It is poorly soluble in water.

  b. Mechanism of action

   (1) Griseofulvin binds to polymerized microtubules, disrupting the mitotic spindle, but its exact mechanism of action is undetermined.

(2) It is **fungistatic**.
c. **Pharmacokinetics**
    (1) Griseofulvin is absorbed in the upper part of the small intestine following oral administration. Most of the drug is eliminated unchanged in the feces.
    (2) Griseofulvin has a particular **affinity for keratin**.
d. **Pharmacologic effects.** Griseofulvin is active against dermatophytes, including *Microsporum, Epidermophyton,* and *Trichophyton* species. It is ineffective against yeasts.
e. **Therapeutic uses.** Because of its affinity for keratin, griseofulvin is useful for treating mycotic diseases of the skin, hair, and nails, such as tinea capitis, pedis (athlete's foot), cruris, corporis, and circinata. It is given orally; topical use has little effect.
f. **Preparations.** Griseofulvin is available as tablets, capsules, and an oral suspension.
g. **Adverse effects.** Extensive clinical use of griseofulvin has revealed relatively low toxicity.

3. **Naftifine and terbinafine**
    a. **Chemistry.** These synthetic antifungal agents are allylamines.
    b. **Mechanism of action.** They decrease the synthesis of ergosterol, an essential component of fungal cell membranes, by inhibiting the enzyme squalene epoxidase.
    c. **Pharmacologic effects and therapeutic uses**
        (1) In vitro, naftifine is fungicidal against dermatophytes and fungistatic against yeasts such as *Candida albicans*. Terbinafine is more active in vitro against dermatophytes that cause tinea infections.
        (2) Clinically, they are used to treat tinea pedis, tinea cruris, and tinea corporis. They are not effective for fungal infections of the hair or nails.
    d. **Preparations and administration**
        (1) Naftifine is available as a 1% cream, which is used topically.
        (2) Terbinafine is available as a solution.
    e. **Adverse effects.** Burning, dryness, redness, and itching have been reported.

4. **Haloprogin and tolnaftate**
    a. **Pharmacologic effects and therapeutic uses**
        (1) Haloprogin is fungicidal to *Epidermophyton, Pityrosporum, Microsporum, Trichophyton,* and *Candida*.
        (2) Tolnaftate is effective for the treatment of most cutaneous mycoses, such as *Trichophyton rubrum* and *Microsporum canis,* but is ineffective against *Candida*.
    b. **Adverse effects.** Unlike tolnaftate, which is free of toxic or allergic reactions, haloprogin can cause irritation, pruritus, and burning sensations.

5. **Miconazole and clotrimazole**
    a. **Pharmacologic effects and therapeutic uses.** These imidazole derivatives are **used primarily as topical agents**.
        (1) They inhibit the growth of common dermatophytes and yeasts, including *Trichophyton* species, *Epidermophyton floccosum, C. albicans,* and *Malassezia furfur*.
        (2) They are used for the treatment of ringworm and other skin infections caused by susceptible organisms, and for vulvovaginal candidiasis.
    b. Miconazole is also available for parenteral administration in the treatment of severe systemic fungal infections, such as candidiasis, coccidioidomycosis, and cryptococcosis. However, toxicity and limited efficacy restrict its usefulness.

B. | **Agents used for systemic fungal infections** (Table 12-6)

1. **Amphotericin B**
    a. **Chemistry.** This drug is a polyene antibiotic.
    b. **Mechanism of action.** The mechanism of action is the same for amphotericin B as for nystatin.
    c. **Pharmacokinetics**
        (1) Amphotericin B is absorbed poorly from the gastrointestinal tract.
        (2) Intravenous administration results in a plasma half-life of approximately 24 hours.
        (3) The drug is excreted very slowly in the urine.

TABLE 12-6. Pharmacologic Properties of Systemic Antifungals

	Amphotericin B	Flucytosine	Ketoconazole	Traconazole	Fluconazole	Miconazole
% Oral bioavailability	< 5	> 80	75	70	> 80	25
Terminal elimination half-life	15 days	3–6 hours	7–10 hours	24–42 hours	22–31 hours	20–24 hours
Unchanged drug in urine (%)	3	> 75	3	< 1	80	1
Mechanism of action	Forms channels in cell membrane	Metabolic inhibitor	Blocks synthesis of ergosterol	Blocks synthesis of ergosterol	Blocks synthesis of ergosterol	Blocks synthesis of ergosterol
Significant adverse effects	Anemia, azotemia, nephrotoxicity, fever, chills	Bone marrow depression, asymptomatic elevation of liver enzymes, confusion, headache	Asymptomatic elevation of liver enzymes, impotence, gynecomastia, menstrual irregularities, photophobia, clinically important drug interactions	Asymptomatic elevation of liver enzymes, hyperkalemia, hypertension, clinically important drug interactions	Asymptomatic elevation of liver enzymes, clinically important drug interactions	Bone marrow depression, hyperlipidemia, hyponatremia, fever, psychosis

d. Pharmacologic effects
   (1) Amphotericin B is a broad-spectrum antifungal agent.
   (2) *Histoplasma capsulatum, Cryptococcus neoformans, Coccidioides immitis, Candida* species, *Blastomyces dermatitidis,* and some strains of *Aspergillus* and *Sporotrichum* are sensitive.
e. Therapeutic uses
   (1) Amphotericin B is the most effective drug available for systemic fungal infections.
   (2) It is frequently used for the treatment of **life-threatening fungal infections** in patients with impaired defense mechanisms (e.g., patients undergoing immuno-suppressive therapy or cancer chemotherapy, and patients with AIDS). Flucyto-sine is sometimes given with amphotericin B for the initial treatment of rapidly progressive, acutely life-threatening fungal infections.
   (3) Amphotericin B is used in the treatment of the following infections:
      (a) Pulmonary, cutaneous, and disseminated forms of blastomycosis
      (b) Acute pulmonary coccidioidomycosis
      (c) Pulmonary histoplasmosis
      (d) *C. neoformans* infections—now the most common life-threatening fungal pathogen associated with AIDS
      (e) Candidiasis, including disseminated forms
   (4) In addition, mucocutaneous lesions of parasitic American leishmaniasis may respond to amphotericin B therapy.
   (5) Intrathecal infusion may be helpful in the treatment of fungal meningitis.
f. Preparations
   (1) Amphotericin B lyophilized powder is available for injection.
   (2) Amphotericin B is also available in topical formulations for treating cutaneous and mucocutaneous candidiasis.
g. Adverse effects. All patients receiving amphotericin B therapy should be hospital-ized, at least during the initiation of therapy.
   (1) **Hypersensitivity reactions** can occur, including anaphylaxis.
   (2) **Fever, chills, headache,** and **gastrointestinal disturbances** are common with intravenous administration. Patients usually develop tolerance to these adverse effects with continuing administration of amphotericin B.
   (3) **Decreased renal function** occurs in over 80% of patients treated with ampho-tericin B, necessitating close observation. The incidence of impaired renal func-tion may increase when amphotericin B is given concurrently with cyclosporine.

2. Flucytosine
   a. Chemistry. This drug is a fluorinated pyrimidine.
   b. Mechanism of action. Flucytosine is converted with fungal cells (but not in the host's cells) to **5-fluorouracil** (see Chapter 11 III D 1), a metabolic antagonist that ultimately leads to inhibition of thymidylate synthetase.
   c. Pharmacokinetics
      (1) Flucytosine is well absorbed from the gastrointestinal tract and is distributed widely throughout the body, including the cerebrospinal fluid.
      (2) It is excreted in the urine, mainly in an unmetabolized form.
   d. Pharmacologic effects
      (1) The drug is effective against *C. neoformans.*
      (2) It is effective against some strains of *Candida,* including some *C. albicans* strains. However, *C. albicans* can become resistant to flucytosine during therapy.
   e. Therapeutic uses
      (1) Flucytosine is not as effective as amphotericin B and is generally not used alone because resistance develops rapidly.
      (2) It is used for systemic infections caused by *C. albicans* and *C. neoformans* (*Cryptococcus meningitidis*), most often in combination with amphotericin B.
   f. Preparations. Flucytosine is available as capsules for oral use.
   g. Adverse effects have included:
      (1) Fatal bone marrow depression

    (2) Gastrointestinal distress, especially when given with amphotericin B

    (3) Skin rash

    (4) Hepatic dysfunction

  3. Ketoconazole

    a. Chemistry. Ketoconazole is a substituted imidazole derivative.

    b. Mechanism of action. Ketoconazole alters membrane permeability by blocking the synthesis of ergosterol, the primary cellular sterol of fungi.

    c. Pharmacokinetics

      (1) Ketoconazole is absorbed from the gastrointestinal tract.

      (2) Because the drug requires an acidic environment for dissolution, agents that increase pH, such as antacids or histamine H_2 blocking agents, can reduce its bioavailability.

    d. Pharmacologic effects and therapeutic uses. Ketoconazole is used for less severe fungal infections.

      (1) Ketoconazole is active in blastomycosis, coccidioidomycosis, histoplasmosis, paracoccidioidomycosis, chronic mucocutaneous candidiasis, and resistant dermatophyte infections.

      (2) Ketoconazole acts more slowly than the other available antifungal agents, requiring long periods of therapy and, thus, is less useful for severe or acute systemic infections.

      (3) It penetrates the cerebrospinal fluid poorly.

    e. Preparations. Ketoconazole is available as tablets for oral use.

    f. Adverse effects. Ketoconazole is much less toxic than amphotericin B.

      (1) Nausea and vomiting are the most common adverse reactions.

      (2) Hepatotoxicity, hypersensitivity reactions (including urticaria or anaphylaxis), and **gynecomastia** are less common untoward effects.

      (3) Ketoconazole **transiently blocks testosterone synthesis and the adrenal response to corticotropin**.

      (4) Ketoconazole blocks several cytochrome P-450–related enzyme steps and, therefore, has the **potential to interact with drugs** metabolized by the microsomal enzyme system (see Chapter 13 II D 5).

  4. Itraconazole

    a. Chemistry. This drug is a synthetic triazole.

    b. Mechanism of action. Itraconazole inhibits cytochrome P-450–dependent enzymes, blocking the synthesis of ergosterol.

    c. Pharmacokinetics

      (1) Oral bioavailability is maximal when taken with food. Drugs that decrease gastric acidity decrease absorption of itraconazole.

      (2) Serum concentrations are lower in patients with AIDS.

      (3) No dosage adjustment is necessary for patients with renal failure.

    d. Pharmacologic effects and therapeutic uses

      (1) Itraconazole is effective oral treatment for histoplasmosis and blastomycosis.

      (2) It is also useful for the treatment of aspergillosis, sporotrichosis, and for some patients with candidiasis, cryptococcosis, and coccidioidomycosis.

    e. Preparation. Itraconazole is available only in an oral formulation.

    f. Adverse effects

      (1) Patients may experience **dose-related nausea** and **abdominal discomfort**.

      (2) Cardiac arrhythmias can occur in patients taking itraconazole and terfenadine.

  5. Fluconazole

    a. Chemistry. This drug is a bis-triazole.

    b. Mechanism of action. It inhibits cytochrome P-450–dependent enzymes, blocking the synthesis of ergosterol.

    c. Pharmacokinetics

      (1) Fluconazole is more water-soluble than ketoconazole and itraconazole, and is highly bioavailable.

(2) Cerebrospinal fluid concentrations approach 50%–90% of simultaneous serum concentrations.

(3) Fluconazole should be discontinued in patients with progressive hepatic dysfunction.

d. Pharmacologic effects and therapeutic uses

(1) Fluconazole is active against several systemic fungal pathogens, including *Aspergillides, B. dermatitides, C. albicans, C. neoformans, C. immitis,* and *H. capsulatum.*

(2) Fluconazole is effective against oropharyngeal and esophageal candidiasis, serious systemic candidal infections, and cryptococcal meningitis.

(3) Fluconazole may be of some value in treating *Candida* peritonitis associated with ambulatory peritoneal dialysis.

e. Preparations. Fluconazole can be administered orally or intravenously.

f. Adverse effects. Fluconazole is less toxic than amphotericin B or flucytosine and better tolerated than ketoconazole.

(1) Gastrointestinal distress and **rash** are the most common adverse effects.

(2) Drug interactions. Though it has a lower binding affinity for cytochrome P-450 enzymes than ketoconazole, it may increase serum concentrations of phenytoin, cyclosporine, and oral hypoglycemic drugs and potentiate the effect of warfarin.

IV. AGENTS USED FOR TREATMENT OF TUBERCULOSIS

A. General considerations

1. Incidence. The incidence of tuberculosis has been increasing because the disease can occur in patients with AIDS and in the homeless.

2. Principles of treatment (Table 12-7)

a. Drugs are used in combination because otherwise microbial resistance rapidly develops.

b. The rising incidence of resistance because of poor compliance may require administration of drugs under direct supervision.

c. First-line drugs for the treatment of tuberculosis include **isoniazid, rifampin, pyrazinamide,** and **ethambutol;** occasionally **streptomycin** is used as well.

(1) Tuberculosis caused by possibly resistant organisms is initially treated with a four-drug regimen of isoniazid, rifampin, pyrazinamide, and either ethambutol or streptomycin.

(2) Tuberculosis resistant to isoniazid only should be treated with rifampin, ethambutol and, in most cases, pyrazinamide for 12 months.

(3) In **patients with human immunodeficiency virus (HIV), disseminated disease,** or **meningitis,** the initial 9-month course of therapy should be continued for 6 months after culture conversion.

(4) For **multiple drug–resistant tuberculosis,** three drugs to which the organism is susceptible should be continued for 12–24 months after culture conversion.

3. Prophylaxis

a. Isoniazid prophylaxis is given to:

(1) Individuals in close contact with the tuberculosis patient, especially children

(2) Any person converting from a negative to a positive skin test

b. Persons exposed to organisms that are resistant to isoniazid should be treated with rifampin (with or without ethambutol) for 12 months. If exposure is to multiple drug–resistant tuberculosis, pyrazinamide should be added.

B. Isoniazid

1. Chemistry. Isoniazid (Figure 12-9) is the hydrazide of isonicotinic acid and is a pyridine.

TABLE 12-7. Regimen Options for the Initial Treatment of Tuberculosis Among Children and Adults

	Tuberculosis Without HIV Infection						Tuberculosis With HIV Infection
	Option A		**Option B**			**Option C**	
		Daily		Daily			Three times/wk	Options A, B, or C
Regimen	Weeks 1–8: Isoniazid + Rifampin + Pyrazinamide	Daily	Weeks 1–2: Isoniazid + Rifampin + Pyrazinamide + Streptomycin OR Ethambutol	Daily		Weeks 1–24: Isoniazid + Rifampin + Pyrazinamide + Ethambutol OR Streptomycin	Three times/wk	
	Weeks 9–24: Isoniazid + Rifampin	Daily OR two to three times/wk	Weeks 3–8: Same drugs	Two times/wk				
			Weeks 9–24: Isoniazid + Rifampin	Two times/wk				
Duration	A total of at least 6 months, continuing for 3 months after culture conversion*		A total of at least 6 months, continuing for 3 months after culture conversion*			A total of at least 6 months, continuing for 3 months after culture conversion*		A total of at least 9 months, continuing for at least 6 months after culture conversion
Comments	In areas where resistance to isoniazid is documented to be greater than 4%, ethambutol or streptomycin should be added to the initial regimen until susceptibility to isoniazid and rifampin is demonstrated.					The strongest evidence from clinical trials indicates that this regimen is most effective if all four drugs are administered for the full 6 months. There is weaker evidence that streptomycin can be discontinued after 4 months if the isolate is susceptible to all drugs. The evidence for stopping pyrazinamide before the end of 6 months is equivocal for the three times/wk regimen. There is no evidence on the effectiveness of this regimen if ethambutol is discontinued before the 6-month course is completed.		

Patients on regimens involving administration of drugs two or three timer per week should be monitored closely to ensure compliance and evaluate response.

Adapted with permission from the Centers for Disease Control and Prevention: Initial therapy for tuberculosis in the era of multidrug resistance: recommendations of the advisory council for the elimination of tuberculosis. JAMA 270(6): 694–698, 1993.

HIV = human immunodeficiency virus.

FIGURE 12-9. Isoniazid.

2. Mechanism of action. Although this is not known, isoniazid probably interferes with cellular metabolism, especially the synthesis of mycolic acid, an important constituent of the mycobacterial cell wall.

3. Pharmacokinetics
   a. The drug is well absorbed from the gastrointestinal tract and diffuses readily into all body tissues and body fluids, including cerebrospinal fluid.
   b. The plasma concentration and the metabolism of isoniazid are affected by whether a given patient is a **fast or a slow acetylator** of the drug, a genetically determined trait.
   c. Isoniazid is excreted mainly in the urine. Slow acetylators have a higher concentration of unchanged (free) isoniazid than fast acetylators.

4. Pharmacologic effects
   a. Isoniazid is effective against most tubercle bacilli.
   b. It is not effective against many atypical mycobacteria.

5. Therapeutic uses. Isoniazid is the most widely used agent in the treatment and prophylaxis of tuberculosis.

6. Preparations. Isoniazid is available as tablets, as syrup, and in injectable form.

7. Adverse effects
   a. Up to 20% of patients taking isoniazid develop **elevated serum aminotransferase levels**.
      (1) Severe hepatic injury occurs more frequently in patients over the age of 35, especially in those who drink alcohol daily.
      (2) Isoniazid is discontinued if symptoms of hepatitis develop or if the aminotransferase activity increases to more than three times normal.
   b. Peripheral and CNS toxicity occur.
      (1) This toxicity probably results from an increased excretion of pyridoxine induced by isoniazid, which produces a pyridoxine deficiency.
      (2) Peripheral neuritis, urinary retention, insomnia, and psychotic episodes can occur.
      (3) Concurrent pyridoxine administration with isoniazid prevents most of these complications.
   c. Isoniazid can also **exacerbate pyridoxine-deficiency anemia** and can produce **blood dyscrasias.**
   d. Isoniazid can **reduce the metabolism of phenytoin,** enhancing its toxicity.
   e. Hypersensitivity reactions (i.e., fever, various rashes) can occur.

C. **Rifampin**

1. Chemistry. Rifampin belongs to the group of complex macrocyclic antibiotics.

2. Mechanism of action. Rifampin **inhibits RNA synthesis** in bacteria and chlamydiae by binding to DNA-dependent RNA polymerase.

3. Pharmacokinetics
   a. Rifampin is well absorbed from the gastrointestinal tract.
   b. It is widely distributed in tissues and is excreted mainly through the liver.

4. Pharmacologic effects
a. Most gram-positive and many gram-negative microorganisms are sensitive to rifampin.
b. Prolonged administration of the drug as the single therapeutic agent promotes the emergence of highly resistant organisms.

5. Therapeutic uses
a. Rifampin is used in the treatment of:
   (1) Tuberculosis (in combination with other agents)
   (2) Atypical mycobacterial infections
   (3) Leprosy

6. Preparations. Rifampin is available in capsules for oral use.

7. Adverse effects
a. **Urine, sweat, tears,** and **contact lenses** may take on an **orange color** because of rifampin administration; this effect is harmless.
b. **Light-chain proteinuria** and **impaired antibody response** may occur.
c. Rifampin induces hepatic microsomal enzymes and, therefore, **affects the half-life of a number of drugs**.
d. When taken erratically in large doses, a **febrile "flu-like" syndrome** can occur.

D. | Pyrazinamide

1. Chemistry. Pyrazinamide is the pyrazine analog of nicotinamide.

2. Mechanism of action. This is unknown.

3. Pharmacokinetics
a. Pyrazinamide is distributed throughout the body after oral administration.
b. It is excreted mainly by glomerular filtration.

4. Therapeutic uses. Pyrazinamide is now widely used in multiagent short-term therapy of uncomplicated pulmonary tuberculosis.

5. Preparations. Pyrazinamide is available as tablets for oral use.

6. Adverse effects
a. **Liver damage** can occur; therefore, liver function studies should be performed before and during therapy.
b. **Hyperuricemia** and **gout** can occur.

E. | Ethambutol

1. Chemistry. The structural formula of ethambutol is shown in Figure 12-10.

2. Mechanism of action. Ethambutol's mechanism of action is unknown. Resistance to the drug occurs rapidly when it is used alone.

3. Pharmacokinetics
a. Ethambutol is well absorbed from the gastrointestinal tract.
b. It is widely distributed in the body, including the cerebrospinal fluid.

4. Pharmacologic effects and therapeutic use. Ethambutol inhibits many strains of *M. tuberculosis*. It is used in combination with other agents for the treatment of tuberculosis.

$$ \underset{\underset{C_2H_5}{|}}{\overset{\overset{CH_2OH}{|}}{H-C}} -NH-CH_2-CH_2-HN-\underset{\underset{CH_2OH}{|}}{\overset{\overset{C_2H_5}{|}}{C}}-H $$

FIGURE 12-10. Ethambutol.

5. **Preparations.** Ethambutol hydrochloride is available in tablet form for oral use.

6. **Adverse effects. Visual disturbances,** including optic neuritis and red–green color-blindness, can occur but are reversible.

F. **Streptomycin** (see Table 12-4)

1. The use of streptomycin in the treatment of tuberculosis has been declining ever since more effective agents became available.

2. When a three-agent combination is used to treat severe forms of tuberculosis (e.g., disseminated or meningeal), streptomycin may be one of the drugs used.

V. AGENTS USED FOR TREATMENT OF LEPROSY

A. **Sulfones**

1. **Chemistry**
   a. The sulfones, the principal class of agents used to treat leprosy, are chemically related to the sulfonamides.
   b. The most important derivatives come from **dapsone** (Figure 12-11).

2. **Mechanism of action**
   a. Dapsone is **bacteriostatic** for *Mycobacterium leprae.*
   b. Its mechanism of action is **similar to that of the sulfonamides** (see II A 2).

3. **Pharmacokinetics**
   a. Dapsone is slowly but completely absorbed from the gastrointestinal tract.
   b. It undergoes intestinal reabsorption from the bile, resulting in a sustained level of the drug in the circulation.

4. **Pharmacologic effects**
   a. Dapsone is effective against *M. leprae,* although resistance to the drug can develop.
   b. It is bacteriostatic for *M. tuberculosis* in vitro.

5. **Therapeutic uses.** Dapsone is the most important drug in the treatment of leprosy. Because of recent resistance to dapsone, it is now usually given with rifampin, with clofazimine, or with both.

6. **Preparations and administration**
   a. Dapsone is administered orally.
   b. Therapy usually is continued for a minimum of 2 years.

7. **Adverse effects**
   a. The most common untoward effects include **hemolysis, methemoglobinemia, nausea, vomiting, rash, transient headache,** and **anorexia.**
   b. The sulfones can cause an **exacerbation of lepromatous leprosy.**
   c. A **fatal infectious mononucleosis–like syndrome** has been reported.

B. **Clofazimine**

1. **Chemistry.** Clofazimine is a phenazine congener.

FIGURE 12-11. Dapsone.

2. **Mechanism of action.** Clofazimine **binds to mycobacteria DNA,** thereby inhibiting template function.

3. **Pharmacokinetics**
   a. Clofazimine is absorbed slowly from the gastrointestinal tract; 50% of an oral dose reaches the systemic circulation.
   b. It is lipophilic and can accumulate in adipose tissue and reticuloendothelial cells.
   c. The elimination half-life after repeated oral dosing is 70 days.

4. **Pharmacologic effects**
   a. Clofazimine exerts a slow **bactericidal** effect on *M. leprae*.
   b. It is also active in vitro against other mycobacteria, including the *M. avium* complex, which can cause disseminated infection in AIDS patients.
   c. It is not active against microorganisms other than mycobacteria.

5. **Therapeutic uses**
   a. Clofazimine is used in combination with dapsone and rifampin in multibacillary leprosy to prevent the emergence of resistance.
   b. Clofazimine in combination with rifampin is effective in treating dapsone-resistant infections.
   c. Clofazimine has an anti-inflammatory effect in erythema nodosum leprosum reactions.

6. **Preparations and administration**
   a. For multibacillary disease, clofazimine is administered orally as part of a three-agent combination for a minimum of 2 years.
   b. For dapsone-resistant leprosy, clofazimine is given first in combination with one or more other agents for 3 years, and then alone.

7. **Adverse effects**
   a. Dose-related abdominal symptoms include **pain, nausea,** and **vomiting**.
   b. A **reddish to dark brown discoloration of the skin, cornea,** and all **body fluids** can occur. This pigmentation may take months or years to disappear after the drug is discontinued.
   c. **Anticholinergic symptoms** can occur.

VI. ANTHELMINTICS (Table 12-8). These drugs are used to treat parasitic infections caused by flatworms and roundworms. The major target is usually the nongrowing adult stage of the parasite's life cycle.

TABLE 12-8. Anthelmintics

Drug	Therapeutic Uses
Diethylcarbamazine	Filaria worms (e.g., *Wuchereria bancrofti, W. malayi, Loa loa, Onchocerca volvulus*)
Praziquantel	Tapeworm infections (*Diphyllobothrium latum, Taenia saginata, Hymenolepis nana*), fluke infections (e.g., schistosomiasis)
Metrifonate	*Schistosoma haematobium*
Niridazole	*S. haematobium*
Mebendazole	Whipworm (*Trichuris trichiura*), hookworm, pinworm, *Ascaris,* echinococcosis
Niclosamide	Tapeworm infections
Pyrantel pamoate	Ascariasis, hookworm, pinworm*
Piperazine	Ascariasis[†], pinworm
Thiabendazole	Cutaneous and visceral larva migrans and strongyloidiasis, trichinosis
Ivermectin	Onchocerciasis (river blindness)

*Pyrantel pamoate produces persistent nicotinic activation, resulting in spastic paralysis of the worms.
[†]Piperazine is thought to block the response of Ascaris muscle cells to acetylcholine; the flaccid worm is then expelled by peristalsis.

VII. **AGENTS USED FOR TREATMENT OF PROTOZOAL INFECTIONS AND MALARIA** (Table 12-9)

VIII. **AGENTS USED FOR TREATMENT OF VIRAL INFECTIONS.** Viruses are obligate intracellular parasites that require the active participation of the metabolic processes of the invaded cell to survive. Thus, agents that are able to kill viruses often injure host cells as well. Despite this interrelationship, there are a growing number of drugs that have substantial therapeutic merit in the treatment of viral infections. Zidovudine (azidothymidine, AZT), used to treat AIDS, is discussed in section X; other antiviral agents are discussed here.

A. | **Acyclovir**

1. **Chemistry.** Acyclovir is a synthetic purine nucleoside analog with an acyclic side chain.

2. **Mechanism of action**
   a. After being converted in vivo to the triphosphate form, acyclovir **inhibits herpes virus DNA synthesis** by two means.
      (1) It interferes with viral DNA polymerase and inhibits viral DNA replication.
      (2) It is incorporated into DNA and leads to premature chain termination.

TABLE 12-9. Agents Used for the Treatment of Protozoal Infections and Malaria

Drug	Therapeutic Use
Metronidazole	Protozoal infections (e.g., trichomoniasis, *Giardia lamblia* infestation, *Entamoeba histolytica* amebiasis) Anaerobic bacterial infections (e.g., those caused by *Bacteroides* species)
Diloxanide furoate	Used to treat asymptomatic passers of amebic cysts
Suramin	African trypanosomiasis (early and late stages) Onchocerciasis*
Nifurtimox	South American trypanosomiasis
Stibogluconate	Leishmaniasis
Pentamidine isethionate	Leishmaniasis (in patients who do not respond to stibogluconate therapy) African trypanosomiasis (early stages) Prophylaxis and treatment of *Pneumocystis carinii* pneumonia
Chloroquine	Uncomplicated acute malaria resulting from *Plasmodium* organisms (except resistant forms) Prophylaxis during residence in an endemic area
Primaquine	Cure and prevent relapses of *P. vivax* and *P. ovale* malaria after departure from endemic areas; given with chloroquine or another schizonticide
Mefloquine	Prophylaxis during travel to areas with chloroquine-resistant malaria
Pyrimethamine, sulfadoxine	Used concurrently for prophylaxis and treatment of chloroquine-resistant strains of *P. falciparum*
Quinine† sulfate	Acute uncomplicated malaria resulting from chloroquine-resistant *P. falciparum*
Dihydrochloride	Severe illness resulting from chloroquine-resistant *P. falciparum*

*Ivermectin is often used instead of suramin in the treatment of onchocerciasis because it is less toxic.
†Quinine sulfate is administered orally, and quinine dihydrochloride is administered parenterally.

b. The drug is several hundred times more toxic for the herpes viruses than for mammalian cells because of the enhanced affinity of the viral enzyme thymidine kinase for acyclovir.

3. Pharmacologic effects. Acyclovir has inhibitory activity in vitro against herpes simplex virus types 1 and 2, varicella-zoster virus, Epstein-Barr virus, and cytomegalovirus. Most acyclovir-resistant herpes simplex virus and varicella-zoster virus isolates have been recovered from treated immunocompromised patients.

4. Therapeutic uses and administration
   a. Intravenous acyclovir is the drug of choice for treatment of **serious infections** caused by herpes simplex virus or varicella-zoster virus.
   b. Oral acyclovir
      (1) Oral acyclovir is effective in treating **primary herpes simplex virus infections**. It is less effective in treating recurrences.
      (2) Acyclovir can be given orally to treat **localized or ophthalmic zoster** if begun within 24 hours.
      (3) In transplant patients, oral acyclovir can be **used prophylactically** to prevent herpes simplex virus and cytomegalovirus.
   c. Topical acyclovir is much less effective than oral acyclovir.

5. Adverse effects
   a. Intravenous therapy can cause **crystalline nephropathy, neurologic reactions, local phlebitis, rash,** and **hives. Encephalopathy** develops in 1% of patients.
   b. Orally, acyclovir is well tolerated; however, **nausea, vomiting, diarrhea,** and **headache** can occur.
   c. Topical applications can cause **local discomfort** and **pruritus**.

B. **Amantadine and rimantadine**

1. Chemistry
   a. Amantadine is a synthetic tricyclic amine with a structure unrelated to that of any other antimicrobial agent.
   b. Rimantadine is the α-methyl derivative of amantadine.

2. Mechanism of action. This is unknown. Amantadine and rimantadine may block either the assembly of influenza A virus or the release of viral nucleic acid in the host cell. Neither drug is active against influenza B.

3. Pharmacokinetics
   a. Amantadine is well absorbed from the gastrointestinal tract and is not metabolized. It is excreted via the kidney.
   b. Rimantadine is well absorbed and extensively metabolized. Its plasma half-life is twice that of amantadine (i.e., 24–36 hours).

4. Therapeutic uses
   a. Antiviral use
      (1) The major anti-infective use for amantadine and rimantadine is for **prophylaxis during influenza A virus epidemics,** at which time unvaccinated patients of all ages who are at high risk are advised to receive one of these drugs.
         (a) Neither drug alters the immune response to influenza A vaccine; thus, vaccination can be given concurrently with the drug.
         (b) Both drugs can help to protect immunodeficient patients and those on dialysis, who may have a poor antibody response to the vaccine.
      (2) Amantadine and rimantadine may also be useful in **shortening the duration of symptoms** when administered after the onset of illness.
   b. The use of amantadine in **parkinsonism** is discussed in Chapter 3 IV D.

5. Preparations and administration. Amantadine and rimantadine are administered orally.

6. Adverse effects. Amantadine causes **dose-related CNS effects** (e.g., confusion, hallucinations, seizures, and coma). Rimantadine has a low risk of CNS effects; however, patients with psychiatric disorders or a history of epilepsy require close monitoring when receiving amantadine or rimantadine.

C. **Ganciclovir**

1. **Chemistry.** Ganciclovir is a synthetic nucleoside analog of 2′-deoxyguanosine.

2. **Mechanism of action.** Ganciclovir **inhibits viral DNA synthesis** in a manner much like that of acyclovir.

3. **Pharmacologic effects**
   a. Ganciclovir inhibits replication of herpes simplex virus types 1 and 2, cytomegalo-virus, Epstein-Barr virus, and varicella-zoster virus.
   b. Ganciclovir is more active against cytomegalovirus, in vitro, than is acyclovir, but resistant strains can develop.

4. **Therapeutic uses.** Ganciclovir is indicated for the treatment of cytomegalovirus retinitis in immunocompromised individuals, including patients with AIDS. However, relapse is common, even with continued treatment.

5. **Preparations and administration.** Ganciclovir is available for intravenous injection. It has also been injected directly into the eye.

6. **Adverse effects**
   a. When administered intramuscularly or subcutaneously, ganciclovir may cause **severe tissue irritation**.
   b. **Granulocytopenia** occurs in 40% and **thrombocytopenia** in 20% of patients treated. These are generally reversible on discontinuation of treatment.
   c. **CNS effects,** from headache to psychosis, convulsions, or coma, can occur in 5%–15% of patients.
   d. **Anemia, fever, rash,** and **abnormal liver function values** can occur.
   e. Ganciclovir is **teratogenic and mutagenic in animals**.

D. **Foscarnet**

1. **Chemistry.** Foscarnet is phosphonoformic acid.

2. **Mechanism of action.** Foscarnet **inhibits DNA polymerase** of human herpes viruses **and the reverse transcriptase of HIV** at a different site from other nucleoside analogs (e.g., ganciclovir, acyclovir, zidovudine).

3. **Therapeutic uses**
   a. Foscarnet is used to treat cytomegalovirus retinitis in AIDS patients, especially in the case of ganciclovir-resistant cytomegalovirus.
   b. Foscarnet is the drug of choice for acyclovir-resistant herpes simplex virus and vari-cella-zoster virus infections.

4. **Preparations and administration.** Foscarnet is available for the intravenous treatment of cytomegalovirus retinitis in AIDS patients.

5. **Adverse effects**
   a. Foscarnet is less well tolerated than ganciclovir; however, it causes less myelosup-pression.
   b. **Dose-limiting nephrotoxicity** is a concern.
   c. Foscarnet binds divalent metal ions, resulting in **metabolic abnormalities**.

E. **Trifluridine**

1. **Chemistry.** Trifluridine is a fluorinated pyrimidine nucleoside.

2. **Mechanism of action.** Trifluridine **inhibits DNA synthesis** but its specific mechanism of action is unknown.

3. **Pharmacologic effects**
   a. Trifluridine is active against herpes simplex virus types 1 and 2 and vacciniavirus.
   b. Some strains of adenovirus are also inhibited.

4. **Therapeutic use.** Trifluridine is indicated for the treatment of primary keratoconjunctivi-tis and recurrent epithelial keratitis resulting from herpes simplex virus types 1 and 2.

5. Preparations and administration. Trifluridine is administered as an ophthalmic solution onto the cornea of the affected eye.

6. Adverse effects include **transient burning and stinging** and **palpebral edema**.

F. **Human interferon**

1. Chemistry
   a. Interferons are naturally occurring glycoproteins that can be produced by almost any mammalian cell type, including lymphocytes and fibroblasts, when the cells are stimulated in the inflammatory process.
   b. Interferons are of three major classes; those used clinically are alpha interferons.

2. Mechanism of action
   a. The antiviral antitumor effects of interferons are thought to result from the **induction of enzymes that inhibit the synthesis of protein and DNA**.
      (1) Interferon-treated cells develop the ability to block viral replication.
      (2) Interferon is able to suppress cell proliferation.
      (3) Interferon also has immunomodulating effects.
         (a) It enhances phagocytosis by macrophages.
         (b) It increases the target-cell–specific cytotoxicity exerted by lymphocytes.
   b. The antiviral state takes several hours to develop after interferon treatment.

3. Therapeutic uses
   a. Interferon preparations are currently used for the treatment of:
      (1) Hairy-cell leukemia
      (2) AIDS-related Kaposi's sarcoma
      (3) Genital (venereal) warts (condylomata acuminata)
   b. In patients with lymphoma, early treatment of a herpes zoster infection with interferon appears to prevent the spread of infection.
   c. Treatment with interferon can induce clinical remission in 30%–40% of patients with **chronic hepatitis B**. Interferon can also cause improvement in patients with hepatitis C or D virus; however, relapse occurs in patients with chronic hepatitis D when treatment is stopped.
   d. Interferon-alpha (IFN-α) has been applied topically in **herpes keratoconjunctivitis** in combination with acyclovir and trifluridine.

4. Preparations and administration
   a. Two recombinantly produced products are available: **interferon alpha-2a** and **interferon alpha-2b;** they differ by only one amino acid residue.
   b. Administration is by the intramuscular or subcutaneous route, or intralesionally into genital warts.

5. Adverse effects
   a. **Influenza-like symptoms** (i.e., fever, chills, myalgias) occur minutes to hours after parenteral administration; they are self-limited.
   b. **Progressive fatigue** is the most common dose-limiting adverse effect when administered chronically.
   c. Interferon **in high doses** acts as an **abortifacient in primates**.
   d. **Bone marrow suppression** with **granulocytopenia** and **thrombocytopenia** is common.
   e. The **plasma concentration of hepatic enzymes increases**.
   f. The **metabolism of other drugs can be reduced** by interferon's action on the cytochrome P-450 system.

G. **Ribavirin**

1. Chemistry. Ribavirin is a synthetic purine nucleoside analog.

2. Mechanism of action. This appears to be multiple:
   a. Ribavirin monophosphate **inhibits enzymes needed for the synthesis of guanine nucleotides**.

    b. Ribavirin triphosphate **inhibits viral RNA polymerase** by competing for substrate sites.

    c. The triphosphate also **interferes with the formation of viral messenger RNA**.

3. Pharmacologic effects. Ribavirin is active in vitro against several DNA and RNA viruses, including herpes simplex, influenza A and B, and respiratory syncytial virus (RSV). High concentrations inhibit replication of the virus that causes AIDS.

4. Therapeutic uses and administration

    a. Ribavirin in aerosol form may decrease morbidity from **severe RSV infection** in infants and young children. It must be administered via a specific small-particle aerosol generator.

    b. Intravenous ribavirin decreases mortality in **Lassa fever** and in **hemorrhagic fever** with renal syndrome. The intravenous use of ribavirin is investigational.

5. Adverse effects

    a. Ribavirin is **contraindicated for patients requiring mechanical ventilation** because the small aerosol particles precipitate on the respirator valves and tubing, causing malfunction that can be lethal.

    b. Rash and **conjunctivitis** have occurred with aerosol use.

    c. Ribavirin is **mutagenic, teratogenic,** and **possibly carcinogenic.**

H. **Vidarabine** (adenine arabinoside, ara-A). Though approved for the treatment of herpes simplex virus and varicella-zoster virus, vidarabine has been largely replaced by acyclovir. Vidarabine may be carcinogenic and should not be used to treat insignificant infections.

IX. **VACCINES AND TOXOIDS.** The information given here concerns the use of these agents in adults. Routine immunization of infants and children is not considered here.

A. **Viral vaccines**

1. Measles virus vaccine

    a. Chemistry. Measles (rubeola) vaccine is made from an attenuated live virus grown in chick fibroblasts.

    b. Therapeutic uses and administration

        (1) Persons born before 1956 presumably have had measles and can be considered immune.

        (2) Persons born after 1956 who did not have measles and were never vaccinated can be considered candidates for immunization.

        (3) The risks associated with revaccination are nil.

            (a) Persons who were vaccinated before age 12 months may require revaccination.

            (b) Revaccination appears safe for immunosuppressed patients.

        (4) Vaccination is not recommended during pregnancy.

    c. Adverse effects. Transient rash occurs in 5% of those vaccinated, and a **low-grade fever** is not uncommon.

2. Rubella (German measles) virus vaccine

    a. Chemistry. Rubella vaccine is made from an attenuated live virus grown in human diploid cells.

    b. Therapeutic uses and administration. Immunization of adults is recommended, especially for unimmunized women of childbearing age. The goal is to prevent fetal rubella infection and consequent fetal damage, which can occur during both the first and second trimesters of pregnancy.

    c. Adverse effects. Adults often experience **joint pain** after vaccination. **Low-grade fever, rash,** and **lymphadenopathy** can also occur.

3. Influenza vaccine

    a. Chemistry

        (1) Influenza vaccine is made from inactivated whole virus or viral subunits grown in chick embryo cells.

       (2) The United States Public Health Service establishes the formulation to be used for each influenza season. The influenza vaccine is available as a whole virus, split virus, or purified surface antigen.

  b. Therapeutic uses and administration

       (1) Immunization decreases morbidity and mortality from influenza, especially in the elderly.

       (2) Influenza usually does not occur before December and peaks in January and February. November is the best time to vaccinate.

       (3) Annual immunization is recommended for:

          (a) Persons with metabolic diseases, severe anemia, cardiopulmonary disorders, or renal disease

          (b) Immunosuppressed patients, including AIDS patients

          (c) Persons older than 65 years of age

          (d) Health personnel who may have contact with high-risk patients

       (4) Influenza vaccine is contraindicated in patients allergic to egg products.

  c. Adverse effects

       (1) **Fever, chills, myalgia,** and **malaise** occasionally occur.

       (2) **Local redness and soreness** at the injection site last a day or two.

  4. Hepatitis B vaccine

    a. Chemistry. Two types are available.

       (1) The earlier vaccine is made from chemically inactivated hepatitis B surface antigen particles.

       (2) A recombinant hepatitis B vaccine is also available.

    b. Therapeutic uses and administration

       (1) Immunization is recommended for **all newborns** and **adolescents**.

       (2) Vaccination is recommended for **persons at increased risk for developing hepatitis B,** such as:

          (a) Susceptible male homosexuals

          (b) Household and sexual contacts of hepatitis B carriers

          (c) Intravenous drug abusers

          (d) Recipients of clotting factors VIII or IX

          (e) Dialysis patients

          (f) Hospital personnel exposed to blood or blood products

          (g) The staff of institutions for the mentally handicapped

       (3) Breakthrough infections are rare, despite the loss of antibody 6–10 years after vaccination.

    c. Adverse effects

       (1) **Soreness at the injection site** is the most common untoward effect.

       (2) The most frequent systemic complaints include **fatigue, headache, fever,** and **malaise**.

  5. Other viral vaccines

    a. Vaccines for **poliomyelitis, pertussis** (whooping cough), and **mumps** are available for routine immunization of infants and children.

    b. Vaccines for immunization against **rabies, yellow fever, equine encephalitis,** and other less common viral diseases are available for use in special high-risk situations.

B. | **Bacterial vaccines and toxoids**

  1. Tetanus and diphtheria toxoids

    a. Chemistry. These are prepared by detoxifying the toxins produced by *C. diphtheriae* and *Clostridium tetani*.

    b. Therapeutic uses and administration

       (1) The toxoids induce levels of antitoxin that are thought to be protective for at least 10 years.

       (2) Primary immunization with these toxoids is often combined with **pertussis vaccine,** but the latter is not recommended for routine use in adults.

       (3) A tetanus–diphtheria toxoid booster should be administered every 10 years.

    c. Adverse effects include **local pain** and **swelling**.
2. **Diphtheria–tetanus–acellular pertussis (DTaP) vaccine**
    a. Chemistry. This vaccine contains much less pertussis toxin and endotoxin than the whole-cell vaccine.
    b. Therapeutic uses. Substituting an acellular pertussis vaccine for the fourth and fifth doses of the diphtheria–pertussis–tetanus vaccine decreases the incidence of local and febrile reactions.

3. **Tetramune**
    a. Chemistry. Tetramune combines the traditional DPT vaccine with a vaccine against influenza B.
    b. Therapeutic use and administration. Tetramune offers the advantage of three to four fewer injections in the first 15 months of life.

4. **Pneumococcal vaccine**
    a. Chemistry. This vaccine contains purified capsular polysaccharides from the 23 types of *S. pneumoniae* that are responsible for 90% of all pneumococcal infections.
    b. Therapeutic uses and administration
      (1) Adult candidates for immunization are quite similar to those for influenza vaccine.
        (a) In general, adults should not be revaccinated with pneumococcal vaccine, because doing so may increase the incidence and severity of adverse reactions.
        (b) Although the vaccine is quite effective in people with normal immune systems, severely immunocompromised patients are not protected.
      (2) The duration of protective antibody titers is not yet known, but titers are expected to persist for up to 9 years. Asplenic patients should be revaccinated after 6 years, because of the high risk of reinfection.
    c. Adverse effects. Erythema and pain at the injection site are the most common untoward effects.

X. AGENTS USED FOR THE TREATMENT OF AIDS AND RELATED OPPORTUNISTIC INFECTIONS

A. General considerations

1. AIDS is caused by HIV, a retrovirus and member of the lentivirus family. Two subtypes, HIV-1 and HIV-2, have been recovered from patients with AIDS.

2. A large number of human cells can be infected by HIV, including macrophages and glial cells. However, the virus preferentially replicates in $CD4^+$ helper T lymphocytes.

B. Antiviral agents

1. **Zidovudine (AZT)**
    a. Chemistry. Zidovudine is a synthetic thymidine analog.
    b. Mechanism of action
      (1) Zidovudine, as the triphosphate, **inhibits the DNA polymerase (reverse transcriptase) of HIV**. HIV reverse transcriptase is 100 times more susceptible to inhibition by zidovudine than is the DNA polymerase of mammalian cells.
      (2) Zidovudine triphosphate is incorporated into viral DNA and **terminates chain growth during DNA synthesis**.
    c. Pharmacokinetics
      (1) Zidovudine is well absorbed from the gastrointestinal tract.
      (2) It is cleared rapidly from the blood (terminal half-life = 1 hour), metabolized in the liver, and excreted by the kidneys.
      (3) Zidovudine penetrates readily into the cerebrospinal fluid.

d. Therapeutic uses

(1) Zidovudine **increases median survival** from less than 9 months to more than 2 years after diagnosis of AIDS.

(2) Its use in symptomatic HIV-infected patients **slows progression to AIDS** and prolongs survival.

(3) Its use in asymptomatic HIV-infected patients may slow progression to the symptomatic condition, but does not impact survival.

e. Preparations and administration. Zidovudine is administered orally every 4 hours around the clock. When anemia develops, therapy is either interrupted or the dose is reduced, or the hematocrit is maintained with transfusions.

f. Adverse effects

(1) **Hematologic toxicity.** Administration of erythropoietin and granulocyte-macrophage colony stimulating factor (GM-CSF) may help alleviate the hematologic effects.

(a) Severe anemia, often with a megaloblastic bone marrow, is the main toxic effect.

(b) Neutropenia is fairly common, especially in patients with AIDS.

(c) Anemia, granulocytopenia, and thrombocytopenia are usually reversible when the dosage is decreased or the drug is stopped.

(2) **Neurotoxicity**

(a) Severe headaches and insomnia are common but are less severe after the first week of therapy.

(b) Seizures and Wernicke's encephalopathy have been reported.

(3) **Other adverse effects.** Nausea and myalgias occur often at the start of therapy.

(4) **Drug interactions**

(a) Ribavirin interferes with the antiviral effect of zidovudine.

(b) Probenecid slows the metabolism and excretion of zidovudine, increasing the risk of hematotoxicity.

(c) Acetaminophen interferes with glucuronidation of zidovudine in the liver.

(5) **Resistance.** With continued use, in-vitro resistance develops and is associated with clinical deterioration.

2. Didanosine (dideoxyinosine)

a. Mechanism of action. Didanosine is a **reverse transcriptase inhibitor**.

b. Therapeutic use. Sequential use of zidovudine and didanosine, rather than continuing zidovudine, appears to delay clinical deterioration.

c. Adverse effects include:

(1) Painful peripheral neuropathy

(2) Acute pancreatitis, hepatic failure

(3) Development of in-vitro resistance

3. Zalcitabine (dideoxycytidine)

a. Mechanism of action. Zalcitabine is a **reverse transcriptase inhibitor**.

b. Therapeutic use. Zalcitabine can be used concurrently with zidovudine in patients with advanced HIV infection.

c. Adverse effect. Peripheral neuropathy can limit dosage.

C. **Treatment of AIDS-related opportunistic infections**

1. *P. carinii* pneumonia

a. General considerations. This infection occurs in 80% of patients with AIDS. Episodes occur when the CD4+ lymphocyte count is less than 200 cells/mm^3. Preventing *P. carinii* delays the first AIDS-related illness by 6–12 months.

b. Therapeutic regimens

(1) **Oral or intravenous trimethoprim–sulfamethoxazole** is the treatment of choice for both pulmonary and extrapulmonary infections.

(a) Trimethoprim–sulfamethoxazole **prophylaxis** can prevent *P. carinii* pneumonia in most patients.

(b) **Adverse effects (rash, nausea,** and **fever)** are frequent in HIV-infected patients, but dose reduction may help alleviate them.

(2) Pentamidine isethionate

 (a) Pentamidine may be administered parenterally to treat *P. carinii* pneumonia. Aerosolized pentamidine is much less effective, but better tolerated, than parenteral pentamidine.

 (b) Adverse effects can be severe and include **hypo-** and **hyperglycemia, renal failure, arrhythmias,** and **orthostatic hypotension**.

(3) Dapsone has been used in combination with oral trimethoprim for treatment of mild or moderate *P. carinii* pneumonia.

(4) Atovaquone is better tolerated than trimethoprim–sulfamethoxazole, but it is less effective for *P. carinii* pneumonia.

2. Mycobacterial infections

a. General considerations. Both tuberculosis and atypical mycobacterial disease (caused by *M. avium* complex) occur in the course of HIV-induced immunosuppression.

 (1) Although the tuberculosis responds excellently to chemotherapy, AIDS patients infected with tuberculosis have a high mortality rate because of the recent increase in multiple-drug–resistant tuberculosis.

 (2) *M. avium* complex is acquired orally or is inhaled as a saprophyte. It progresses to a continuous bacteremia, infecting multiple organs. Concurrent infections with *Cryptosporidium* can occur; they present as gastrointestinal symptoms.

b. Therapeutic regimens

 (1) Therapeutic regimens for tuberculosis are discussed in IV A 2 c (4).

 (2) Rifampin (see IV C) is used in the treatment of atypical mycobacterial disease caused by *M. avium* complex.

3. Cytomegalovirus infections

a. General considerations. These are also common superinfections in patients with AIDS. Retinitis is a frequent manifestation.

b. Therapeutic regimens. Ganciclovir and foscarnet (see VIII C, D) are often used to treat cytomegalovirus in AIDS patients.

4. Toxoplasmosis

a. General considerations. The protozoan *Toxoplasma gondii* produces most intracranial mass lesions in AIDS patients; the lesions present as a global encephalitis.

b. Therapeutic regimens

 (1) The most effective available treatment is **pyrimethamine plus sulfadiazine**. However, the tissue–cyst form is resistant to these and other currently available agents.

 (2) Clindamycin with pyrimethamine is an alternative treatment for cerebral toxoplasmosis.

c. Prophylactic regimens. Trimethoprim–sulfamethoxazole appears to be effective.

5. Cryptococcosis

a. General considerations. *C. neoformans,* a fungus, is acquired by inhaling the organism. However, 80% of AIDS patients with cryptococcal disease develop cryptococcal meningitis.

b. Therapeutic regimens. Amphotericin B is currently the treatment of choice (see III B 1).

6. Herpes simplex virus and varicella-zoster virus

a. General considerations. Mucocutaneous herpes simplex virus infections can occur in HIV-infected patients.

b. Therapeutic regimens are discussed in VIII A and D.

DIRECTIONS: Each of the numbered items or incomplete statements in this section is followed by answers or by completions of the statement. Select the **one** numbered answer or completion that is **best** in each case.

1. A patient is being treated with an antibiotic for an acute uncomplicated urinary tract infection. A significant skin reaction occurs, leading to an exfoliative dermatitis. The mechanism of action of the antibiotic causing this condition is

(A) inactivation of transpeptidase
(B) interference with messenger RNA and ribosomal function
(C) prevention of the incorporation of para-aminobenzoic acid (PABA) into folic acid
(D) interference with DNA polymerase
(E) inhibition of reverse transcriptase

2. An intravenous drug addict enters the emergency room with a fever of 103° F and chills. It is determined that the patient has endocarditis. Blood cultures confirm the presence of methicillin-resistant *Staphylococcus aureus*. Correct parenteral therapy would include which drug?

(A) Amoxicillin
(B) Vancomycin
(C) Gentamicin
(D) Ampicillin
(E) Piperacillin

3. Which of the following agents is used to treat tapeworm infestations?

(A) Niclosamide
(B) Niridazole
(C) Piperazine
(D) Diloxanide
(E) Pentamidine

DIRECTIONS: Each of the numbered items or incomplete statements in this section is negatively phrased, as indicated by a capitalized word such as NOT, LEAST, or EXCEPT. Select the ONE lettered answer or completion that is BEST in each case.

4. Correct statements about vaccines include all of the following EXCEPT

(A) individuals vaccinated before age 12 months may require measles revaccination
(B) rubella vaccine is recommended for women of childbearing age
(C) influenza vaccine decreases influenza mortality among the elderly
(D) pneumococcal vaccine is recommended for people who are severely immunocompromised
(E) hepatitis B vaccine is recommended for individuals at high risk for hepatitis B (e.g., homosexuals, intravenous drug abusers)

5. All of the following statements about antiviral agents are true EXCEPT

(A) acyclovir may be given orally for primary herpes simplex virus infections
(B) foscarnet is the drug of choice for acyclovir-resistant herpes simplex and varicella-zoster virus
(C) amantadine may be given orally in conjunction with influenza vaccine
(D) relapse is common with continued treatment with ganciclovir for cytomegalovirus retinitis in AIDS patients
(E) treatment with interferon has proven unsuccessful in inducing remission in patients with chronic hepatitis B

6. All of the following statements regarding the treatment of tuberculosis are true EXCEPT

(A) drugs are used in combination to minimize resistance development
(B) the treatment of uncomplicated tuberculosis includes the use of isoniazid and rifampin daily for 6 months
(C) cloniazid continues to be the most widely used agent in the treatment and prophylaxis of tuberculosis
(D) urine, sweat, and tears can take on an orange color because of ethambutol administration
(E) the lack of compliance by patients being treated can lead to the development of resistance

7. A patient was recently diagnosed with Legionnaires' disease after returning from a cruise to Bermuda. The patient responds to antimicrobial therapy. The drug used to cure this individual has all of the following characteristics EXCEPT

(A) it is effective in children in curing *Streptococcus* impetigo
(B) it may cause epigastric distress
(C) it is also useful for the treatment of *Mycobacterium avium*
(D) it may cause thrombophlebitis when administered intravenously
(E) it is also effective against pneumonia resulting from *Mycoplasma*

8. All of the statements regarding clavulanic acid are true EXCEPT

(A) it is an irreversible lactamase inhibitor
(B) it is structurally related to the penicillins
(C) it is often combined with ciprofloxacin to treat infections caused by beta-lactamase–producing strains of *Haemophilus influenzae*
(D) it is often combined with amoxicillin to treat infections caused by beta-lactamase–producing strains of *Staphylococcus aureus*

9. A 14-year-old adolescent steps on a rusty nail. One month later, the diagnosis of *Staphylococcus aureus* osteomyelitis is made by x-ray and bone biopsy. Drugs that would be considered effective therapy include all of the following EXCEPT

(A) oxacillin
(B) norfloxacin
(C) cloxacillin
(D) nafcillin
(E) cefazolin

DIRECTIONS: Each set of matching questions in this section consists of a list of four to twenty-six lettered options (some of which may be in figures) followed by several numbered items. For each numbered item, select the ONE lettered option that is most closely associated with it. To avoid spending too much time on matching sets with large numbers of options, it is generally advisable to begin each set by reading the list of options. Then, for each item in the set, try to generate the correct answer and locate it in the option list, rather than evaluating each option individually. Each lettered option may be selected once, more than once, or not at all.

Questions 10–12

Match each description with the drug it best describes.

(A) Gentamicin
(B) Loracarbef
(C) Aztreonam
(D) Neomycin
(E) Tetracycline

10. An aminoglycoside that is often combined with polymixin and bacitracin for the treatment of topical infections

11. Can be substituted for gentamicin in the treatment of urinary tract infections

12. Has limited usefulness against gram-positive bacteria, because of the development of resistance

Questions 13–16

Match each statement with the drug it best describes.

(A) Amphotericin B
(B) Flucytosine
(C) Ketoconazole
(D) Itraconazole
(E) Fluconazole

13. Its mechanism of action is similar to nystatin

14. It is the most effective drug for treating systemic fungal infections in AIDS patients

15. The only fungicidal agent listed

16. Fever, chills, and decreased renal function can occur with intravenous administration

Questions 17–19

For each illness presented below, select the best combination therapy.

(A) Clofazimine plus dapsone plus rifampin
(B) Nafcillin plus gentamicin
(C) Zidovudine (AZT) plus didanosine (dideoxyinosine)
(D) Zidovudine (AZT) plus zalcitabine (dideoxycytidine)
(E) Pentamidine plus amantadine

17. A neutropenic patient is hospitalized with a fever of 104° F; blood cultures are drawn

18. A patient is diagnosed as having multibacillary leprosy

19. A patient was recently diagnosed with AIDS; an effort is made to delay clinical deterioration

1. The answer is C *[II A 2 a, 5 a (1), 7 a (1)].* Sulfonamides are the preferred agents for the treatment of acute uncomplicated urinary tract infections. Approximately 75% of untoward effects involve the skin. The mechanism of action for sulfonamides is the prevention of the incorporation of para-aminobenzoic acid (PABA) into folic acid. Penicillin combines with and inactivates transpeptidase. Aminoglycosides inhibit protein biosynthesis by acting directly on the ribosome; they interfere with the proper attachment of messenger RNA to ribosomes during the initiation of protein synthesis. Acyclovir interferes with DNA polymerase and inhibits viral DNA replication. Zidovudine (AZT) inhibits reverse transcriptase.

2. The answer is B *[II H 5 a].* Vancomycin is the drug of first choice in serious infection caused by methicillin-resistant *Staphylococcus aureus*. Amoxicillin, ampicillin, and piperacillin are penicillinase-sensitive antibiotics like methicillin and would not be indicated. Gentamicin, an aminoglycoside, is bactericidal against a wide variety of gram-negative organisms and some strains of *S. aureus*, but is not the drug of first choice.

3. The answer is A *[Table 12-8; Table 12-9].* Niclosamide is the drug of choice for the treatment of most tapeworms. Niridazole is used to treat schistosomiasis. Piperazine is used to treat ascariasis and pinworms. Diloxanide is an amebicide. Pentamidine is used in leishmaniasis and trypanosomiasis. Pentamidine is also used to treat *Pneumocystis carinii* pneumonia, which occurs in AIDS patients and in other immunosuppressed patients.

4. The answer is D *[IX A 1 b (3) (a), 2 b, 3 b (1), 4 b, B 4 b (1) (b)].* Pneumococcal vaccine is most effective in individuals with normal immune systems; it does not protect severely immunocompromised patients. Individuals born before 1956 are likely to be immune to measles and, thus, would not need the vaccine. However, revaccination is recommended for individuals vaccinated before age 12 months. Immunization with rubella vaccine is recommended for unimmunized women of childbearing age, because the aim is to prevent rubella infection in the fetus. Influenza vaccine decreases morbidity and mortality in the elderly. Hepatitis B vaccine is now made chemically via recombinant technology.

Homosexuals, hemophiliacs, intravenous drug abusers, and dialysis patients are all at high risk, and immunization is recommended.

5. The answer is E *[VIII A 3, 4 b, B 4 a (1) (a), C 4, D 3 b, F 3 c].* Treatment with interferon can induce clinical remission in 30%–40% of patients with chronic hepatitis B. Acyclovir has an enhanced affinity for the viral enzyme thymidine kinase, which makes it several hundredfold more toxic to herpes viruses than to mammalian cells. Acyclovir is effective against both type 1 and type 2 herpes simplex viruses. Foscarnet is the drug of choice for acyclovir-resistant herpes. Amantadine is given orally for prophylaxis of influenza A; it does not alter the immune response to influenza A vaccine and, therefore, can be given concurrently. Ganciclovir is indicated for the treatment of cytomegalovirus retinitis in AIDS patients; however, relapse has been reported with continued treatment.

6. The answer is D *[IV A 2, C 7 a; Table 12-7].* Urine, sweat, and tears can take on a harmless orange color as the result of rifampin administration. Reversible visual disturbances, including optic neuritis and red–green color-blindness, can occur with ethambutol administration. Drugs are used in combination to minimize resistance development. Lack of patient compliancy is a key factor in the development of resistant strains; administration of drugs under supervision may become necessary to minimize the development of resistant microorganisms. Isoniazid continues to be one of the most widely used agents, and along with rifampin, is used in the treatment of uncomplicated tuberculosis.

7. The answer is C *[II F 5, 7 a (2)–(3)].* The erythromycin macrolide "cousins," clarithromycin and azithromycin, have shown promise for the treatment of *Mycobacterium avium* in AIDS patients; however, erythromycin is not effective against this pathogen. Erythromycin is effective in treating Legionnaires' disease. Adverse effects of erythromycin include epigastric upset and, when administered intravenously, thrombophlebitis. *Mycoplasma* pneumonia is also effectively treated with erythromycin.

8. The answer is C *[II B 1 c, e (4) (a)].* Clavulanic acid is an irreversible beta-lactamase inhibitor that is structurally related to the penicillins. It extends the spectrum of beta-lactamase antibiotics such as amoxicillin, but is not combined with quinolones (e.g., cipro-floxacin).

9. The answer is B *[II B 2 g (2), 3 f (1); Table 12-5]*. Norfloxacin is a quinolone antiinfective, and is used only for urinary tract infections. Nafcillin, oxacillin, and cloxacillin are all penicillinase-resistant penicillins that would effectively treat the osteomyelitis. Cefazolin, a first-generation cephalosporin, would also be effective.

10–12. The answers are: 10-D *[II C 7 d (1)]*, **11-C** *[II B 5 e (1)]*, **12-E** *[II D 4 a]*. Neomycin is often combined with polymyxin and baci-tracin for topical use as a broad-spectrum antibiotic.

Aztreonam, a monobactam, can be substituted for aminoglycosides in the treatment of urinary tract infections.

The use of tetracyclines for treatment of infectious disease has declined because of increasing bacterial resistance.

13–16. The answers are: 13-A *[III B 1 b]*, **14-A** *[III B 1 e (1)]*, **15-A** *[III A 1 b, B 1 b]*, **16-A** *[III B 1 g]*. Amphotericin B, which has a mechanism of action similar to that of nystatin, is the only fungicidal agent listed. It is the most effective drug available for systemic fungal infections; however, toxicity (fever, chills, and nephrotoxicity) limits its use to life-threatening infections. Flucytosine is sometimes given with amphotericin B for the initial treatment of rapidly progressive fungal infections. Keto-conazole, itraconazole, and fluconazole are fungistatic agents that have a better safety profile than amphotericin B, but they are not as effective in life-threatening fungal infections.

17–19. The answers are: 17-B *[I C 3 a (2)]*, **18-A** *[V B 4 a, 5 a]*, **19-C** *[X B 2 b, 3 b]*. Initial (blind) therapy, using nafcillin and gentamicin, should be administered to a seriously ill individual after blood cultures are taken. These drugs will provide complete gram-positive and gram-negative coverage until the results of cultures are available.

Clofazimine exerts a slow bactericidal effect on *Mycobacterium leprae*. It is used in combination with dapsone and rifampin in multi-bacillary leprosy to prevent the emergence of resistance.

In AIDS patients, the sequential use of zidovudine (AZT) and didanosine (dideoxyino-sine) appears to delay clinical deterioration. Zidovudine (AZT) and zalcitabine (dideoxycy-tidine) is a more appropriate therapy for patients with advanced HIV infection.

Chapter 13
Principles of Drug Interactions

I. INTRODUCTION

A. **Definition.** A **drug interaction** occurs whenever the pharmacologic action of a drug is altered by a second substance. Theoretically, this change may be related to:

1. **Pharmacokinetic interactions**—that is, differences in the **plasma levels** of a drug achieved with a given dose of that drug

2. **Pharmacodynamic interactions**—that is, differences in **effects** produced by a given plasma level of a drug

B. **General considerations**

1. Although many examples of drug interactions are known, many are *not* clinically important. Clinically important changes often are seen with agents having a low therapeutic index (e.g., cardiac glycosides) or a poorly defined therapeutic endpoint (e.g., antipsychotic agents).

2. Often drug interactions can be avoided by using a different drug that has the desired pharmacologic effect, but not the unwanted interaction.

II. PHARMACOKINETIC INTERACTIONS

A. **General considerations**

1. The duration and intensity of a drug's action are a function of the plasma level of the drug, which is related directly to the drug's rates of absorption, distribution, metabolism, and excretion. One or more of these rates may be altered by the following:
   a. Concomitant or previous drug therapy
   b. Dietary factors
   c. Exposure to environmental chemicals; that is, to chemicals not used for therapeutic purposes

2. Physical factors, such as the ambient temperature, and effects of disease (e.g., fever) can also alter the pharmacokinetic properties of drugs but will not be considered here.

B. **Interactions affecting the systemic delivery of drugs**

1. **Drug interactions in vitro.** Some drugs are **incompatible** with intravenous infusion fluids.
   a. Ampicillin, ascorbic acid, chlorpromazine, barbiturates, and promethazine react **with dextran solutions**. The drugs break down or form chemical complexes.
   b. Benzylpenicillin (penicillin G), chlorpromazine, erythromycin, gentamicin, hydrocortisone, kanamycin, methicillin, promazine, streptomycin, and tetracyclines react **with heparin solutions**. Chemical complexes form.

2. Drug absorption interactions in vivo

a. Altered absorption after parenteral administration is not common but can occur.

(1) For example, a subcutaneous or intramuscular injection of epinephrine or methacholine given concomitantly with another drug will alter the entry of the other drug into nearby capillaries.

(2) This occurs because of the vasoconstricting or vasodilating effects of the accompanying adrenergic or cholinergic agonist.

b. Altered absorption after oral administration is more commonly observed.

(1) Complexes can be formed. For example:

(a) Tetracycline and cations, such as calcium (e.g., in milk and some antacids) or aluminum ion (e.g., in some antacids), combine to produce an insoluble salt, which results in very poor and erratic tetracycline blood levels.

(b) Cholestyramine binds acidic compounds, cardiac glycosides, and thyroxine, blocking their absorption.

(2) Intestinal motility can be altered. The ultimate effect on drug absorption in this case depends upon the site at which the drug is primarily absorbed (small intestine, stomach).

(a) For example, anticholinergic agents (e.g., atropine) and opiate-like agents delay gastric emptying and slow the absorption of some drugs, such as acetaminophen, which are absorbed in the intestine.

(b) Stimulation of gastrointestinal motility can reduce drug absorption. For example, metoclopramide decreases absorption of cimetidine, which is absorbed primarily in the stomach.

(3) Absorption can be blocked. For example:

(a) Phenytoin and oral contraceptives inhibit the hydrolysis of folic acid (to the monoglutamate) in the gut, and thus, they reduce its absorption.

(b) Colchicine produces malabsorption of vitamin B_{12}.

(c) Milk products and antacids may decrease fluoroquinolone absorption.

(4) Diet may influence drug absorption.

(a) The presence of food in the stomach may exert a nonspecific effect in reducing or slowing the absorption of some drugs.

(b) A fatty meal will increase the absorption of lipid-soluble drugs (e.g., griseofulvin).

(5) Changes in gastric pH can alter absorption.

(a) Weak acids, such as salicylates, are not absorbed well when the gastric pH is elevated with antacids.

(b) Ketoconazole is poorly absorbed in the absence of gastric acidity.

c. Monoamine oxidase (MAO) inhibitors block oxidative deamination of naturally occurring monoamines, including tyramine.

(1) Many fermented foods contain tyramine, which is formed as a bacterial breakdown product of tyrosine.

(2) Exogenous tyramine can result in the release of norepinephrine and epinephrine, resulting in severe headache and hypertensive crisis.

C. Interactions affecting drug distribution

1. Competition for plasma protein–binding sites. Many drugs, especially acidic ones, bind to plasma proteins. Drugs, and also other substances, can compete for plasma protein–binding sites.

a. The effect is often to release more free drug and, thus, enhance its pharmacologic effect.

b. This mechanism is especially significant when a high percentage of the drug (over 90%) is normally protein-bound, as is the case with coumarin anticoagulants, sulfonamides, salicylates, indomethacin, and most other nonsteroidal anti-inflammatory agents. For example:

(1) Sulfisoxazole in premature infants increases the likelihood of fatal kernicterus because the sulfonamide displaces bilirubin from protein-binding sites.

(2) Phenylbutazone potentiates the anticoagulant actions of warfarin by this mechanism and may cause excessive bleeding.

2. Displacement of a plasma protein–bound drug can result in complex changes in the pharmacologic effects of the drug that can be difficult to predict.
   a. There is a transient rise in the plasma levels of free drug, but the plasma half-life is frequently reduced.
   b. A marked increase in the pharmacologic effect can occur if the normal route of drug elimination is impaired by disease (e.g., cirrhosis) or by saturation of metabolizing enzymes required for drug elimination.

D. | **Interactions affecting drug metabolism**

   1. Rate of biotransformation. The most common and most important cause for differences in plasma levels of a drug is a change in the rate of biotransformation of the drug.

   2. Rate of first-pass metabolism. Variations in a person's plasma drug levels are more common with drugs that undergo extensive gastrointestinal metabolism or first-pass hepatic metabolism (e.g., propranolol).

   3. Inhibition of metabolism. Many drugs that are inactivated by biotransformation can have a prolonged duration of action if their metabolism is inhibited by other agents. For example, fluoroquinolones (especially enoxacin) inhibit the biotransformation of methylxanthines and may cause theophylline and caffeine toxicity.

   4. Inhibition of nonmicrosomal enzymes [see Chapter 1 II D 2 a (2)]
   a. Drugs that can inhibit MAO, such as the antitumor agent procarbazine and the antidepressant tranylcypromine, can retard the metabolism of various drugs, such as barbiturates and benzodiazepines, and of amines, such as serotonin and norepinephrine. All selective serotonin reuptake inhibitors, including paroxetine, can cause a life-threatening reaction characterized by hyperthermia, rigidity, and coma if administered concurrently with an MAO inhibitor. After stopping paroxetine therapy, patients should not take an MAO inhibitor for at least 2 weeks, and vice versa.
   b. Because 6-mercaptopurine is inactivated in part by xanthine oxidase, the concurrent administration of the xanthine oxidase inhibitor, allopurinol, can result in an accumulation of 6-mercaptopurine with a consequent increase in bone marrow depression.
   c. Disulfiram inhibits acetaldehyde dehydrogenase and, thus, prevents acetaldehyde, the oxidation product of ethanol, from being further metabolized. The resultant accumulation of acetaldehyde causes flushing, nausea, vomiting, and tachycardia.
   d. Any drug that inhibits hepatic metabolism may increase the risk of arrhythmias in patients taking terfenadine.

   5. Induction or inhibition of microsomal enzymes (mixed-function oxygenases, or the cytochrome P-450 system) can also affect drug metabolism [see Chapter 1 II D 2 a (1)].
   a. Inducers. More than 200 drugs and a large number of dietary and environmental chemicals are known inducers of this enzyme system.
      (1) Induction of mixed-function oxygenases results in an accelerated metabolism of substrates.
      (2) The induction is due to new protein synthesis. The pattern of the newly synthesized proteins and the rate of appearance of new mixed-function oxygenase activities differ with different inducers.
      (3) Some inducers of mixed-function oxygenases are:
         (a) Barbiturates, glutethimide, phenytoin
         (b) Polycyclic aromatic hydrocarbons, such as benzopyrene
         (c) Halogenated hydrocarbon insecticides (e.g., DDT)
         (d) Nicotine
         (e) Ethanol, when ingested chronically
      (4) Some inducers stimulate their own metabolism.

    b. Inhibitors. There are also a number of inhibitors of mixed-function oxygenases, including:
      (1) Organophosphorus insecticides
      (2) Carbon tetrachloride
      (3) Ozone
      (4) Carbon monoxide
      (5) Cimetidine
      (6) Omeprazole

E. **Interactions affecting drug excretion**

    1. Reduction in urinary elimination. Many weak organic acids (e.g., aspirin, penicillin, methotrexate) are excreted by a common **transport system** in the proximal tubules. Competition for this transport system by weak acids can result in a reduction in the urinary elimination of the competing drugs. (Comparable interactions between weak organic bases have not been well characterized in humans.) For example:
      a. Probenecid can block the excretion of penicillin, indomethacin, cefazolin, and methotrexate.
      b. Aspirin can block the excretion of methotrexate and, thus, cause serious adverse effects.
      c. Angiotensin-converting enzyme (ACE) inhibitors may decrease renal excretion of lithium.

    2. Changes in urinary pH can influence the elimination of weak acids and bases because their passive reabsorption requires that they be un-ionized. This mechanism can be important in the treatment of overdoses of weak acids and bases (e.g., aspirin or amphetamines).
      a. Agents that alkalinize the urine (e.g., acetazolamide or sodium bicarbonate) will increase the excretion of weak acids.
      b. Agents that acidify the urine (e.g., ammonium chloride) will enhance the elimination of weak bases.

    3. Changes in urinary volume, such as with diuretics, often can reduce the renal toxicity of chemicals and drugs, presumably by reducing the tubular concentration of the toxin. For example, mannitol reduces cisplatin toxicity.

    4. Stimulation of biliary excretion by some drugs can alter the elimination of other drugs.
      a. For example, phenobarbital enhances the biliary excretion of many drugs by increasing both bile flow and the synthesis of proteins that function in the biliary conjugation–excretion mechanism.
      b. Activated charcoal and cholestyramine increase the excretion of drugs that undergo extensive enterohepatic recirculation by binding to them in the gastrointestinal tract.

III. PHARMACODYNAMIC INTERACTIONS

A. **Receptor interactions.** Drug interactions can occur at the level of the **drug receptor**. For example, the H_2-receptor antagonist cimetidine blocks the action of histamine-like agonists, such as betazole, by this mechanism.

B. **Physiologic interactions.** Agents can reduce the effect of other drugs by acting via different cellular mechanisms (**physiologic antagonism**). For example, acetylcholine and norepinephrine have opposing effects on heart rate (see Chapter 1 III A 1 b, D 4).

C. **Drug interactions**

1. Agents can **enhance the action of other drugs** although they act via different cellular mechanisms. For example, ethanol can enhance the central nervous system depression caused by opioids or tranquilizers.

2. The action of one drug can be influenced by **changes in the intracellular or extracellular environment** that are caused by another drug. For example, diuretic-induced hypokalemia can increase the possibility of digitalis-induced cardiac toxicity.

3. **Chemical inactivation** can occur systemically to reduce a drug's action. For example, protamine binds to heparin, thereby neutralizing it.

STUDY QUESTIONS

DIRECTIONS: Each of the numbered items or incomplete statements in this section is followed by answers or by completions of the statement. Select the ONE numbered answer or completion that is BEST in each case.

1. A classic example of the inhibition of renal secretion of a drug is the interaction between probenecid and

(A) streptomycin
(B) chloramphenicol
(C) chlortetracycline
(D) penicillin
(E) neomycin

2. The concomitant administration of antacids with tetracycline will reduce the effectiveness of the antibiotic because

(A) antacids inhibit the absorption of tetracycline
(B) antacids stimulate the drug microsomal metabolizing system, so that the tetracycline is metabolized more rapidly
(C) ions in antacids solubilize the tetracycline
(D) antacids enhance the renal excretion of tetracycline
(E) high blood levels of tetracycline result in increased protein binding

3. Drinking beer after taking disulfiram causes flushing, nausea, and tachycardia. This occurs because disulfiram inhibits the

(A) accumulation of acetaldehyde
(B) metabolism of acetaldehyde
(C) excretion of acetaldehyde
(D) intestinal transport of acetaldehyde
(E) protein binding of acetaldehyde

DIRECTIONS: Each of the numbered items or incomplete statements in this section is negatively phrased, as indicated by a capitalized word such as NOT, LEAST, or EXCEPT. Select the ONE lettered answer or completion that is BEST in each case.

4. Pharmacokinetic drug interactions can result from all of the following EXCEPT

(A) impaired absorption
(B) induction of the drug microsomal enzyme metabolizing system
(C) inhibition of the drug microsomal enzyme metabolizing system
(D) inhibition of renal excretion
(E) the combination of a bacteriostatic antibiotic and a bactericidal antibiotic

5. A depressed patient has been taking a monoamine oxidase (MAO) inhibitor for years. She consults a new psychiatrist, but does not tell him about her psychoactive therapy. The psychiatrist initiates paroxetine therapy. All of the following may occur EXCEPT

(A) hyperthermia
(B) rigidity
(C) hemorrhage
(D) coma
(E) death

6. All of the following statements concerning interactions that affect renal drug excretion are correct EXCEPT

(A) aspirin blocks the excretion of methotrexate
(B) probenecid blocks the excretion of indomethacin
(C) captopril increases the excretion of lithium
(D) sodium bicarbonate increases the excretion of aspirin
(E) probenecid blocks the excretion of methotrexate

7. All of the following are drug interactions that affect absorption EXCEPT

(A) tetracycline—milk
(B) tetracycline—antacids containing aluminum
(C) tetracycline—cimetidine
(D) cholestyramine—cardiac glycosides
(E) cholestyramine—thyroxine

8. All of the following agents would be capable of inducing the cytochrome P-450 metabolizing system EXCEPT

(A) barbiturates
(B) cimetidine
(C) DDT
(D) glutethimide
(E) phenytoin

DIRECTIONS: Each set of matching questions in this section consists of a list of four to twenty-six lettered options (some of which may be in figures) followed by several items. For each numbered item, select the ONE lettered option that is most closely associated with it. To avoid spending too much time on matching sets with large numbers of options, it is generally advisable to begin each set by reading the list of options. Then, for each item in the set, try to generate the correct answer and locate it in the option list, rather than evaluating each option individually. Each lettered option may be selected once, more than once, or not at all.

Questions 9–13

Barbiturates can be involved in drug interactions with many other drugs. For each drug listed below, select the mechanism that is the most likely cause of an interaction with a barbiturate.

(A) Incompatibility in vitro
(B) Induction of microsomal enzymes
(C) Inhibition of nonmicrosomal enzymes
(D) Enhancement of pharmacologic effects
(E) Interference with renal excretion

 9. Warfarin

10. Dextran

11. Tranylcypromine

12. Digitoxin

13. Phenothiazines

ANSWERS AND EXPLANATIONS

1. The answer is D *[II E 1 a]*. Probenecid is capable of blocking the renal tubular excretion of penicillin G, thereby prolonging its half-life. In fact, probenecid was originally developed for this purpose, in the days when penicillin was in short supply. Probenecid also blocks the renal excretion of many other drugs. However, the renal excretion of streptomycin, chloramphenicol, chlortetracycline, oxytetracycline, or neomycin would not be significantly affected by the coadministration of probenecid.

2. The answer is A *[II B 2 b]*. Low blood levels of tetracycline result from the concomitant administration of antacids. Antacids inhibit the absorption of tetracycline because ions, such as calcium and aluminum, in the antacids chelate the tetracycline. Antacids do not stimulate or inhibit the drug microsomal metabolizing system, nor do they enhance the renal excretion of tetracycline. Antacids would decrease, not increase, blood levels of tetracycline.

3. The answer is B *[II D 4 c]*. Disulfiram inhibits the enzyme acetaldehyde dehydrogenase and consequently inhibits the metabolism of acetaldehyde, the oxidation product of ethanol. The resulting accumulation of acetaldehyde causes flushing, nausea, and tachycardia.

4. The answer is E *[II A 1, B 2, D 5, E]*. Pharmacokinetic drug interactions are those that involve altered plasma levels of a drug. All of the factors in the question can result in altered plasma levels of a drug after its administration except for the combination of a bacteriostatic antibiotic with a bactericidal one. The latter is a pharmacodynamic type of drug interaction because plasma drug levels are not altered. Instead, the bacteriostatic agent can block the desirable actions of the bactericidal antibiotic by preventing cell replication.

5. The answer is C *[II D 4]*. Hemorrhage does not occur when a serotonin reuptake inhibitor (e.g., paroxetine) is administered concurrently with a monoamine oxidase (MAO) inhibitor. The resultant reaction is, however, potentially life-threatening and is characterized by hyperthermia, rigidity, and coma.

6. The answer is C *[II E 1–2]*. Angiotensin-converting enzyme (ACE) inhibitors (e.g., captopril) decrease, not increase, the renal excretion of lithium. Many weak organic acids are excreted by a common transport system in the proximal tubule. Probenecid blocks the renal excretion of indomethacin, methotrexate, penicillin, and other agents secreted in the proximal tubule. Aspirin can block the excretion of methotrexate. Sodium bicarbonate, which alkalinizes the urine, increases the excretion of aspirin.

7. The answer is C *[II B 2 b (1)]*. Tetracyclines do not interact with the H_2-receptor antagonist cimetidine. Tetracyclines do form insoluble complexes with cations, such as the calcium in milk and aluminum in antacids. The anion-exchange resin, cholestyramine, binds both cardiac glycosides and thyroxine, thus blocking their absorption.

8. The answer is B *[II D 5 a]*. Barbiturates, glutethimide, phenytoin, and DDT are capable of inducing the cytochrome P-450 metabolizing system, so that they all would enhance the metabolism of other agents degraded by this system. The induction of mixed-function oxygenases results from new protein synthesis. Cimetidine inhibits the activity of cytochrome P-450, thereby slowing the metabolism of many drugs that are substrates for hepatic mixed-function oxidases.

9–13. The answers are: 9-B *[Chapter 3 II A 5 g]*, **10-A** *[Chapter 13 II B 1 a]*, **11-C** *[Chapter 13 II D 4 a]*, **12-B** *[Chapter 3 II A 5 g]*, **13-D** *[Chapter 3 II A 5 a]*. Most drug interactions involving the barbiturates result from induction of hepatic microsomal enzymes by the barbiturate; this causes accelerated metabolism of the other drug (e.g., warfarin, digitoxin, corticosteroids, and β blockers, to name only a few).

Dextran solutions are incompatible with various drugs, including barbiturates.

Tranylcypromine is an inhibitor of monoamine oxidase (MAO), a nonmicrosomal enzyme, and this can retard the metabolism of a barbiturate.

A barbiturate plus another CNS depressant (e.g., a phenothiazide, ethanol, or an antihistamine) can cause marked depression.

Chapter 14
Poisons and Antidotes

I. INTRODUCTION

A. **Definition. Toxicology** is the study of poisons, including their actions, adverse effects, and treatment of the conditions that they produce. These poisons include household, environmental, industrial, or pharmacologic substances.

B. **Subdivisions of toxicology**

1. **Experimental toxicology** involves the investigation of the toxic effects of chemicals on biologic systems.

2. **Clinical toxicology** involves the diagnosis and treatment of poisonings.

3. **Environmental toxicology** involves the identification and elimination of environmental poisons.

C. **Poisons and their antidotes**

1. A variety of industrial solvents, heavy metals, gases, and common household chemicals can be dangerous poisons. Drugs that are used clinically may also be poisons in high doses.

2. Acute exposure to a toxic substance is likely to produce different symptoms than symptoms produced by chronic exposure to lower concentrations.

3. Antidotes have been developed for some poisons. These act either by preventing absorption or by inactivating or antagonizing the actions of the poisons.

D. **Quantitative toxicity**

1. **Median lethal dose (LD$_{50}$)** is the smallest dose of a given chemical that will kill 50% of a test group of animals. The LD$_{50}$ is used to extrapolate the toxic potential of a compound to humans. It is used with all routes of poisoning except inhalation.

2. **Median lethal concentration (LC$_{50}$)** is the smallest concentration of a given chemical that will kill 50% of a test group of animals. It is applicable to chemicals that are inhaled. The LC$_{50}$ is expressed relative to the duration of exposure.

3. **Threshold limit value (TLV)** is the maximal amount of a chemical that is considered safe. Industrial and governmental hygienists provide an official listing of the TLV levels of airborne poisons to which workers may safely be exposed for an 8-hour period.

II. SPECIFIC POISONS

A. **Gaseous poisons**

1. **Simple asphyxiants** are usually inert industrial gases, such as **nitrogen** (N_2), **carbon dioxide** (CO_2), and **methane** (CH_4). Asphyxiants decrease the oxygen available to the lungs and cause hypoxia.

2. **Irritants** that affect the respiratory tract can cause asphyxia.
   a. **Water-soluble irritants** affect the eyes and upper respiratory tract. They can affect the lungs and can be corrosive. Examples include **hydrochloric acid** (HCl), **hydrofluoric acid** (HF), **sulfur dioxide** (SO_2), and **ammonia** (NH_3).
   b. **Water-insoluble irritants** can be trapped in nasopharyngeal secretions and can descend into the alveoli, causing pneumonitis and pulmonary edema. Examples include **chlorine gas** and **ozone**.

3. **Systemic toxicants** are absorbed by inhalation or percutaneously.
   a. **Cyanide** (hydrocyanic acid, HCN) is one of the most rapidly acting poisons.
      (1) **Mechanism of action.** Cyanide anions form complexes with ferric ions of the cytochrome oxidase system, interfering with electron transfer in the **cytochrome a–a₃ complex**. This leads to a blockage in oxygen transfer to tissues and causes a cytotoxic hypoxia.
      (2) **Diagnosis.** The patient's breath has the characteristic odor of oil of bitter almond, which should assist in diagnosis.
      (3) **Treatment** must be rapid and is designed to prevent or reverse the cyanide–ferric ion binding in the cytochrome oxidase system.
         (a) **Amyl nitrite** is administered by inhalation, accompanied by **intravenous sodium nitrite**.
            (i) Nitrite oxidizes a limited amount of hemoglobin to methemoglobin, which has a greater affinity for cyanide ion than does cytochrome a–a₃.
            (ii) The cyanide–cytochrome complex, therefore, dissociates, and normal oxidative metabolism resumes.
         (b) **Thiosulfate.** A mitochondrial trans-sulfurase can convert cyanide to thiocyanate, which is relatively nontoxic. This detoxification can be increased by the intravenous administration of thiosulfate.
         (c) **Gastric lavage.** If the cyanide has been ingested, gastric lavage should follow the above-mentioned treatment procedures.
   b. **Carbon monoxide** is the most common cause of accidental and suicidal poisoning.
      (1) **General considerations**
         (a) Carbon monoxide is an odorless, colorless, and tasteless gas.
         (b) Two common sources of carbon monoxide are houses with inadequate ventilation and automobile exhaust systems.
      (2) **Pharmacokinetics and mechanism of action**
         (a) Carbon monoxide is absorbed and excreted by the lungs.
         (b) The affinity of hemoglobin for carbon monoxide is about 220 times greater than its affinity for oxygen.
            (i) Exposure to very high ambient concentrations of carbon monoxide can result in rapid death with no premonitory signs.
            (ii) Exposure to lower concentrations of carbon monoxide will cause unconsciousness, then coma, followed by convulsions and death.
      (3) **Diagnosis.** Usually the circumstances surrounding acute carbon monoxide poisoning, such as a running automobile engine, combined with the patient's "cherry red" cyanosis, will make the diagnosis obvious.
      (4) **Treatment**
         (a) The patient should be removed from the air containing carbon monoxide and may require resuscitation.
         (b) **Oxygen (100%)** should be administered, which reduces the half-life of carboxyhemoglobin from 5 hours to 1 hour.
            (i) When the poisoning is severe, hypobaric oxygen therapy at a pressure of 2–3 atm is recommended, which reduces the half-life of carboxyhemoglobin to 20 minutes.
            (ii) Oxygen should be given until the level of carboxyhemoglobin decreases to at least 10%.
         (c) Patients may also require treatment for hypotension, metabolic acidosis, and cardiac effects.

4. Organic solvents
   a. General considerations
   (1) Organic solvents have an appreciable vapor pressure, are volatile, and can become an inhalation hazard, especially in an industrial environment.
   (2) They are fat-soluble and can be absorbed through the skin, accumulating in both fat and nervous tissue.
   b. Classification. Classes of toxic organic solvents include:
   (1) Saturated hydrocarbons, such as pentane, hexane, heptane, and octane
   (2) Unsaturated hydrocarbons, such as kerosene
   (3) Aromatic compounds, such as benzene and toluene
   (4) Halogenated hydrocarbons, such as methylene dichloride, dichloromethane, chloroform, and carbon tetrachloride
   c. Adverse effects. The toxic manifestations of organic solvents vary with the individual substance.
   d. Treatment. In general, the best and only therapy is to remove the individual from the exposure to the solvent.

B. Heavy metal intoxication

1. Mechanism of action
   a. All of the heavy metals bind to a wide variety of macromolecules in membranes and the cytosol. Because heavy metals are not metabolized, they may accumulate in the body.
   b. The heavy metals can inactivate important enzyme activities, and disrupt membranes.
   c. Because of the diverse affinities for the multiple organic ligands, it has been difficult to identify a single molecular target for the toxicity of these substances.

2. Specific intoxicants
   a. Arsenic poisoning can be produced by absorption from lungs, gastrointestinal tract, and skin.
   (1) Pharmacokinetics and mechanism of action
   (a) Arsenic is often used in household plant-spray pesticides as lead arsenate.
   (b) The trivalent form (As^{3-}) is toxic and binds to thiol groups of enzymes and other proteins in tissue.
   (c) Tolerance to chronic arsenic poisoning can develop.
   (2) Adverse effects
   (a) Acute poisoning causes hypotension, capillary transudation, muscle spasms, vertigo, delirium, and interference with kidney function.
   (b) Chronic poisoning results in persistent capillary dilation, malaise, and fatigue. Encephalopathy, peripheral neuritis, and sensory loss can occur.
   (3) Diagnosis. Sulfhydryl-rich tissues—namely, nails and hair—take up arsenic, producing pale bands in the fingernails and toenails that are useful in diagnosis.
   (4) Treatment. The **antidote** for arsenic poisoning is **dimercaprol** (see II B 3 a). Dimercaprol contains sulfhydryl groups, which compete with sulfhydryl moieties on proteins for the arsenic.
   b. Lead is the most common cause of heavy metal poisoning, especially in large urban areas.
   (1) Pharmacokinetics and mechanism of action
   (a) Acute poisoning is rare. Exposure has been markedly reduced because of stringent regulations on the use of lead in paints and other products. The most common routes of absorption of lead are the gastrointestinal tract and respiratory system.
   (b) Organic lead poisoning
   (i) This is rare, except among "gasoline sniffers."
   (ii) Tetraethyl lead is found in some gasoline and can be absorbed when inhaled.
   (iii) Penetration can also occur via the skin because tetraethyl lead is fat-soluble.

(iv) Eventually, the organic lead is converted in the body to inorganic lead, producing the symptoms of chronic lead poisoning.

(2) **Diagnosis**

(a) Wristdrop and to a lesser extent footdrop occur as a result of degenerative changes in motor neurons.

(b) An abdominal syndrome, consisting of constipation, anorexia, and a persistent metallic taste, appears early in the course of lead poisoning.

(c) A black "lead line" can occur on the gums but may be absent if the intoxicated person practices good dental hygiene.

(d) Because the distribution of lead is similar to that of calcium, lead is deposited in and mobilized from bone.

(e) Lead is a potent inhibitor of hemoglobin synthesis and produces a normocytic hypochromic anemia. A reticulocytosis can also occur.

(f) A characteristic basophilic stippling of red blood cells often occurs.

(g) Increased coproporphyrin and δ-aminolevulinic acid levels are found in the urine.

(h) The most serious manifestation is **lead encephalopathy**.

(i) The patient will often demonstrate clumsiness, irritability, vertigo, and projectile vomiting.

(ii) The condition must be differentiated from meningitis.

(iii) A fatality rate as high as 25% has been reported. In addition, 40% of the survivors demonstrate various neurologic abnormalities, including seizures, cerebral palsy, optic atrophy, and mental retardation.

(3) **Treatment** consists of intravenous infusions of calcium disodium ethylenediamine tetraacetic acid (edetate calcium disodium, $CaNa_2EDTA$; see II B 3 b).

(a) Initially (for 3–5 days), $CaNa_2EDTA$ is given in combination with dimercaprol.

(b) Oral penicillamine, which is a good chelator of lead, can be given as long-term therapy (for 3–6 months) after the initial dimercaprol and $CaNa_2EDTA$ therapy.

c. **Mercury**

(1) **Pharmacokinetics and mechanism of action**

(a) Toxicity can occur by inhalation, skin penetration, or ingestion of substances containing mercury.

(i) Mercurial fungicides are present in some latex paints and can be inhaled.

(ii) Dermal application of methylmercury ointments can result in absorption through the skin.

(iii) Inorganic mercury preparations can be ingested, resulting in acute poisoning, in contrast to the two instances above, which usually produce chronic poisoning.

(b) Mercurous (Hg^+) salts are less toxic than mercuric (Hg^{2+}) salts because they are less soluble, resulting in decreased skin penetration.

(c) Mercury is capable of attaching to sulfhydryl groups of enzymes and other proteins. In addition, it concentrates in the kidney.

(2) **Diagnosis**

(a) Acute intoxication can result in cardiovascular collapse and anuria.

(b) Chronic intoxication resulting from inhalation or skin penetration can produce:

(i) Neurologic manifestations, including irritability, tremors, and psychosis

(ii) Mercuria lentis, a brown discoloration of the anterior portion of the optic lens

(iii) Gingivitis and stomatitis

(iv) Progressive renal damage

(3) **Treatment.** Dimercaprol is used in the treatment of mercury poisoning. Diaphoresis can be used adjunctively.

d. **Other metals**

(1) **Antimony** produces effects similar to those of arsenic. Chronic poisoning can result in myocardial damage.

(2) Gold produces effects similar to those of arsenic.

(3) Nickel is a sensitizing agent and causes a dermatitis known as "nickel itch."

(4) Beryllium is an industrial hazard capable of causing a chronic granulomatous condition somewhat similar to sarcoidosis. In some instances, lung carcinoma can occur.

(5) Zinc intoxication can occur from inhalation of fresh fumes in smelting, causing a condition known as "metal-fume fever." Delayed chills with fever lasting up to 36 hours can occur. Tolerance develops with chronic exposure.

3. **Chelating agents as antidotes** (Table 14-1)

  a. Dimercaprol (2,3-dimercaptopropanol, British antilewisite, **BAL**)

    (1) Mechanism of action. Dimercaprol forms stable chelates, enhancing their excretion.

    (2) Preparations and administration. Dimercaprol cannot be administered orally. It is administered intramuscularly as a 10% solution of dimercaprol in oil. It is most effective when administered within 1–2 hours after toxic ingestion.

    (3) Therapeutic uses. Dimercaprol is indicated for the treatment of arsenic, antimony, gold, lead, and mercury poisoning.

    (4) Adverse effects include a dose-related rise in blood pressure and tachycardia. Nausea, vomiting, and headache, as well as a burning sensation of the lips and mouth, have been reported. The drug is potentially nephrotoxic.

  b. CaNa$_2$EDTA

    (1) Mechanism of action. CaNa$_2$EDTA forms stable, soluble metal chelates.

    (2) Preparations and administration

      (a) The calcium disodium derivative of EDTA (CaNa$_2$EDTA) is recommended rather than Na$_2$EDTA because CaNa$_2$EDTA is less likely to cause hypocalcemia tetany.

      (b) Because of poor oral absorption, it is administered intramuscularly. Pain occurs at the site of intramuscular injection.

      (c) It is not metabolized and is rapidly excreted.

    (3) Therapeutic uses. CaNa$_2$EDTA is used principally for lead poisoning but has been used for iron, copper, and zinc poisoning as well.

    (4) Adverse effects. Hydropic degeneration of the proximal tubule has been reported, but generally CaNa$_2$EDTA has a low toxicity potential.

  c. Penicillamine and N-acetylpenicillamine

    (1) Mechanism of action. Penicillamine forms stable, soluble metal chelates. The *l*-isomer is a pyridoxine antagonist.

    (2) Therapeutic uses. These orally administered agents are used for the treatment of heavy-metal poisoning. It is particularly effective in chelating copper.

    (3) Adverse effects. D-Penicillamine has caused serious allergic, hematologic, and renal toxicity.

TABLE 14-1. Antidotes for Heavy Metal Intoxication

Toxicant	Antidote
Arsenic	Dimercaprol
Lead	CaNa$_2$EDTA (initial) Penicillamine (chronic)
Mercury	Dimercaprol
Antimony	Dimercaprol
Gold	Dimercaprol
Copper	Penicillamine
Iron	Deferoxamine

CaNa$_2$EDTA = calcium disodium ethylenediamine tetraacetic acid.

    d. Deferoxamine

      (1) Mechanism of action

        (a) Deferoxamine exhibits a high affinity for the ferric ion.

        (b) It competes with the iron of ferritin and hemosiderin, while the iron of transferrin and of cytochromes is not affected.

      (2) Preparations and administration. Because oral absorption of deferoxamine is poor, it is given parenterally to chelate iron that has been absorbed.

      (3) Therapeutic uses. Deferoxamine is used to treat acute iron poisoning.

      (4) Adverse effects include hypotension and allergic reactions. Anuria, renal disease, and pregnancy are contraindications.

C. **Commonly occurring overdoses**

    1. Ethanol accounts for approximately one-fourth of all drug poisonings each year.

      a. The **lethal blood level** of ethanol is considered to be **0.5 g/dl;** however, it varies from patient to patient.

      b. Diagnosis

        (1) A microdiffusion test is a simple screening test for the presence of blood ethanol.

        (2) Gas chromatography, a procedure used to separate out volatile substances, allows one to differentiate between ethanol and methanol. In addition, blood ethanol concentrations can be determined.

      c. Treatment of ethanol overdosage consists of intensive supportive care with special attention to preventing hypoglycemia and ketoacidosis.

    2. Barbiturate overdosage is a common form of poisoning in adults; treatment is mainly supportive. Maintenance of cardiopulmonary stability is of prime importance.

      a. Lavage or emesis can be attempted if proper precaution has been taken to avoid aspiration. Gastric lavage is contraindicated in the comatose patient.

      b. Because barbiturates are acidic, alkalinization of the urine and the promotion of diuresis is often beneficial.

      c. Hemodialysis is the most effective means of treating severe barbiturate overdosage. It tends to be more effective in removing short-acting barbiturates rather than long-acting ones because the degree of protein binding is considerably less.

      d. Analeptic agents are contraindicated.

    3. Salicylate intoxication primarily occurs in children.

      a. Frequently observed signs and symptoms of salicylate intoxication are discussed in Chapter 9 II A 6.

      b. Plasma salicylate levels are often good indicators of the severity of salicylate poisoning.

        (1) Plasma levels below 50 mg/dl produce no major symptoms, and treatment is to induce emesis or administer gastric lavage.

        (2) With plasma levels between 50 and 100 mg/dl, the patient often presents with hyperpnea due to salicylate stimulation of the respiratory center. Increased blood glucose levels and hyperpyrexia may be seen.

          (a) Treatment is by inducing emesis or using gastric lavage.

          (b) The administration of sodium bicarbonate to alkalinize the urine may be advisable, but must be performed with caution.

          (c) Correction of hyperthermia with ice blankets is often needed.

          (d) The blood salicylate level is rechecked within a few hours.

        (3) With plasma levels over 110 mg/dl, the same procedures as above are performed; however, hemodialysis or peritoneal dialysis may be needed.

        (4) Plasma levels over 160 mg/dl are usually lethal, death being caused by respiratory arrest.

    4. Acetaminophen overdose can result in liver toxicity (see Chapter 9 II B 6 b).

    5. Acids (e.g., hydrochloric, nitric, sulfuric, sodium bisulfate) are found in home products, such as cleaning agents and automobile batteries.

      a. If swallowed, severe mucous membrane burns can occur. Respiratory distress resulting from glottal edema and gastrointestinal scarring can occur.

b. Emetics and lavages are contraindicated.

c. Dilution with water or milk following ingestion is the treatment of choice.

6. **Alkalies** (e.g., sodium hypochlorite, sodium hydroxide, potassium hydroxide) are substances that are found in household products, such as Drano.
   a. Severe burns of the skin, mucous membranes, and eyes can occur on contact.
   b. They tend to be more severe injuries than seen with acid caustic ingestion.
   c. Immediate and extensive irrigation of affected areas is recommended.
   d. Oral ingestion requires dilution with water or milk.
   e. Steroid therapy for a 3-week course has been used when esophageal burns occur.

7. **Benzodiazepine overdose** (see Chapter 3 VI C 4 b)

8. **Narcotics overdose.** Naloxone and naltrexone (see Chapter 3 IX E 5, 6) are used along with general support measures to treat narcotics overdose.

III. MANAGEMENT OF POISONING

A. General principles

1. The **exposure** of the patient to the toxic substance **should be avoided or reduced**.
   a. The individual should be removed from the contaminated air if the toxic substance is air-borne.
   b. The individual's clothing should be removed immediately if the clothing is soaked in the poison.
   c. When the poison has been ingested, vomiting should be induced or gastric lavage should be used except when that is contraindicated, as in the case of caustic poisons or a comatose patient.

2. **Supportive therapy** should be given to maintain basic respiratory and cardiovascular function.

3. **Telephone management.** Personnel at poisoning "hotlines" field the majority of calls concerning poisonings in the pediatric population. Most ingestions in children under the age of 5 years are accidental.

4. Although few poisons have specific antidotes, the most common substance that is effective and generally available in a household is **milk**.
   a. Milk is amphoteric, and both acids and bases are compatible.
   b. Both the calcium and protein can serve as chelators.
   c. Milk coats the stomach, thereby protecting it and delaying absorption.

B. Induction of vomiting

1. **Syrup of ipecac** is the preferred emetic for inducing vomiting.
   a. It is best administered with a glass of warm water, which dilutes the toxicant and solubilizes the stomach contents.
   b. Syrup of ipecac (or any emetic) must be used with particular caution when central nervous system (CNS) integrity is compromised because of the risk of aspiration pneumonia.

2. **Salt water** and **using a finger to promote emesis** are both **dangerous**.

3. **Contraindications to induced emesis** include:
   a. Caustic poisons, such as lye
   b. Petroleum distillates, such as lighter fluid or gasoline
   c. A comatose patient
   d. A patient in whom convulsions may be imminent, as with ingestion of a large dose of aspirin

4. **Alternatives to emesis.** The major alternatives to emesis include the following:
   a. **Gastric lavage** is especially useful in treating poisoning by aromatic substances, such as perfume, or when some contraindication for emesis exists.
   b. **Activated charcoal** adsorbs the poison or toxin and delays gastrointestinal absorption. It is especially helpful in the treatment of poisoning from aromatic and alkaloid compounds.
   c. **Cathartics** are used to hasten the removal of a toxic substance and are useful for ingestion of hydrocarbons and enteric-coated tablets. **Sodium sulfate** is a frequently used cathartic.
   d. **Dialysis** is most effective if the poison has a small volume of distribution and has low protein binding. Peritoneal dialysis and hemodialysis have limited use in the treatment of intoxication with chemicals.
   e. **Pharmacologic antagonism** can be effective with compounds that act at specific receptors, but stimulation of physiologic mechanisms may be deleterious (physiologic antagonism); for example, CNS stimulants used in respiratory depression can cause convulsions.

STUDY QUESTIONS

DIRECTIONS: Each of the numbered items or incomplete statements in this section is followed by answers or by completions of the statement. Select the **one** lettered answer or completion that is **best** in each case.

---

1. The therapeutic efficacy of sodium nitrite in the treatment of patients with cyanide poisoning is based on

(A) the formation of methemoglobin
(B) an increase in oxidative phosphorylation
(C) an increase in coronary arterial blood flow
(D) a decrease in intracranial pressure
(E) relaxation of the nonvascular smooth muscle

2. Mercury is toxic because it

(A) complexes with hemoglobin to form methemoglobin
(B) inhibits hemoglobin synthesis, producing anemia
(C) binds to ferric ions of the cytochrome a–a$_3$ complex
(D) inhibits anaerobic glycolysis
(E) binds to sulfhydryl groups

3. Which of the following statements about lead poisoning is true?

(A) Lead poisoning is the least common cause of heavy metal poisoning
(B) Acute lead poisoning is more common than chronic exposure
(C) The most common route of absorption is through the skin
(D) Footdrop is the most common sign of lead poisoning
(E) A black "lead line" can occur on the gums

DIRECTIONS: Each of the numbered items or incomplete statements in this section is negatively phrased, as indicated by a capitalized word such as NOT, LEAST, or EXCEPT. Select the ONE lettered answer or completion that is BEST in each case.

---

4. A 2-year-old toddler accidentally ingests Drano. All of the following statements are true EXCEPT

(A) ingestion of alkalies tends to cause more severe injury than ingestion of acids
(B) extensive irrigation is indicated
(C) milk as a dilutant is contraindicated
(D) steroid therapy may be effective in the presence of esophageal burns
(E) the child may have respiratory distress

5. A comatose patient is brought to the emergency room after taking an overdose of secobarbital. Proper therapy would include all of the following EXCEPT

(A) ventilatory support
(B) frequent monitoring of blood pressure
(C) placement of an intravenous catheter
(D) an emetic agent
(E) monitoring urinary volume

6. All of the following statements about arsenic poisoning are true EXCEPT

(A) arsenic is used in household plant-spray pesticides
(B) the trivalent form is toxic and binds to sulfhydryl groups
(C) the antidote is dimercaprol
(D) a characteristic basophilic stippling of red blood cells often occurs
(E) tolerance to chronic arsenic poisoning can develop

7. All of the following statements about toxicology are true EXCEPT

(A) certain heavy metals can be considered hazardous poisons
(B) chronic exposure to a toxic substance is likely to produce the same symptoms as acute exposure
(C) antidotes of poisons can act by preventing absorption of the poison
(D) antidotes of poisons can act by antagonizing the actions of poisons
(E) activated charcoal is a management alternative to syrup of ipecac

ANSWERS AND EXPLANATIONS

1. The answer is A *[II A 3 a (3)]*. The inhalation of amyl nitrite and the intravenous administration of sodium nitrite cause the oxidation of hemoglobin to methemoglobin. Methemoglobin competes with cytochrome oxidase for the cyanide ion, allowing the cytochrome oxidase to function in normal oxidative metabolism.

2. The answer is E *[II B 1, 2 c (1) (c)]*. Mercury, like arsenic, binds to sulfhydryl groups of proteins, frequently inactivating those proteins that are enzymes or producing structural damage. Interaction with the ferric ions of the cytochrome oxidase system is the principal mechanism of cyanide damage. Hemoglobin synthesis is disrupted by lead, which causes a microcytic hypochromic anemia. A number of substances can cause methemoglobinemia (e.g., nitrites, nitrates, chlorates, quinones), but mercury is not one of them.

3. The answer is E *[II B 2 b (1), (2)]*. Lead poisoning is the most common heavy metal poisoning. Chronic exposure is much more common than acute poisoning. The gastrointestinal and respiratory tracts are the most common routes of absorption. Wristdrop is seen more frequently than footdrop. The black "lead line" often seen on the gums may be missing in a person who practices good dental hygiene.

4. The answer is C *[III A 4]*. Milk and water are effective dilutants and can be used as part of an extensive irrigation process in a patient who ingests Drano. Alkalies tend to cause more severe injury than acid ingestion, and steroid therapy may help with esophageal burns. Patients may present with or develop respiratory distress.

5. The answer is D *[II C 2]*. Treatment for an overdose of secobarbital, a barbiturate, would focus on maintaining basic life functions, including placement of an intravenous catheter and ventilatory support if indicated. Maintenance of cardiopulmonary stability is of prime importance, and alkalinization of the urine and promotion of diuresis is often beneficial. There are no specific antagonists for barbiturates, and generalized central nervous system (CNS) stimulants such as amphetamines are not indicated. Hemodialysis is the most effective means of treating a severe barbiturate overdose. If the patient were conscious, emesis would indeed be indicated, but it should not be used in a comatose patient.

6. The answer is D *[II B 2 a, b (2) (f)]*. Lead arsenate is often used as a household plant-spray pesticide. The trivalent form of arsenic (As^{3-}) is toxic and binds to sulfhydryl groups. Dimercaprol can be used as an antidote because it contains sulfhydryl groups, which compete with sulfhydryl moieties on proteins for arsenic. Tolerance to chronic arsenic poisoning can develop (e.g., in agricultural workers). Basophilic stippling of red blood cells is seen with lead poisoning, not with arsenic poisoning.

7. The answer is B *[I C; II B; III B 4 b]*. Acute exposure to a toxic substance is likely to produce different symptoms than are seen with chronic exposure to lower concentrations. Antidotes act by both preventing the absorption and antagonizing the actions of poisons. Certain heavy metals can be dangerous poisons. Activated charcoal is a useful alternative to inducing vomiting with syrup of ipecac when a person has ingested a poison. It adsorbs the poison and delays gastrointestinal absorption.

COMPREHENSIVE EXAM

QUESTIONS

DIRECTIONS: Each of the numbered items or incomplete statements in this section is followed by answers or by completions of the statement. Select the ONE lettered answer or completion that is BEST in each case.

1. A patient complaining of abnormal movements is found to have a parkinsonian tremor and tardive dyskinesia. Chronic use of which of the following drugs would cause these symptoms?

(A) Flurazepam
(B) Codeine
(C) Chloral hydrate
(D) Triflupromazine
(E) Carbamazepine

2. In patients with congestive heart failure (CHF), digitalis glycosides are used because they produce a positive inotropic effect that can best be defined as an increase in

(A) the force of myocardial contraction
(B) cardiac filling pressure
(C) the heart rate
(D) venous pressure
(E) cardiac conduction velocity

3. A 67-year-old man is diagnosed with acute pulmonary coccidioidomycosis. Proper therapy includes

(A) high doses of penicillin G
(B) griseofulvin
(C) flucytosine
(D) amphotericin B
(E) pentamidine

4. Which of the following statements best characterizes potentiation?

(A) Potentiation occurs if a drug lacking an effect of its own increases the effect of a second, active drug
(B) Potentiation occurs if two drugs with the same effect, when given together, produce an effect that is equal in magnitude to the sum of the effects when the drugs are given individually
(C) Potentiation occurs if two drugs with the same effect, when given together, produce an effect that is greater in magnitude than the sum of the effects when the drugs are given individually
(D) Potentiation occurs if two drugs with the same effect, when given together, produce an effect that is equal in magnitude to the effect of each drug given alone
(E) None of the above statements correctly characterizes potentiation

5. A 57-year-old man with known coronary heart disease is taking terfenadine for allergic rhinitis. Concurrent use of which one of the following could increase his risk of arrhythmia?

(A) Phenobarbital
(B) Alcohol
(C) Phenytoin
(D) Glutethimide
(E) Cimetidine

6. Which of the following antiarrhythmic agents is incorrectly matched by class?

(A) Mexiletine—class IB
(B) Encainide—class IC
(C) Esmolol—class IV
(D) Propranolol—class II
(E) Verapamil—class IV

7. Terfenadine and astemizole differ by which important property when compared to classic antihistamines?

(A) They are ineffective for the treatment of seasonal rhinitis
(B) They produce less sedation
(C) They are available for topical use
(D) They have greater adverse anticholinergic effects
(E) They have very short half-lives

8. The pharmacologic actions of scopolamine most closely resemble those of

(A) hexamethonium
(B) atropine
(C) succinylcholine
(D) acetylcholine
(E) curare

9. The local anesthetic with the shortest duration of action is

(A) procaine
(B) bupivacaine
(C) lidocaine
(D) mepivacaine
(E) tetracaine

10. Which of the following drugs, if given concomitantly with warfarin, would require an increase in warfarin dosage?

(A) Aspirin
(B) Barbiturates
(C) Disulfiram
(D) Phenylbutazone
(E) Trimethoprim-sulfamethoxazole

11. A 62-year-old patient who is known to have glaucoma is scheduled for a cholecystectomy. Which neuromuscular blocking agent is contraindicated?

(A) Tubocurarine
(B) Pancuronium
(C) Succinylcholine
(D) Gallamine
(E) Metocurine

12. A 47-year-old man has been treated for essential hypertension for 6 months. The patient's hypertension is under control; however, he now complains of impotence, vertigo, and difficulty in doing mental work. Laboratory results reveal a positive Coombs' test. Which antihypertensive agent is capable of causing these effects?

(A) Captopril
(B) Hydralazine
(C) Lisinopril
(D) Methyldopa
(E) Prazosin

13. A patient with renal failure is to undergo abdominal surgery. Which competitive neuromuscular blocking agent could be used in this patient as an adjunct to the surgery?

(A) Pipercuronium
(B) Gallamine
(C) Atracurium
(D) Succinylcholine
(E) Decamethonium

14. A 3-month-old infant is brought to the emergency room with seizures of the tonic–clonic type. His mother reports that these seizures have been occurring for the past 50 minutes. The treatment of choice is

(A) a benzodiazepine
(B) a barbiturate
(C) phenytoin
(D) carbamazepine
(E) valproate

15. A patient has undergone knee replacement surgery. He has chronic obstructive pulmonary disease with documented decreased pulmonary function. Postoperatively, he complains of severe pain, but nausea precludes the oral administration of analgesics. Which drug would be the best option?

(A) Meperidine, intramuscularly
(B) Acetaminophen, rectally
(C) Morphine, intramuscularly
(D) Morphine, intravenously
(E) Ketorolac, intramuscularly

16. The following pairs consist of a chelating agent and a heavy metal. Which pair is correctly matched?

(A) Dimercaprol—iron
(B) Calcium disodium EDTA—arsenic
(C) Penicillamine—copper
(D) Deferoxamine—lead

17. Which antineoplastic drug acts during a specific phase of the cell cycle?

(A) Methotrexate
(B) 5-Fluorouracil
(C) Mechlorethamine
(D) Cyclophosphamide
(E) Melphalan

18. A diabetic patient presents with cough, hemoptysis, and a single shaking chill. His temperature is 101°F, and a chest x-ray demonstrates lobar pneumonia. Gram staining reveals gram-positive diplococci. Correct therapy would be to administer

(A) gentamicin
(B) penicillin G
(C) carbenicillin and gentamicin
(D) ampicillin
(E) ciprofloxacin

19. Oral contraceptives containing an estrogen and norethindrone act mainly by which of the following mechanisms?

(A) Accelerating the growth of ovarian follicles
(B) Increasing the secretion of follicle-stimulating hormone (FSH)
(C) Hastening the release of luteinizing hormone (LH)
(D) Suppressing ovulation
(E) Thickening the consistency of the cervical mucus

20. Which of the following agents used to treat gout could actually increase the frequency of acute gouty attacks during initial therapy?

(A) Sulfinpyrazone
(B) Allopurinol
(C) Colchicine
(D) Probenecid
(E) Indomethacin

21. A hypertensive crisis might be seen with which of the drug classes listed below?

(A) Tricyclic antidepressants
(B) Barbiturates
(C) Narcotic analgesics
(D) Monoamine oxidase (MAO) inhibitors
(E) Phenothiazines

22. Agents that produce neuromuscular blockade act by inhibiting which of the following events?

(A) Synthesis of acetylcholine from acetyl coenzyme A and choline
(B) Release of acetylcholine from the pre-junctional membrane
(C) Packaging of acetylcholine into synaptic vesicles
(D) Interaction of acetylcholine with cholinergic receptors
(E) Re-uptake of acetylcholine into the nerve ending

23. Which of the following agents is a selective β_1-adrenergic antagonist that is also available as a topical formulation for the treatment of glaucoma?

(A) Betaxolol
(B) Carteolol
(C) Labetalol
(D) Nadolol
(E) Timolol

Questions 24–27

A 29-year-old black man presents to the clinic for a routine examination. His family history is significant for cardiovascular disease, including a father who died of a myocardial infarction at 49 years of age and a grandfather who is presently 70 years old and has severe congestive heart failure (CHF). Physical examination is unremarkable except that the patient is 20 pounds heavier than ideal body weight, and his blood pressure is 160/100. Repeat blood pressure evaluation confirms this reading.

24. First line therapy for this patient should be

(A) initiation of captopril therapy
(B) initiation of propranolol therapy
(C) initiation of verapamil therapy
(D) dietary restriction
(E) initiation of hydralazine therapy

25. The recommended therapy made little difference. Which therapy should be tried next?

(A) Reserpine
(B) Dietary restriction
(C) Methyldopa
(D) Thiazide diuretic
(E) Diltiazem

26. Two months later, the patient's blood pressure is 156/98. The physician discontinues previous therapy and initiates therapy with a selective β blocker, such as

(A) atenolol
(B) propranolol
(C) nadolol
(D) timolol
(E) labetalol

27. One month later, the patient's blood pressure is 140/86. However, the patient reports persistent dizziness. The physician stops the current therapy and initiates therapy that was initially well tolerated but ultimately caused bronchospasm and cough. An agent capable of producing these effects is

(A) methyldopa
(B) captopril
(C) diltiazem
(D) reserpine
(E) propranolol

28. A patient being treated for endogenous depression also has an obsessive–compulsive disorder. The psychiatrist treats the patient with an agent that is a selective inhibitor of serotonin reuptake in the central nervous system (CNS). This agent is most apt to be

(A) bupropion
(B) fluoxetine
(C) tranylcypromine
(D) amitriptyline
(E) deprenyl

29. A patient with arthritis presents with a sore throat, fever, and dependent edema. The patient had been in good health previously. A complete blood count reveals a white cell count of 500 (normal = 5000–8000). A drug capable of causing this effect is

(A) aspirin
(B) indomethacin
(C) sulindac
(D) phenylbutazone
(E) diclofenac

30. An 18-year-old woman presents with urgency, frequency, and burning urination. She is afebrile. Urinalysis reveals the presence of red blood cells. Appropriate therapy after urine culture would include which of the following agents?

(A) Aztreonam
(B) Carbenicillin
(C) Gentamicin
(D) Trimethoprim-sulfamethoxazole

31. How does terazosin rapidly improve urine flow in patients with benign prostatic hypertrophy?

(A) It blocks postsynaptic α_1 adrenoreceptors
(B) It rapidly constricts smooth muscle in the prostate capsule
(C) It rapidly constricts smooth muscle in the urethra
(D) It reduces the size of the prostate

32. A 57-year-old farmer of Swedish descent presents with several hard, gray lesions on his nose. After suitable diagnostic studies, a topical preparation is prescribed, which is most likely to contain

(A) cisplatin
(B) mercaptopurine
(C) vincristine
(D) 5-fluorouracil
(E) mitotane

33. Which of the following antibiotics should be administered to a patient whose renal function is severely compromised?

(A) Erythromycin
(B) Tobramycin
(C) Piperacillin
(D) Cefazolin
(E) Norfloxacin

34. Allopurinol is most likely to potentiate the pharmacologic action of

(A) 5-fluorouracil
(B) bleomycin
(C) 6-mercaptopurine
(D) doxorubicin
(E) methotrexate

35. A teenager overdoses on heroin. In the emergency room, the patient's blood pressure is 100/60, but his respiratory rate is 4/min, and he is comatose. Which of the following would be most important to this patient's management?

(A) Syrup of ipecac
(B) Direct respiratory stimulant
(C) Pharmacologic antagonist (e.g., naltrexone)
(D) Use of a cathartic
(E) Gastric lavage

36. A teenaged girl presents with a pruritic dermatitis on her earlobes. The cause is found to be a recently purchased set of earrings. She should be advised to avoid jewelry containing which of the following metals?

(A) Gold
(B) Nickel
(C) Platinum
(D) Silver
(E) Zinc

37. A patient with severe hypertension is being treated with an agent that stimulates presynaptic α_2 receptors in the vasomotor center of the brain. The patient might be taking

(A) guanethidine
(B) reserpine
(C) clonidine
(D) prazosin
(E) minoxidil

38. The diuretic of choice for a patient receiving the nephrotoxic antitumor agent cisplatin is

(A) ethacrynic acid
(B) mercaptomerin
(C) acetazolamide
(D) chlorothiazide
(E) mannitol

39. Which cancer chemotherapeutic agent could be used for a patient with rheumatoid arthritis who did not respond to nonsteroidal anti-inflammatory agents?

(A) Cyclophosphamide
(B) Pentostatin
(C) Cytarabine
(D) Methotrexate
(E) Doxorubicin

Questions 40–41

A 10-year-old boy is admitted to the hospital with an initial diagnosis of acute lymphoblastic leukemia. His liver, spleen, and lymph nodes are extensively infiltrated.

40. Which of the following drug combinations would be most appropriate for inducing remission?

(A) Prednisone and vincristine
(B) Cyclophosphamide and methotrexate
(C) Cyclophosphamide and vinblastine
(D) 6-Mercaptopurine and methotrexate
(E) Cytarabine and 5-fluorouracil

41. The patient is given allopurinol to reduce the complications of his cancer chemotherapy. The rationale underlying the allopurinol therapy is that

(A) allopurinol increases the renal clearance of uric acid
(B) the most effective therapeutic regimens interfere with purine biosynthesis
(C) rapid lympholysis produces large quantities of uric acid
(D) lower doses of the remission-inducing drugs can be given
(E) allopurinol inhibits the metabolism of pyrimidine analogs

42. A 67-year-old man is found to have tachypnea, pitting edema, and audible S_3 and S_4 heart sounds. A chest x-ray supports the diagnosis of congestive heart failure (CHF). Which of the following is an appropriate diuretic?

(A) Mannitol
(B) Hydrochlorothiazide
(C) Bumetanide
(D) Triamterene
(E) Spironolactone

DIRECTIONS: Each of the numbered items or incomplete statements in this section is negatively phrased, as indicated by a capitalized word such as NOT, LEAST, or EXCEPT. Select the ONE lettered answer or completion that is BEST in each case.

---

43. Therapeutic uses for propranolol include all of the following EXCEPT

(A) atrial fibrillation
(B) atrial flutter
(C) paroxysmal atrial tachycardia
(D) ventricular arrhythmias
(E) low-output congestive heart failure

44. A 55-year-old salesman with mild type II diabetes spends a significant amount of time traveling. He has trouble maintaining a suitable diet with restaurant meals and cannot take insulin easily because of sterilization problems. All of the following agents could be tried in this patient EXCEPT

(A) acetohexamide
(B) chlorpropamide
(C) glyburide
(D) sulfanilamide
(E) tolbutamide

45. Substances that act as inhibitors of the mixed-function oxygenase system include all of the following EXCEPT

(A) carbon monoxide
(B) cimetidine
(C) carbon tetrachloride
(D) organophosphorous insecticides
(E) phenobarbital

46. Adverse effects of cardiac glycosides include all of the following EXCEPT

(A) they have a low margin of safety
(B) intoxication is often precipitated by the depletion of Na^+
(C) they can cause vision changes
(D) decreased renal function can predispose to toxicity
(E) they can cause ventricular tachycardia

47. Synonyms for sympathetic antagonists include all of the following EXCEPT

(A) adrenergic blocking agents
(B) antiadrenergic agents
(C) sympatholytics
(D) cholinomimetics

48. Characteristics of aspirin include all of the following EXCEPT

(A) its analgesic, antipyretic, and anti-inflammatory actions are due to inhibition of prostaglandin synthesis
(B) toxic doses are capable of producing respiratory and metabolic acidosis
(C) it can increase mean bleeding time
(D) excretion can be increased by alkalinizing urine
(E) low doses increase urate excretion

49. When used intravenously, lidocaine has all of the following effects EXCEPT

(A) it suppresses premature ventricular contractions
(B) it reverses atrial arrhythmias
(C) it decreases Na^+ conductance in automatic cells
(D) it has no effect on sinus nodal pacemaker discharge
(E) it is rapidly metabolized by the hepatic microsomal enzyme system

50. Drugs that are likely to aggravate bronchial asthma include all of the following EXCEPT

(A) morphine
(B) tubocurarine
(C) propranolol
(D) amphetamine
(E) meperidine

51. A 67-year-old man is started on warfarin sodium therapy for the prophylactic treatment of venous thrombosis. The patient asks for full disclosure of possible adverse effects. All of the following drugs or adverse effects are correctly matched with causes or results EXCEPT

(A) major bleeding—2% of patients treated
(B) warfarin necrosis—occurs 3–10 days after initiation of therapy
(C) purple toe syndrome—caused by venous emboli
(D) cimetidine—increases anticoagulant action
(E) phenobarbital—decreases anticoagulant action

52. All of the following drugs are correctly matched with a form of cancer that they are used to treat EXCEPT

(A) busulfan—colon cancer
(B) cisplatin—testicular cancer
(C) cyclophosphamide—Hodgkin's disease
(D) 5-fluorouracil—breast cancer
(E) methotrexate—lymphoblastic leukemia

53. Digitalis glycosides are used with all of the following conditions EXCEPT

(A) atrial fibrillation
(B) high-output cardiac failure
(C) paroxysmal atrial tachycardia
(D) atrial flutter

54. A patient who recently had prostate surgery develops a urinary tract infection. *Pseudomonas aeruginosa* is cultured. Suitable therapy would include all of the following agents EXCEPT

(A) amoxicillin and clavulanate
(B) aztreonam
(C) ceftazidime
(D) ciprofloxacin
(E) tobramycin

55. All of the following statements about the therapeutic index (TI) are true EXCEPT

(A) it is used to evaluate the safety of a drug
(B) a low TI indicates that the drug is dangerous to use therapeutically
(C) a high TI indicates that the ED_{50} far exceeds the LD_{50}
(D) aspirin has a high TI
(E) the TI may be a less useful indicator than the standard margin of safety

56. A 48-year-old woman who is being treated with propranolol for essential hypertension experiences a worsening of her chronic obstructive pulmonary disease. Acceptable alternate therapy could include all of the following EXCEPT

(A) diltiazem
(B) verapamil
(C) nicardipine
(D) nadolol
(E) thiazide diuretic

57. Correct statements concerning procaine include all of the following EXCEPT

(A) it has an ester linkage
(B) it interferes with sodium influx during depolarization
(C) it is relatively short acting
(D) it can produce a lupus-like syndrome
(E) its metabolic product can inhibit the action of sulfonamides

58. True statements about cimetidine include all of the following EXCEPT

(A) it is a competitive H_2-receptor antagonist
(B) it is useful for the treatment of duodenal ulcers
(C) it is used in the treatment of Zollinger-Ellison syndrome
(D) it causes somnolence
(E) it reduces blood flow in the liver

59. All of the following statements about therapeutic iron preparations are true EXCEPT that

(A) ferrous sulfate is the drug of first choice for iron-deficiency anemia
(B) ferrous sulfate contains about 20% elemental iron
(C) adverse effects of ferrous sulfate are often inversely related to the amount of soluble iron in the upper gastrointestinal tract
(D) iron dextran is useful in treating patients with malabsorption syndromes
(E) reticuloendothelial cells phagocytize iron dextran

60. Metoclopramide can be used to treat all of the following conditions EXCEPT

(A) diabetic gastroparesis
(B) chemotherapy-induced vomiting
(C) gastroesophageal reflux disease
(D) peptic ulcer disease
(E) radiation-induced vomiting

61. The thrombolytic agent streptokinase has all of the following properties EXCEPT

(A) it is obtained from group C β-hemolytic streptococci
(B) it can produce significant hypertension, especially on reperfusion
(C) it has been used to treat acute pulmonary embolism
(D) it stimulates the conversion of endogenous plasminogen to plasmin
(E) it can produce gastrointestinal bleeding in 5%–10% of patients

62. Pharmacologic doses of glucocorticoids can result in all of the following effects EXCEPT

(A) stimulation of leukocyte migration
(B) stabilization of lysosomal membranes
(C) reduced activity of fibroblasts
(D) reversal of a histamine-stimulated increase in capillary permeability
(E) inhibited antibody synthesis

63. Pharmacologic effects of the classic antihistamines (H_1-receptor antagonists) include all of the following EXCEPT

(A) sedation with low doses
(B) convulsions with high doses
(C) prevention of motion sickness
(D) inhibition of gastric acid secretion
(E) an antipruritic effect

64. Disadvantages of alimentary administration include all of the following EXCEPT

(A) the rate of absorption is variable
(B) irritation of the mucosal surfaces can occur
(C) the compliance of the patient is not ensured
(D) it is the least safe route of administration
(E) hepatic metabolism may occur before the drug reaches its site of action

65. A patient with progressive rheumatoid arthritis is no longer benefiting from the administration of nonsteroidal anti-inflammatory agents, and auranofin is prescribed. All of the following statements about auranofin are true EXCEPT

(A) it may be somewhat less effective than injectable gold for the treatment of rheumatoid arthritis
(B) it is more likely to cause renal or mucocutaneous toxicity than injectable gold
(C) a high incidence of diarrhea is associated with its use
(D) eosinophilia and proteinuria often occur with its use
(E) cutaneous reactions are often seen

66. A young woman is diagnosed as having candidal vaginitis. Her past medical history reveals that she has just completed a 10-day course of antibiotic therapy for streptococcal pharyngitis. Antibiotics capable of producing this untoward effect include all of the following EXCEPT

(A) amoxicillin
(B) ampicillin
(C) cefaclor
(D) cephalexin
(E) erythromycin

67. All of the following statements concerning cyclosporine are true EXCEPT

(A) it is a highly selective inhibitor of B lymphocytes
(B) it inhibits the production of interleukin-2 by helper T cells
(C) it is often used in combination with prednisone to sustain transplanted organs
(D) it can be administered orally
(E) its major adverse effect is nephrotoxicity

68. Characteristics of ergot alkaloids include all of the following EXCEPT

(A) they stimulate smooth muscle
(B) they are agonists at tryptamine receptors
(C) they show central nervous system (CNS) stimulating effects
(D) they can produce vasoconstriction
(E) they can be blocked by propranolol

69. Quinidine can produce all of the following effects on the heart EXCEPT

(A) a reduction in the maximal rate of rise ($\dot{V}_{max}$) of depolarization
(B) an increase in the effective refractory period
(C) a decrease in automaticity
(D) an increase in inotropic action
(E) a decrease in conduction velocity

70. All of the following statements about erythropoietin are true EXCEPT

(A) erythropoietin administration could decrease the need for transfusion
(B) erythropoietin is used to correct acute severe anemia
(C) erythropoietin works by stimulating the proliferation of immature erythroid progenitor cells
(D) erythropoietin cannot be administered orally
(E) erythropoietin's pharmacokinetics are not affected by dialysis

71. Diisopropyl fluorophosphate (DFP) increases all of the following effects EXCEPT

(A) lacrimation
(B) bronchodilation
(C) salivation
(D) muscle twitching
(E) muscle weakness

72. The response to a dose of an oral anticoagulant is often changed by concomitant administration of other drugs, which affect the dose–response by different mechanisms. True statements about such drugs and their mechanisms include all of the following EXCEPT

(A) phenylbutazone impairs platelet aggregation
(B) phenobarbital induces the drug microsomal metabolizing system
(C) acetylsalicylic acid impairs platelet aggregation
(D) glutethimide inhibits the drug microsomal metabolizing system
(E) cimetidine inhibits the drug microsomal metabolizing system

73. All of the following statements regarding disease-modifying antirheumatic drugs (DMARDs) are true EXCEPT

(A) they are often used in combination with nonsteroidal anti-inflammatory drugs (NSAIDs)
(B) they affect the immunologic response
(C) they interfere with the pathogenesis of rheumatoid arthritis
(D) they produce regression of degenerative lesions
(E) they do not provide rapid, symptomatic relief of joint pain

74. Isoniazid is the most widely used agent in the treatment of tuberculosis. True statements regarding this agent include all of the following EXCEPT

(A) it is used in conjunction with other agents in the treatment of tuberculosis
(B) its metabolism is partly under genetic control
(C) it is ineffective against many atypical mycobacteria
(D) it can be administered as a prophylactic agent to children or young adults who have converted from a tuberculin-negative to tuberculin-positive skin test
(E) fast acetylators have a higher concentration of free isoniazid

75. Pairs of compounds with opposing effects on blood glucose concentrations include all of the following EXCEPT

(A) tolbutamide and diazoxide
(B) insulin and cortisol
(C) insulin and glucagon
(D) glucagon and isoproterenol
(E) glucagon and propranolol

76. Each of the following antiarrhythmic agents is correctly matched with an appropriate adverse effect EXCEPT

(A) quinidine—cinchonism
(B) procainamide—hypotension with intravenous administration
(C) lidocaine—systemic lupus erythematosus–like syndrome
(D) disopyramide—untoward anticholinergic effects
(E) flecainide—excessive mortality and nonfatal cardiac arrest

Questions 77–78

A 70-year-old woman with a history of congestive heart failure, for which she takes digoxin and a diuretic agent, is seen because of an arrhythmia. Electrolyte determination reveals a serum potassium level of 2.8 mEq/L.

77. Diuretics capable of producing this patient's hypokalemia include all of the following EXCEPT

(A) bumetanide
(B) ethacrynic acid
(C) hydrochlorothiazide
(D) furosemide
(E) amiloride

78. Immediate therapy for this patient should include

(A) high doses of spironolactone
(B) insulin and glucose administration
(C) high doses of amiloride
(D) potassium supplementation
(E) high doses of triamterene

79. Aspirin, phenylbutazone, and sulfamethoxazole have all of the following characteristics in common EXCEPT

(A) they are all highly protein bound
(B) they can all cause agranulocytosis
(C) they all interact with warfarin
(D) they can all affect platelet function
(E) they all cause hypersensitivity reactions

80. All of the following points should be kept in mind when considering long-term corticosteroid therapy EXCEPT

(A) abrupt withdrawal may cause signs of adrenal insufficiency
(B) therapy may precipitate peptic ulcers
(C) patients may become intolerant to stressful situations for as long as 1 year after therapy is stopped
(D) therapy may lead to increased infections
(E) hypoglycemia may occur

81. Fluconazole is a popular systemic antifungal agent. Reasons for this include all of the following EXCEPT

(A) when administered orally, it is highly bioavailable
(B) its mechanism of action is unique in that it does not block the synthesis of ergosterol
(C) it is active against acquired immune deficiency syndrome–related *Cryptococcus neoformans*
(D) it penetrates the blood–brain barrier
(E) it is less toxic than amphotericin B

82. All of the following anesthetic drugs and descriptions are correctly matched EXCEPT

(A) lidocaine—an ester but metabolized in the liver
(B) mepivacaine—an amide metabolized in the liver
(C) procaine—a short-acting local anesthetic that lacks topical activity
(D) tetracaine—a good spinal anesthetic
(E) bupivacaine—in certain situations a duration of action that can exceed 24 hours

83. Correct statements concerning vitamin B_{12} deficiency include all of the following EXCEPT

(A) it can be caused by intrinsic factor deficiency
(B) dietary vitamin B_{12} deficiency is uncommon
(C) pernicious anemia requires parenteral vitamin B_{12} therapy
(D) vitamin B_{12} will reverse the neurologic changes of pernicious anemia

84. A 19-year-old attempts suicide by ingesting 60 aspirin tablets (approximately 20 grams). When he is brought to the emergency room, he is convulsing. Appropriate treatment of this patient might include all of the following EXCEPT

(A) induced emesis with syrup of ipecac
(B) correction of abnormal electrolyte balance
(C) alkalization of urine
(D) dialysis
(E) ventilatory support

85. Enalapril is an antihypertensive agent that acts by competitive inhibition of angiotensin-converting enzyme (ACE). Properties of enalapril include all of the following EXCEPT

(A) it reduces total peripheral resistance and mean arterial pressure
(B) it is used alone and in combination therapy
(C) it decreases renin secretion by inhibiting angiotensin II production
(D) its blood pressure–lowering effects appear to be additive with thiazide diuretics
(E) it has a longer duration of action than captopril

DIRECTIONS: Each group of items in this section consists of lettered options followed by a set of numbered items. For each item, select the **one** lettered option that is **most** closely associated with it. Each lettered option may be selected once, more than once, or not at all.

Questions 86–89

Match each description that follows with the anti-infective agent most likely to be associated with it.

(A) Clindamycin
(B) Gentamicin
(C) Nafcillin
(D) Tetracycline
(E) Rifampin

86. This agent is very effective in the treatment of *Chlamydia* infections.

87. This agent is often administered along with isoniazid and ethambutol.

88. This agent is the drug of choice for *Bacteroides fragilis* infection.

89. This agent is poorly absorbed orally because it is polycationic.

Questions 90–94

Match each diuretic with its site of action on the diagram below.

90. Mannitol

91. Spironolactone

92. Hydrochlorothiazide

93. Amiloride

94. Furosemide

Questions 95–97

For each diuretic agent that follows, select its major mechanism of action.

(A) Inhibits carbonic anhydrase
(B) Inhibits electrolyte reabsorption in the ascending limb of the loop of Henle
(C) Competitively antagonizes aldosterone
(D) Binds to sulfhydryl enzymes
(E) Inhibits active Na^+ secretion, decreasing K^+ excretion in the distal nephron

95. Ethacrynic acid

96. Acetazolamide

97. Triamterene

Questions 98–102

Barbiturates can be involved in drug interactions with many other drugs. For each drug listed below, select the mechanism that is the most likely cause of an interaction with a barbiturate.

(A) Incompatibility in vitro
(B) Induction of microsomal enzymes
(C) Inhibition of nonmicrosomal enzymes
(D) Enhancement of pharmacologic effects
(E) Interference with renal excretion

98. Warfarin

99. Dextran

100. Tranylcypromine

101. Digitoxin

102. Phenothiazines

Questions 103–106

Match each of the following autacoid antagonists to the enzyme that it inhibits.

(A) Cyclooxygenase
(B) Peptidyl dipeptidase
(C) Phospholipase A_2
(D) Thromboxane synthetase
(E) Cystathionine synthetase

103. Captopril

104. Hydralazine

105. Ibuprofen

106. Prednisolone

Questions 107–109

Match the correct propionic acid derivative with the statement that best describes it.

(A) Ibuprofen
(B) Naproxen
(C) Fenoprofen
(D) Ketoprofen
(E) Flubiprofen

107. A more effective analgesic than aspirin, it is available "over the counter" in low doses.

108. When treated concurrently with methotrexate, the patient can develop life-threatening hepatotoxicity.

109. It is available in ophthalmic dosage form for the treatment of postoperative meiosis.

Questions 110–114

For each clinical condition, select the drug that is most likely to be used in its management.

(A) Carmustine
(B) Cyclophosphamide
(C) Dacarbazine
(D) Methotrexate
(E) Mitotane

110. Adrenal carcinoma

111. Brain tumor

112. Malignant melanoma

113. Psoriasis

114. Renal transplants

Questions 115–117

Match each statement about drug action with the drug that is most likely to be associated with it.

(A) Cyclophosphamide
(B) 5-Fluorouracil
(C) Cytarabine
(D) Vincristine
(E) Mitomycin

115. In addition to being a natural product, this drug is an alkylating agent because it is reduced intracellularly and alkylates DNA.

116. This drug inhibits DNA polymerase and can be incorporated into DNA and RNA.

117. This drug is a phase-specific agent, producing metaphase arrest.

Questions 118–121

For each of the following descriptions of drug actions, select the agent with which it is most likely to be associated.

(A) Phenylephrine
(B) Amphetamine
(C) Diisopropyl fluorophosphate (DFP)
(D) Neostigmine
(E) Methacholine

118. Purely muscarinic in its action

119. Irreversible cholinesterase inhibitor

120. Closely resembles norepinephrine in its cardiovascular actions

121. Enzyme inhibitor as well as receptor agonist

Questions 122–125

Match each untoward effect with the anti-infective agent associated with it.

(A) Trimethoprim–sulfamethoxazole
(B) Gentamicin
(C) Tetracycline
(D) Chloramphenicol
(E) Ciprofloxacin

122. Stevens-Johnson syndrome

123. Gray-baby syndrome

124. Ototoxicity and nephrotoxicity

125. Tooth discoloration

ANSWERS AND EXPLANATIONS

1. The answer is D *[Chapter 3 V A 3, B 5 a].* The presenting symptoms of this patient are compatible with chronic use of a phenothiazine, such as triflupromazine. Patients who develop extrapyramidal side effects often display rigidity and tremor at rest as well as sucking and smacking of the lips. Flurazepam, codeine, chloral hydrate, and carbamazepine do not produce extrapyramidal side effects.

2. The answer is A *[Chapter 5 I B 3 a, b].* The most important property of the cardiac glycosides is to increase the force of myocardial contraction (positive inotropic effect). In patients with congestive heart failure (CHF), this leads to an increase in cardiac output, a decrease in cardiac filling pressures, and decreases in heart size and venous and capillary pressures. Digitalis also tends to slow the heart rate in patients with CHF; this negative chronotropic effect is the result of a decrease in sympathetic activity brought about by increased cardiac output. Digitalis also decreases conduction velocity through the atrioventricular (AV) node; this effect is unrelated to the positive inotropic effect.

3. The answer is D *[Chapter 12 III A 2 e, B 1 e (3) (b), 5 d (1)].* Amphotericin B is effective in the treatment of acute pulmonary coccidioidomycosis. The other agents listed would be ineffective. Griseofulvin is used for mycotic diseases of the skin, hair, and nails. Flucytosine is used for systemic infections caused by *Candida albicans* or *Cryptococcus meningitidis*. Penicillin G has no antifungal activity. Pentamidine is most useful for the prophylaxis and treatment of *Pneumocystis carinii* pneumonia. It has no antifungal activity.

4. The answer is A *[Chapter 1 III B 5 c].* Potentiation occurs if a drug lacking an effect of its own increases the effect of a second, active drug. If two drugs with the same effect, when given together, produce an effect that is equal in magnitude to the sum of the effects when the drugs are given individually, the effects of the two drugs are additive. If two drugs with the same effect, when given together, produce an effect that is greater in magnitude than the sum of the effects when the drugs are given individually, synergism has occurred. If two drugs with the same effect, when given together, produce an effect that is less than the combined effect of the two drugs individually, antagonism has occurred.

5. The answer is E *[Chapter 13 II D 4 d].* Cimetidine inhibits nonmicrosomal enzymes, which may increase the risk of arrhythmia in patients taking terfenadine. Barbiturates (e.g., phenobarbital, glutethimide, and phenytoin) and chronic alcohol use induce microsomal enzymes and could reduce blood levels of terfenadine.

6. The answer is C *[Table 5-4].* Esmolol, like propranolol, is a class II antiarrhythmic agent. These agents act by β-adrenergic blockade. Class I agents (e.g., mexiletine, encainide) depress phase 0 of the action potential by blocking Na^+ channels. Class III agents (e.g., amiodarone, bretylium) prolong repolarization and lengthen phase 2. Class IV agents (e.g., verapamil, diltiazem) are Ca^{2+} antagonists.

7. The answer is B *[Chapter 8 V A 1 g (2) (b)].* Both terfenadine and astemizole lack significant central nervous system (CNS)-sedating effects. Both agents are effective for seasonal rhinitis, and both agents are administered orally. Astemizole has a half-life of 9 days. Because astemizole is extremely long-acting, adverse effects may be a problem. Terfenadine lacks significant adverse anticholinergic effects.

8. The answer is B *[Chapter 2 VI B].* Scopolamine is a competitive muscarinic blocker and, therefore, most closely resembles atropine in its mechanism of action. It is more potent than atropine in decreasing bronchial, salivary, and sweat gland secretions, in its sedative effect, and in producing mydriasis and cycloplegia. It is less potent than atropine in its effects on the heart, bronchial muscle, and intestines.

9. The answer is A *[Chapter 4 II C 2].* From shortest to longest duration of action, the local anesthetics are procaine, lidocaine, tetracaine, mepivacaine, and bupivacaine. Procaine is rapidly metabolized by pseudocholinesterase and lacks topical activity.

10. The answer is B *[Chapter 7 V A 2; Table 7-1].* Warfarin, a coumarin-derived anticoagulant, acts by interfering with the vitamin K–dependent synthesis of active coagulation factors II, VII, IX, and X. Disulfiram, aspirin, trimethoprim-sulfamethoxazole, and phenylbutazone increase the response to warfarin and other oral anticoagulants; thus, their use would probably require a reduction in warfarin dosage. Disulfiram affects warfarin activity by prolonging the half-life of levowarfarin, and this effect increases hypoprothrombinemia. Aspirin and phenylbutazone both impair platelet aggregation. Barbiturates and glutethimide have the reverse effects on anticoagulation. These drugs reduce the response to warfarin and, thus, would probably require an increase in warfarin dosage, because they induce the hepatic enzyme system that increases drug metabolism.

11. The answer is C *[Chapter 2 VIII A 1, D 2 c].* Because succinylcholine can depolarize cholinergic skeletal muscle receptors, it affects the extraocular muscles and, therefore, can cause an increase in intraocular pressure. Therefore, succinylcholine would be contraindicated in a glaucoma patient.

12. The answer is D *[Chapter 5 IV G 2 f].* Methyldopa is an antihypertensive agent capable of producing impotence, vertigo, and decreased mental acuity. In addition, methyldopa can cause sedation, extrapyramidal signs, postural hypotension, and hepatic dysfunction; rebound hypertension can occur with sudden withdrawal of methyldopa therapy. A positive Coombs' test develops in as many as 25% of patients taking methyldopa.

13. The answer is C *[Chapter 2 VIII C 2; Table 2-5].* Atracurium can be used in patients with renal failure because it does not rely on the kidney for excretion; rather, it is largely dependent on a nonenzymatic process known as Hoffmann elimination. Succinylcholine and decamethonium are depolarizing, not competitive agents. The competitive blocking agents gallamine and pipercuronium are excreted via the kidney and, therefore, would be contraindicated in patients with renal failure.

14. The answer is B *[Chapter 3 III A 1, 2, C 1, E, F 1 a, 2 a].* Barbiturates are the drugs of choice for infantile tonic–clonic seizures. It should be noted, however, that they are no longer the treatment of choice for the prophylactic control of generalized seizure states. The various benzodiazepines differ in the types of seizures that they control. Diazepam, given intravenously, is the drug of choice for status epilepticus in adults, but not in children. Phenytoin and carbamazepine are also used for tonic–clonic seizures, but neither of these

agents would be the treatment of choice in the situation described. Valproate is more useful for absence seizures, although it is also used for grand mal seizures.

15. The answer is E *[Chapter 3 IX B 1 d (1), C 1 c; Chapter 9 II M 3].* Ketorolac administered intramuscularly would be the best option for relieving pain in this patient. Because the patient has chronic obstructive pulmonary disease, the use of a narcotic (e.g., meperidine, morphine) would be a risk because of the potential for respiratory depression. Acetaminophen is not effective against severe pain, such as this patient is experiencing. Ketorolac provides good analgesic activity without the respiratory depression associated with the use of narcotic analgesics.

16. The answer is C *[Chapter 14 II B 3 a–d].* Penicillamine is an orally effective treatment for copper and lead poisoning. Calcium disodium EDTA is useful in the treatment of lead, iron, copper, and zinc poisoning, but not in arsenic poisoning. Dimercaprol is useful in the treatment of mercury poisoning, as well as in poisoning by arsenic, antimony, gold, and lead. Deferoxamine exhibits a high affinity for the ferric ion and is used in iron poisoning.

17. The answer is A *[Chapter 11 I C 3; II B 2 c; III B 1 c, D 1 b (5)].* Methotrexate acts during the DNA synthetic phase of the cell cycle. Although 5-fluorouracil is proliferation-dependent, it is phase-nonspecific, perhaps due to its RNA actions. Alkylating agents, such as mechlorethamine, cyclophosphamide, or melphalan, are not phase-specific.

18. The answer is B *[Chapter 12 II B 2 f (1), C 6 b (1)].* The diabetic patient described in the question most likely has pneumococcal pneumonia, for which the drug of first choice would be penicillin G. Gentamicin is not active against pneumococcal pneumonia, while carbenicillin and ampicillin, although effective, are not the drugs of first choice. Ciprofloxacin has only modest activity against many streptococci.

19. The answer is D *[Chapter 10 III D 2 a (1) (b)].* Oral contraceptives that combine an estrogen and a progestin act by blocking the surge of luteinizing hormone (LH) and follicle-stimulating hormone (FSH) that normally occurs in the middle of the menstrual cycle. In this way, they suppress ovulation and ovarian follicle growth. The "minipill," which contains progestin alone, acts by thickening the consistency of the cervical mucus, forming a barrier to the entry of sperm.

20. The answer is B *[Chapter 9 IV E 4 b]*. Acute attacks of gout occur more frequently during initial therapy with allopurinol. This effect may be explained by the active dissolution of microcrystalline deposits of sodium urate (tophi) in subcutaneous tissue, which results in brief episodes of hyperuricemia and crystal deposition in joints. Simultaneous administration of colchicine decreases the frequency of these attacks.

21. The answer is D *[Chapter 3 VII B 2 d (2) (b)]*. Tricyclic antidepressants, barbiturates, narcotic analgesics, and phenothiazines can be associated with hypotension, not hypertension. Monoamine oxidase (MAO) inhibitors can interact with sympathomimetic amines, especially indirectly acting ones (e.g., amphetamine, tyramine), and with certain foods (e.g., cheese, beer), which have a high tyramine content. Catecholamines are released from nerve terminals, producing the hypertensive crisis.

22. The answer is D *[Chapter 2 VIII A]*. Both competitive and noncompetitive neuromuscular blocking agents interact with cholinergic receptors to produce neuromuscular blockade. Competitive agents, such as tubocurarine, act at the skeletal muscle cholinergic receptor in a reversible fashion. Succinylcholine, however, acts at this site in a more complex manner, and metabolism is required for the termination of its action.

23. The answer is A *[Chapter 2 III B 10]*. Betaxolol is a selective β_1-adrenergic antagonist that is available as a topical formulation for the treatment of glaucoma. Nadolol and carteolol are nonselective β blockers. Carteolol also possesses intrinsic sympathomimetic activity. Labetalol is a nonselective β blocker with selective α_1-blocking activity. Timolol is used topically for the treatment of glaucoma but is a nonselective β blocker.

24–27. The answers are 24-D *[Chapter 5 IV A 1]*, **25-D** *[Chapter 5 IV A 2, B 1]*, **26-A** *[Chapter 5 IV C 3 a]*, **27-B** *[Chapter 5 IV I 1 g (6), (7)]*. Because the patient described in the question did not have severe hypertension and the physical examination was unremarkable, dietary restriction was indicated. However, the patient was asked to return for a checkup in 1 month.

After 1 month, no perceptible difference was seen in the blood pressure reading. First-line therapy for black hypertensive men should include thiazide diuretics. In general, black individuals respond better to volume loss as opposed to β blockers, but this is a generalization.

After 2 months of thiazide diuretics, the patient was switched to atenolol. In low doses, the only cardioselective β blocker listed is atenolol. All of the other agents are nonselective.

One month later, the patient's blood pressure is 140/86; however, the patient reports feeling dizzy. The physician stops the atenolol and initiates captopril, which was initially well tolerated but ultimately caused cough and bronchospasm. Captopril is a competitive inhibitor of peptidyl dipeptidase, an angiotensin-converting enzyme (ACE). ACE inhibitors are frequently used for the treatment of mild to moderate hypertension.

28. The answer is B *[Chapter 3 VII B 4 a (1), (4) (a), (b)]*. Fluoxetine selectively inhibits serotonin reuptake in the central nervous system (CNS) and produces little effect on central norepinephrine or dopamine function. It is used to treat endogenous depression and obsessive–compulsive disorder. Bupropion weakly blocks dopamine reuptake. Tranylcypromine and deprenyl work by inhibiting monoamine oxidase. Amitriptyline inactivates the reuptake of amines after release from the presynaptic neuron.

29. The answer is D *[Chapter 9 II A 3 h (1), C 7, D 6, K 5, L 5]*. Phenylbutazone, by directly affecting the renal tubules, can cause significant salt and water retention, leading to edema. Phenylbutazone can also cause agranulocytosis or aplastic anemia. Although indomethacin also can cause blood dyscrasias, its salt-retaining properties are much less significant than those occurring with phenylbutazone. The properties of sulindac are similar to those of indomethacin. Aspirin would not affect the leukocyte count or cause edema. Gastrointestinal symptoms and elevated hepatic transaminases are the most frequent adverse effects associated with diclofenac use.

30. The answer is D *[Chapter 12 II A 5 a (1)]*. The major indication for the use of sulfa drugs such as trimethoprim-sulfamethoxazole is the treatment of acute uncomplicated urinary tract infections. Carbenicillin and gentamicin represent broad-spectrum therapy, which is unnecessary for the treatment of an uncomplicated cystitis. Aztreonam, a monobactam, is often substituted for parenteral aminoglycoside therapy and would not be used for the treatment of uncomplicated cystitis.

31. The answer is A *[Chapter 5 IV F 2].*
Terazosin is a postsynaptic α_1-adrenoreceptor blocker that relaxes smooth muscle tone in the bladder neck, prostate capsule, and prostatic urethra. Terazosin has no effect on the size of the prostate.

32. The answer is D *[Chapter 11 III D 1 e (4)].*
The patient described in the question has actinic keratoses—premalignant skin lesions that develop most often in fair-skinned persons who are chronically exposed to sunlight. 5-Fluorouracil, an antimetabolite type of antineoplastic agent, has proved very successful in treating actinic keratoses, although the lesions are apt to recur. Cisplatin, mercaptopurine, vincristine, and mitotane are also antineoplastic agents, but they are used parenterally, and not for this form of cancer.

33. The answer is A *[Chapter 12 II C 3 b (3), F 3 a (2)].* In a patient with renal disease, any antibiotic that is renally excreted should be administered with caution. Erythromycin is concentrated in the liver and is excreted primarily in bile and feces and, thus, may be useful in the treatment of infections in renally compromised patients. Tobramycin, piperacillin, cefazolin, and norfloxacin are principally excreted via the kidney.

34. The answer is C *[Chapter 11 III C 1 g (4)].*
Attempts to inhibit the degradation of 6-mercaptopurine (and thus enhance its effects) led to the development of the xanthine oxidase inhibitor, allopurinol. Allopurinol blocks not only the metabolism of 6-mercaptopurine but also the formation of uric acid from hypoxanthine and xanthine. Therefore, allopurinol can inhibit the hyperuricemia and hyperuricosuria that occurs with 6-mercaptopurine therapy. Because allopurinol prevents the inactivation of 6-mercaptopurine, the dose of 6-mercaptopurine must be reduced when a patient is also given allopurinol.

35. The answer is C *[Chapter 3 IX E 6 a; Chapter 14 III B 1 b].* A pharmacologic antago-

nist (e.g., naltrexone) is the drug of choice for heroin overdose. Syrup of ipecac should not be used if central nervous system (CNS) integrity is compromised. A physiologic antagonist (direct respiratory stimulant) is not useful and could induce convulsions. Gastric lavage is not indicated, while use of a cathartic is best reserved for hydrocarbons and enteric-coated tablets.

36. The answer is B *[Chapter 14 II B 2 d (3)].*
Nickel is sensitizing and can cause a pruritic dermatitis. Nickel is often used in inexpensive jewelry and as components of wearing apparel, such as the buckles on bra or slip straps. Of all the metals listed in the question, nickel is the most likely to cause a contact dermatitis.

37. The answer is C *[Chapter 5 IV G 1].*
Clonidine, by stimulating presynaptic α_2 receptors in the vasomotor center of the brain, decreases sympathetic outflow to the peripheral vessels. Both guanethidine and reserpine are agents that block postganglionic adrenergic neurons. Prazosin is a selective postsynaptic α_1-adrenergic receptor blocker. Minoxidil directly relaxes arteriolar smooth muscle.

38. The answer is E *[Chapter 6 VIII D 4; Chapter 11 VI D 5; Chapter 13 II E 3].*
The antitumor agent cisplatin causes severe nephrotoxicity if it is given without concomitant hydration or a diuretic. The osmotic diuretic mannitol is most commonly employed to reduce this side effect. Mannitol is also useful prophylactically to reduce the risk of acute renal failure in conditions such as cardiovascular operations and severe trauma. Ethacrynic acid, mercaptomerin, acetazolamide, and chlorothiazide are not as effective as mannitol in these situations.

39. The answer is D *[Chapter 11 III B 4 d].*
Methotrexate is considered by some rheumatologists to be "first-line" therapy for the treatment of rheumatoid arthritis. The drug has also been used in the treatment of psoriasis. Methotrexate is used in combination with a number of agents for a variety of cancers.

40–41. The answers are 40-A *[Chapter 11 IV C 5 b (5)],* **41-C** *[Chapter 9 IV A 3 a, E 2].*
Vincristine is far superior to vinblastine in the treatment of lymphocytic leukemia. When combined with prednisone, it is the treatment of choice for inducing remission in acute

lymphoblastic leukemia in children.

Rapid lympholysis produces large quantities of uric acid via nucleic acid release and catabolism. The xanthine oxidase inhibitor allopurinol is given because it inhibits uric acid formation and, thus, is effective in preventing acute gouty arthritis attacks during antineoplastic therapy. Because allopurinol is an inhibitor of xanthine oxidase, it increases the renal excretion of xanthine and hypoxanthine. Because allopurinol is an analog of hypoxanthine, it inhibits the metabolism of purines, not pyrimidines.

42. The answer is C *[Chapter 6 VII D 1, 2].*
A rapid-acting, potent "loop" diuretic is needed in a patient presenting with acute congestive heart failure (CHF). Bumetanide is such a diuretic. Mannitol, hydrochlorothiazide, triamterene, and spironolactone would not give the immediate diuretic response that is needed.

43. The answer is E *[Chapter 5 II E 1 d; Table 5-5].* Propranolol administration can exacerbate congestive heart failure (CHF), asthma, and chronic obstructive pulmonary disease. Propranolol is used to control supraventricular tachyarrhythmias, including atrial fibrillation, atrial flutter, and paroxysmal supraventricular tachycardia. It is useful in ventricular arrhythmias that result from enhanced adrenergic stimulation (e.g., from emotional stress). It is also sometimes used to abolish digitalis-induced ventricular arrhythmias, but it can cause conduction problems, resulting in atrioventricular (AV) dissociation.

44. The answer is D *[Chapter 10 V B, C; Chapter 12 II A].* The patient in the question is a candidate for therapy with an oral hypoglycemic agent. These drugs, the sulfonylureas, are used to treat non–insulin-dependent (type II) diabetes in patients who cannot be treated by dietary control or insulin therapy. Sulfanilamide is one of the sulfonamides, which are antimicrobial agents. The sulfonylureas were developed in the 1940s after the discovery that some sulfonamide drugs had a hypoglycemic effect. Today's antimicrobial sulfonamides are not likely to cause hypoglycemia, but they may increase the hypoglycemic effects of the sulfonylureas.

45. The answer is E *[Chapter 13 II D 5 b].*
Inhibitors of the mixed-function oxygenase system include carbon monoxide, ozone,

cimetidine, carbon tetrachloride, and organophosphorous insecticides. Inhibition of the microsomal enzymes causes the metabolism of certain drugs to be reduced, resulting in higher systemic levels of the drug. Thus, poisoning by any of these toxic substances might cause an increased drug effect as well as the effects of the poison itself. Phenobarbital is capable of inducing the hepatic microsomal drug-metabolizing enzyme system.

46. The answer is B *[Chapter 5 I B 6 a–e].*
Digitalis glycosides have a low margin of safety. In most patients, the lethal dose is likely to be only 5–10 times the minimal effective dose. Intoxication can be precipitated by depletion of K^+, not Na^+. The hypokalemia is often the result of diuretic therapy but can also be the result of protracted vomiting or diarrhea. Other signs of toxicity include abnormal color perception, anorexia, nausea, and, more importantly, ventricular tachycardia. When the serum digoxin level rises above 2 ng/ml, therapy with the glycoside should be discontinued until the level falls below the concentration.

47. The answer is D *[Chapter 2 III].* Synonyms abound for drugs acting on the autonomic nervous system. Drugs that mimic the actions of the sympathetic nervous system are called sympathomimetics or adrenergic agents. Drugs with the opposite effect are known as sympathetic antagonists, sympatholytics, adrenergic blocking agents, and antiadrenergic agents, while subsets of this class are called α blockers and β blockers. Drugs that mimic the actions of the parasympathetic nervous system and the effects of acetylcholine are called parasympathetic, parasympathomimetic, cholinomimetic, or cholinergic agents. Drugs that mimic atropine are known as antimuscarinic agents. To complicate the terminology further, the catecholamines are not cholinergic but adrenergic, so termed because epinephrine was originally called adrenaline and norepinephrine was originally called noradrenaline.

48. The answer is E *[Chapter 9 I A 1; II A 3 a–d, h, i, 6 d].* Low doses of aspirin decrease urate excretion and could produce a gout attack in predisposed patients. All of the other statements in the question are true. Aspirin has analgesic, antipyretic, and anti-inflammatory actions, all of which are mediated by an inhibition of prostaglandin synthesis. Aspirin can increase mean bleeding time, and toxic doses can produce respiratory and metabolic acidosis. Excretion is increased by alkalinizing the urine.

49. The answer is B *[Chapter 5 II C 1 b, c].* Lidocaine is an effective antiarrhythmic agent and is the drug of choice for premature ventricular contractions, although it is ineffective in reversing atrial arrhythmias. It decreases Na^+ but not K^+ conductance in automatic cells. It does not affect sinus nodal pacemaker discharge. Lidocaine is rapidly metabolized by the hepatic microsomal enzyme system.

50. The answer is D *[Chapter 2 II G; III B 1 d (3); VIII D 3; Chapter 3 VIII A 1 a; IX B 1 d (6), C 1 d].* Morphine, meperidine, and tubocurarine are capable of releasing histamine and, thus, aggravate bronchial asthma. Since propranolol is a nonselective β-adrenergic blocker, it too can aggravate bronchial asthma. Amphetamine, being a sympathomimetic agent, does not aggravate bronchial asthma.

51. The answer is C *[Chapter 7 V B 6 a–c; Table 7-1]* All of the drugs or adverse effects are correctly matched with the causes or results listed except the purple toe syndrome, which is caused by cholesterol emboli from atheromatous plaques, following bleeding into the plaque. It can occur 3–8 weeks after starting warfarin therapy. Two percent of patients treated with warfarin experience major bleeding. Warfarin necrosis may occur 3–10 days after initiation of therapy. Concurrent use of cimetidine increases warfarin's anticoagulant action, and phenobarbital decreases its anticoagulant action.

52. The answer is A *[Chapter 11 II B 4 c, D 4; III B 4 a, D 1 e (1); VI D 4 b].* Busulfan, an alkyl sulfonate alkylating agent, is a myelosuppressive drug and is used to treat chronic granulocytic leukemia, not colon cancer. Cisplatin has a mechanism of action similar to that of the alkylating agents. It is one of the most effective agents against solid tumors. Cyclophosphamide, a nitrogen mustard, is also an alkylating agent and is used to treat a variety of cancers; it is also useful as an immunosuppressant for organ transplantation. 5-Fluorouracil and methotrexate are both antimetabolites and are used to treat a number of solid tumors. 5-Fluorouracil is also used topically for certain premalignant and malignant skin cancers. Methotrexate is also used in the therapy of acute lymphoblastic leukemia in children and in the treatment of psoriasis.

53. The answer is B *[Chapter 5 II B 4].* Cardiac glycosides are contraindicated in cardiac tamponade, high-output congestive heart failure, constrictive pericarditis, and idiopathic hypertrophic subaortic stenosis with outlet obstruction. In all of these conditions, a high-pressure system is involved, and a positive inotropic effect in such circumstances is undesirable. Cardiac glycosides are very useful in supraventricular arrhythmia, such as atrial fibrillation, atrial flutter, and paroxysmal atrial tachycardia. Cardiac glycosides are of greatest value for treating low-output cardiac failure.

54. The answer is A *[Chapter 12 II B 2 e (4) (a) (ii), 5 d (3), C 6 b (1) (a), I 4 b; Table 12-3].* Ceftazidime, a third-generation cephalosporin, has greater activity against *Pseudomonas aeruginosa* than other third-generation cephalosporins. Tobramycin is an aminoglycoside with excellent activity against *P. aeruginosa*. Both agents are administered parenterally. Aztreonam is also administered parenterally and is effective against gram-negative pathogens but has poor activity against gram-positive cocci and anaerobic bacteria. Ciprofloxacin is highly active against bacteria that cause enteritis and against staphylococci. It is somewhat less active against *P. aeruginosa* but is indicated for both complicated and uncomplicated urinary tract infections. Amoxicillin and clavulanate have no activity against *P. aeruginosa*.

55. The answer is C *[Chapter 1 III B 6].* The therapeutic index (TI) is a measure that is used in evaluating the safety and usefulness of a drug. The formula for the TI is:

$$TI = \frac{LD_{50}}{ED_{50}}$$

where LD_{50} is the minimum dose that is **lethal** for 50% of the population, and ED_{50} is the minimum dose that is **effective** for 50% of the population. Therapeutically, the standard margin of safety has been considered more useful because the numerator is more restrictive. The standard margin of safety $[(LD_1/ED_{99}) - 1 \times 100]$ shows how much the dose that is effective for 99% of the population must be increased to be toxic for 1% of the population.

56. The answer is D *[Chapter 5 IV A 2, C 4 a, D]*. Nadolol, which is similar to propranolol, is a nonselective β-blocker and could exacerbate chronic obstructive pulmonary disease. Diltiazem, verapamil, and nicardipine are all Ca^{2+}-channel blocking agents and do not worsen chronic obstructive pulmonary disease. The use of a thiazide diuretic would be an acceptable alternative to propranolol.

57. The answer is D *[Chapter 4 II B 1 b, C 2; Chapter 5 II B 2 f (4) (c)]*. Unlike procainamide, procaine does not cause a lupus-like syndrome. Procaine is an ester of diethylaminoethanol and para-amino benzoic acid (PABA), which can inhibit the action of sulfonamides. It does interfere with sodium influx during depolarization. It has a short duration of action and is metabolized by pseudocholinesterase.

58. The answer is D *[Chapter 8 V A 2 a]*. Cimetidine is the prototype H_2-receptor antagonist. It is used in the treatment of duodenal ulcers and hypersecretory states such as Zollinger-Ellison syndrome. The H_2-blockers are not sedating and would not cause somnolence, in contrast to H_1 blockers. Because cimetidine reduces liver blood flow, it can markedly decrease the hepatic clearance of drugs whose metabolism is dependent on liver blood flow.

59. The answer is C *[Chapter 7 I C, D]*. Ferrous sulfate, which contains 20% elemental iron, is the drug of first choice for iron-deficiency anemia. The adverse effects seen with ferrous sulfate are directly, not inversely, related to the amount of soluble iron in the upper gastrointestinal tract. Iron dextran, which is parenterally administered, is useful in patients with malabsorption syndromes. The iron is split off from the sugar molecule of iron dextran by phagocytization in the reticuloendothelial cells.

60. The answer is D *[Chapter 2 IV F, G]*. Metoclopramide, a parasympathetic (cholinergic) agonist, has proved useful for the treatment of delayed gastric emptying (gastroparesis) due to diabetes, for gastroesophageal reflux disease, and as an antiemetic in vomiting induced by certain types of radiation and cancer chemotherapy. Because it is a parasympathetic drug, it could exacerbate peptic ulcer disease.

61. The answer is B *[Chapter 7 IV C 2 a]*. Intravenous administration of streptokinase reduces blood pressure, total peripheral resistance, and cardiac afterload, which can result in hypotension. All of the other statements about this thrombolytic agent are correct. Streptokinase is a protein without known enzymatic activity that is obtained from group C β-hemolytic streptococci. Its interaction with a proactivator of plasminogen results in a proteolytic activity that converts plasminogen to plasmin, which is then capable of hydrolyzing fibrin clots. This property is the basis for the use of streptokinase in treating acute pulmonary embolism. Gastrointestinal bleeding occurs in 5%–10% of patients.

62. The answer is A *[Chapter 10 III G 3 d (2)]*. Leukocyte migration is suppressed, not stimulated, by glucocorticoids. This effect is thought to be one component of the overall anti-inflammatory effect of corticosteroids. Pharmacologic doses of glucocorticoids can result in stabilization of lysosomal membranes, reduced activity of fibroblasts, reversal of a histamine-stimulated increase in capillary permeability, and inhibited antibody synthesis—all of the other effects listed in the question.

63. The answer is D *[Chapter 8 V A 1 d, e, g]*. All of the pharmacologic effects listed in the question, with the exception of inhibition of gastric acid secretion, are associated with the classic antihistamines (H_1-receptor antagonists). They are used prophylactically for motion sickness and for vestibular disturbances, such as Meniere's disease. Overdosage can lead to convulsions, while low (therapeutic) doses cause sedation. The principal pharmacologic effect of the H_2-receptor antagonists, not the H_1-receptor antagonists, is inhibition of histamine-stimulated gastric acid secretion.

64. The answer is D *[Chapter 1 II B 1 a (3)]*. The oral route of administration is considered to be a relatively safe route. However, several disadvantages are associated with oral administration. Drugs that are orally administered will have variable rates of absorption. Compliance is not ensured, and irritation of the mucosal surfaces can occur with some drugs [e.g., nonsteroidal anti-inflammatory drugs (NSAIDs)]. First-pass metabolism results when hepatic metabolism occurs before the drug reaches its site of action.

65. The answer is B *[Chapter 9 III B 5 c (3), 6]*. Auranofin is a recently approved analog of gold thioglucose that can be administered orally. Although it may be less effective than injectable gold for the treatment of arthritis, it is less toxic than injectable gold, which can cause renal or mucocutaneous toxicity. Auranofin is associated with a high incidence of diarrhea, but this is often self-limiting and rarely requires discontinuation of therapy. Cutaneous reactions, mucosal lesions, eosinophilia, and proteinuria are other common side effects.

66. The answer is E *[Chapter 12 II B 2 h (2) (c) (ii)]*. All of the antibiotics listed in the question with the exception of erythromycin (i.e., amoxicillin, ampicillin, cefaclor, cephalexin) are broad-spectrum agents and, therefore, can produce fungal superinfections. Local application of an appropriate antifungal agent is often sufficient therapy for the treatment of a fungal vaginitis.

67. The answer is A *[Chapter 9 III E]*. Cyclosporine is not a selective inhibitor of B lymphocytes. Rather, it inhibits the production of interleukin-2 by helper T cells. Cyclosporine is often used in combination with steroids to reduce transplant rejection. Nephrotoxicity, its major adverse effect, is dose-related and occurs in 25%–75% of treated patients.

68. The answer is E *[Chapter 2 III A 4]*. Ergot alkaloids are tryptaminergic and dopaminergic agonists; in addition, they interact at α-adrenergic receptors. Their chemical structure resembles lysergic acid diethylamide, and thus, central nervous system (CNS) stimulation can occur. They also directly stimulate smooth muscle. Ergot alkaloids are weak α blockers and partial α agonists; they would not be blocked by propranolol, which is a nonselective β blocker.

69. The answer is D *[Chapter 5 II B 1 c, f]*. Quinidine reduces the maximal rate of rise (V_{max}) of depolarization during phase 0. It increases the effective refractory period but decreases automaticity and conduction velocity in ventricular tissue. Quinidine depresses myocardial contractility, and caution must, therefore, be used if quinidine is administered to patients with any degree of congestive heart failure (CHF).

70. The answer is B *[Chapter 7 III A 2, B 1, C 1–3]*. Erythropoietin is not intended for patients needing immediate correction of severe anemia. It is better suited for patients with chronic anemia secondary to chronic renal failure. By stimulating erythroid progenitor cells, it elevates or maintains red blood cell levels, decreasing the need for transfu-

sions. It must be administered parenterally because peptidases inactivate it in the gastrointestinal tract. Erythropoietin's pharmacokinetics are not affected by dialysis.

71. The answer is B *[Chapter 2 V E 1 a, 2]*. Diisopropyl fluorophosphate (DFP) is an irreversible cholinesterase inhibitor, which increases acetylcholine levels. Increased lacrimation, salivation, muscle twitching, and weakness are cholinergic (cholinomimetic) effects; increased bronchodilation is not.

72. The answer is D *[Table 7-1]*. Both phenylbutazone and aspirin affect platelet aggregation. These two drugs **increase** the response to oral anticoagulants, which can cause severe hemorrhage. Phenylbutazone, in addition, can displace warfarin from albumin, which increases the warfarin blood level. Glutethimide, like phenobarbital and other barbiturates, induces the drug microsomal metabolizing system. This **decreases** the response to oral anticoagulants, so that higher doses are required to produce the desired anticoagulant effect. Cimetidine inhibits the drug microsomal metabolizing system, increasing blood levels of oral anticoagulants.

73. The answer is D *[Chapter 9 III A; Figure 9-6]*. Disease-modifying antirheumatic drugs (DMARDs) do not cause degenerative lesions to regress once they are formed; rather, they interfere with the pathogenesis of rheumatoid arthritis by modifying the immunological response thought to be associated with the disease. Because DMARDs do not produce rapid, symptomatic relief of joint pain, they are often used in combination with nonsteroidal anti-inflammatory agents (NSAIDs).

74. The answer is E *[Chapter 12 IV B 3 b, c, 4 b]*. Isoniazid is the most widely used agent in the treatment of tuberculosis. To prevent the development of mycobacterial resistance, isoniazid is used in conjunction with rifampin or other agents in the treatment of active disease. It can be used alone as prophylaxis in persons who have converted from tuberculin-negative to tuberculin-positive and also in close contacts of patients who have newly diagnosed active disease. Isoniazid is not effective against atypical mycobacteria. Its metabolism depends in part on genetically determined acetyl transferase activity. Patients who are fast acetylators will have lower, not higher, concentrations of unchanged (free) isoniazid.

75. The answer is D *[Chapter 2 II B 2 g; Chapter 5 IV E 4 b (1); Chapter 10 III G 3; IV E, I 1 c; V].* The oral hypoglycemic agent tolbutamide decreases blood glucose concentrations, while the antihypertensive agent diazoxide increases them. Insulin decreases blood glucose concentrations, while cortisol, glucagon, and isoproterenol all increase blood glucose concentrations. Propranolol decreases blood sugar.

76. The answer is C *[Chapter 5 II B 1 f (3), 2 f (4) (c), (5), 3 d (2), C 1 f, D 2].* A syndrome resembling systemic lupus erythematosus can occur with procainamide, not lidocaine. This syndrome is reversible on discontinuation of therapy but can develop in as many as 30% of patients taking procainamide for long periods of time. Quinidine can cause cinchonism. Intravenous administration of procainamide can cause hypotension. Untoward anticholinergic effects may occur with disopyramide. Excessive mortality and nonfatal cardiac arrest can occur following flecainide administration.

77–78. The answers are 77-E *[Chapter 6 VI F 1, VII E 1, IX A 4 a],* **78-D** *[Chapter 5 I B 7 b; Chapter 6 VI F 1; IX].* Amiloride is a potassium (K+)-sparing diuretic; therefore, it is not likely to cause hypokalemia. Hypokalemia is a potential complication of furosemide, ethacrynic acid, bumetanide, and hydrochlorothiazide therapy. If a patient is concurrently receiving digoxin therapy, aggravated toxicity of this cardiac glycoside can become a major therapeutic problem.

Immediate potassium supplementation with oral preparations is indicated. Spironolactone, triamterene, and amiloride are used as adjunct diuretics for preventing hypokalemia, but they are not used for the treatment of hypokalemia once it occurs. Insulin and glucose are used for the treatment of hyperkalemia.

79. The answer is B *[Table 7-1; Chapter 9 II B 6 a].* Aspirin does not affect the leukocyte count, whereas phenylbutazone and sulfonamides can cause agranulocytosis. Aspirin, phenylbutazone, and sulfamethoxazole all are highly protein bound, affect platelet function, and interact with warfarin. They are all capable of producing hypersensitivity reactions.

80. The answer is E *[Chapter 10 III G 3 i].* Hyperglycemia, not hypoglycemia, can result from prolonged therapy. Because cortico-

steroids alter the mucosal defense mechanisms, peptic ulceration can result from prolonged therapy. The immunosuppressive effects of corticosteroids increase susceptibility to infection. Sudden withdrawal of corticosteroids can result in signs of adrenal insufficiency. The patient may have to be protected during stressful situations for 1 year or more after withdrawal.

81. The answer is B *[Chapter 12 III B 5 b, c (1), d (2), f].* Fluconazole is highly bioavailable. It penetrates the blood–brain barrier and is active against *Cryptococcus neoformans*. It is less toxic than amphotericin B and flucytosine, but its mechanism of action is similar to most antifungal agents. It inhibits cytochrome P-450–dependent enzymes, blocking the synthesis of ergosterol.

82. The answer is A *[Chapter 4 II C 2–4, 7].* Lidocaine is an amide, not an ester. Like mepivacaine, it is metabolized in the liver. Procaine is rapidly metabolized by pseudocholinesterase and is short-acting. It has no topical activity and is given parenterally. Tetracaine is the most frequently used spinal anesthetic agent. Bupivacaine is an amide local anesthetic, is more potent and has a longer duration of action than mepivacaine, and its effects can last more than 24 hours in some situations.

83. The answer is D *[Chapter 7 II C 2, 4].* Vitamin B_{12} is so prevalent in foodstuffs from animal sources that a dietary deficiency of the vitamin is very uncommon. The usual cause of vitamin B_{12} deficiency is a lack of intrinsic factor, as occurs in pernicious anemia and following gastrectomy. In such cases, parenteral vitamin B_{12} therapy is given, because oral B_{12} alone will not be absorbed, and oral combinations of vitamin B_{12} plus intrinsic factor are too unreliable. Antibodies to intrinsic factor can develop, preventing absorption of the vitamin; also, patients can eventually become refractory to oral intrinsic factor. Because the neurologic damage that results from vitamin B_{12} deficiency is **not** reversible, prompt, adequate therapy with parenteral vitamin B_{12} is important, to prevent further neurologic damage from occurring.

84. The answer is A *[Chapter 9 II A 2 d; Chapter 14 III B 1 b].* Because this patient is convulsing, syrup of ipecac would be contraindicated because of the risk of aspiration pneumonia. If the patient were alert, emesis could be induced. Alkalinizing the urine promotes the renal excretion of aspirin. Correction of abnormal electrolyte balance, dialysis, and ventilatory support all may be required in this case.

85. The answer is C *[Chapter 5 IV I 1 b–d, f (1) (b); Chapter 8 V C 2 c].* Enalapril decreases the secretion of aldosterone, not renin, by inhibiting the production of angiotensin II. In addition, vasoconstrictor properties associated with angiotensin II are inhibited. Enalapril is a specific competitive inhibitor of peptidyl dipeptidase [angiotensin-converting enzyme (ACE)], the enzyme that converts angiotensin I to angiotensin II. Enalapril is more potent and has a longer duration of action than captopril.

86–89. The answers are 86-D *[Chapter 12 II D 5 b],* **87-E** *[Chapter 12 IV C 5 a (1), 7 a],* **88-A** *[Chapter 12 II G 4 b, 7],* **89-B** *[Chapter 12 II C 3 a, 6 b, 8].* Tetracyclines (e.g., demeclocycline) are effective in the treatment of *Chlamydia* infections. Agents such as demeclocycline can produce a severe phototoxic skin reaction.

Rifampin, which is used in combination with isoniazid and ethambutol for the treatment of tuberculosis, may cause urine, sweat, tears, and contact lenses to have a harmless orange color.

 Clindamycin is the drug of first choice for *Bacteroides fragilis* infections. It can produce pseudomembranous colitis as an untoward effect.

The aminoglycosides (e.g., gentamicin) are polycations, which accounts for their pharmacokinetic properties, including poor oral absorption. These agents have a predilection for causing both ototoxicity and nephrotoxicity.

90–94. The answers are 90-A *[Chapter 6 I A 7; Figure 6-2],* **91-D** *[Chapter 6 I A 8; Figure 6-2],* **92-C** *[Chapter 6 I A 5; Figure 6-2],* **93-D** *[Chapter 6 I A 8; Figure 6-2],* **94-C** *[Chapter 6 I A 6; Figure 6-2].* Mannitol is a sugar alcohol osmotic diuretic that is filtered at the glomerulus but is poorly absorbed because of its molecular size. The solute in the proximal tubule decreases the reabsorption of sodium and water, resulting in a large volume of urine.

Spironolactone is a competitive antagonist of aldosterone that interferes with aldosterone-mediated sodium–potassium exchange. Thus, it increases sodium loss at the distal tubular site while decreasing potassium loss.

Hydrochlorothiazide inhibits chloride reabsorption in the distal portion of the ascending limb of the loop of Henle, resulting in the renal excretion of sodium, chloride, bicarbonate, and potassium.

Amiloride inhibits active sodium reabsorption at the distal convoluted tubule by disrupting normal sodium transport, which in turn reduces the net driving force for potassium secretion.

Furosemide inhibits electrolyte reabsorption in the thick ascending limb of the loop of Henle. Because it acts at the luminal surface of the nephron, furosemide must reach the urine to exert a diuretic effect.

95–97. The answers are 95-B *[Chapter 6 VII A],* **96-A** *[Chapter 6 IV A 1],* **97-E** *[Chapter 6 IX A 1 a].* Ethacrynic acid inhibits electrolyte reabsorption in the ascending limb of the loop of Henle, producing an increased urinary excretion of Na^+, Cl^-, and K^+.

Acetazolamide is a carbonic anhydrase inhibitor. It inhibits this enzyme at both the proximal and distal convoluted tubule. Carbon dioxide reabsorption from the glomerular filtrate is suppressed, and HCO_3^- excretion is increased. Due to a decrease in the reabsorption of Na^+ in exchange for H^+, the Na^+–K^+ exchange in the distal convoluted tubule increases. The result is an alkaline urine.

Triamterene inhibits active Na^+ reabsorption and, thus, increases the excretion of Na^+ and Cl^-. There is a net change in the electrogenic force across tubular membranes, which reduces the net driving force for K^+ secretion, resulting in the decreased excretion of K^+. The major site of action is the distal nephron.

98–102. The answers are 98-B *[Chapter 3 II A 5 g; Table 7-1],* **99-A** *[Chapter 13 II B 1 a],* **100-C** *[Chapter 13 II D 4 a],* **101-B** *[Chapter 13 II D 5],* **102-D** *[Chapter 3 V B 3 b (9)].* Most drug interactions involving the barbiturates result from induction of hepatic microsomal enzymes by the barbiturate; this causes accelerated metabolism of the other drug (e.g., warfarin, digitoxin, corticosteroids, and β blockers, to name only a few). However, other mechanisms can also be involved. Thus, a barbiturate plus another central nervous system (CNS) depressant (e.g., a phenothiazine, ethanol, or an antihistamine) can cause marked depression. Tranylcypromine is an inhibitor of monoamine oxidase (MAO), a nonmicrosomal enzyme. Inhibition of MAO can retard the metabolism of a barbiturate. Dextran solutions are incompatible with various drugs, including barbiturates. Barbiturates can also interfere with the absorption of some drugs (e.g., dicumarol, griseofulvin), and some barbiturates compete with other drugs (e.g., aspirin) for plasma protein binding sites.

103–106. The answers are 103-B *[Chapter 8 V C 2]*, **104-D** *[Chapter 8 IV C 3 a]*, **105-A** *[Chapter 9 II G 2 d (3)]*, **106-C** *[Chapter 8 V D 1 a, b]*. Captopril belongs to the class of drugs known as angiotensin-converting enzyme (ACE) inhibitors because they inhibit peptidyl dipeptidase, the ACE that normally converts angiotensin I to angiotensin II. The autacoid angiotensin II is a potent vasoconstrictor that raises blood pressure, and thus, ACE inhibitors are used clinically to treat hypertension.

Hydralazine inhibits thromboxane synthetase, the enzyme involved in the formation of thromboxanes from prostaglandin H. Thromboxane A_2 is, like angiotensin II, a potent vasoconstrictor, and hydralazine is used clinically as an antihypertensive vasodilator.

Ibuprofen is a nonsteroidal anti-inflammatory drug (NSAID). These agents act by inhibiting cyclooxygenase; and thus, they inhibit the synthesis of both prostaglandins and thromboxanes. Several prostaglandins serve as mediators of the inflammatory response. Some NSAIDs inhibit 15-lipoxygenase as well as cyclooxygenase; and aspirin, by inhibiting platelet cyclooxygenase, also interrupts the thromboxane synthetase pathway.

Prednisolone and other glucocorticoids inhibit phospholipase in a number of tissues, thereby blocking all eicosanoid formation in these tissues. Thus, glucocorticoids block the synthesis of prostaglandins, leukotrienes, and thromboxanes, which probably explains their potent anti-inflammatory effects. Moreover, since leukotrienes play a role in hypersensitivity reactions, their suppression may explain the efficacy of glucocorticoids in allergic disorders.

107–109. The answers are 107-A *[Chapter 9 II G 2 b]*, **108-D** *[Chapter 9 II G 5 c (3)]*, **109-E** *[Chapter 9 II G 6 b (2)]*. Ibuprofen is equal to aspirin in its anti-inflammatory effect but is a more effective analgesic than aspirin or acetaminophen.

Ketoprofen exhibits a profile similar to ibuprofen, but if it is used concurrently with methotrexate, the patient can develop life-threatening methotrexate hepatotoxicity.

Flubiprofen is the only nonsteroidal anti-inflammatory drug (NSAID) approved for ophthalmic use. It decreases meiosis without affecting intraocular pressure.

110–114. The answers are 110-E *[Chapter 11 VI C 4]*, **111-A** *[Chapter 11 II C 3 c]*, **112-C** *[Chapter 11 II E 4]*, **113-D** *[Chapter 11 III B 4 b]*, **114-B** *[Chapter 11 II B 4 b (2)]*. Mitotane is a derivative of the insecticide DDT that shows selective activity against cells of the adrenal cortex, both normal and neoplastic. It is, therefore, used in the management of inoperable adrenal carcinoma.

Carmustine, a nitrosourea, is lipid-soluble and crosses the blood–brain barrier. Thus, it is useful in treating brain tumors.

Dacarbazine, an alkylating agent, is one of the most useful drugs for malignant melanoma.

Methotrexate, a folic acid analog, can be given orally or parenterally. It has proved useful for the treatment of severe psoriasis, a nonmalignant condition characterized by overproliferation of epidermal cells.

Cyclophosphamide is a nitrogen mustard that can be given orally as well as parenterally. Because of its potent immunosuppressant properties, it is used to control rejection of transplanted organs.

115–117. The answers are 115-E *[Chapter 11 IV B 4 b]*, **116-C** *[Chapter 11 III D 2 b]*, **117-D** *[Chapter 11 IV C 2 b]*. Mitomycin is both a natural product and an alkylating agent. Isolated from a *Streptomyces* species, mitomycin C is reduced by a reduced nicotinamide adenine dinucleotide phosphate (NADPH)–dependent reductase and alkylates DNA.

Cytarabine inhibits DNA polymerase and, thus, kills cells in S phase. Cytarabine nucleotides can be incorporated into DNA and RNA, but the significance of this is not known.

Vincristine, a natural product, is an M-phase–specific agent that blocks proliferating cells as they enter metaphase.

118–121. The answers are 118-E *[Chapter 2 IV B 1 b]*, **119-C** *[Chapter 2 V E 1 a]*, **120-A** *[Chapter 2 II E 1]*, **121-D** *[Chapter 2 V B]*. Methacholine, because of the addition of the β-methyl group, is purely muscarinic in action.

Diisopropyl fluorophosphate (DFP) is an irreversible organophosphate cholinesterase inhibitor.

Phenylephrine, though less potent, resembles norepinephrine in its cardiovascular effects.

Neostigmine, besides being a reversible cholinesterase inhibitor, also stimulates nicotinic receptors.

122–125. The answers are 122-A *[Chapter 12 II A 7 a (2)],* **123-D** *[Chapter 12 II E 7 e],* **124-B** *[Chapter 12 II C 8 a],* **125-C** *[Chapter 12 II D 8 f].* Sulfonamides, such as trimethoprim–sulfamethoxazole, may cause Stevens-Johnson syndrome (characterized by fever, malaise, and erythema multiforme). However, this is a rare adverse effect.

Gray-baby syndrome can develop in neonates, especially premature infants, who have been administered large doses of chloramphenicol. Immaturity of the hepatic and renal systems impairs the infant's ability to metabolize and excrete the drug, leading to cyanosis, respiratory irregularities, and vascular motor collapse. The characteristic ashen hue of the skin is the source of the name for this often fatal syndrome.

Administration of gentamicin can produce labyrinthine damage and vestibular disturbances that are dose- and duration-dependent. Gentamicin can also produce acute renal insufficiency and tubular necrosis. The dosage must be adjusted when any degree of renal failure is present.

Administration of tetracycline to children may cause the teeth to turn yellow or brown. Discoloration is total dose- and time-related, and occurs most frequently when tetracycline is given to infants prior to their first dentition. Discoloration of permanent teeth can result if the child is between 2 months and 7 years of age, or if prenatal exposure occurs.

Index

Note: Page numbers in *italic* denote illustrations; those followed by (t) denote tables; those followed by Q denote questions; and those followed by E denote explanations.